DATE DUE

M

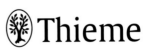

An Evidence-based Approach to Vitamins and Minerals

Health Benefits and Intake Recommendations

Jane Higdon, PhD †
Linus Pauling Institute
Oregon State University
Corvallis, Oregon, USA

Victoria J. Drake, PhD
Manager
Micronutrient Information Center
Linus Pauling Institute
Oregon State University
Corvallis, Oregon, USA

2nd edition

20 illustrations

Thieme
Stuttgart · New York

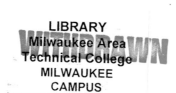

Library of Congress Cataloging-in-Publication Data

Higdon, Jane.
  An evidence-based approach to vitamins and minerals / Jane Higdon, Victoria Drake. -- 2nd ed.
    p. ; cm.
  Includes bibliographical references and index.
  ISBN 978-3-13-132452-8 (alk. paper)
  1. Vitamins in human nutrition--Handbooks, manuals, etc. 2. Trace elements in nutrition--Handbooks, manuals, etc. I. Drake, Victoria (Victoria J.) II. Title.
  [DNLM: 1. Vitamins--therapeutic use. 2. Avitaminosis--prevention & control. 3. Dietary Supplements. 4. Nutritional Requirements. QU 160]
  QP771.H54 2011
  613.2'86--dc23
                              2011015798

Important note: Medicine is an ever-changing science undergoing continual development. Research and clinical experience are continually expanding our knowledge, in particular our knowledge of proper treatment and drug therapy. Insofar as this book mentions any dosage or application, readers may rest assured that the authors, editors, and publishers have made every effort to ensure that such references are in accordance with **the state of knowledge at the time of production of the book.**

Nevertheless, this does not involve, imply, or express any guarantee or responsibility on the part of the publishers in respect to any dosage instructions and forms of applications stated in the book.

Every user is requested to examine carefully the manufacturers' leaflets accompanying each drug and to check, if necessary in consultation with a physician or specialist, whether the dosage schedules mentioned therein or the contraindications stated by the manufacturers differ from the statements made in the present book. Such examination is particularly important with drugs that are either rarely used or have been newly released on the market. Every dosage schedule or every form of application used is entirely at the user's own risk and responsibility. The authors and publishers request every user to report to the publishers any discrepancies or inaccuracies noticed. If errors in this work are found after publication, errata will be posted at www.thieme.com on the product description page.

© 2012 Georg Thieme Verlag,
Rüdigerstrasse 14,
70469 Stuttgart, Germany
http://www.thieme.de
Thieme New York, 333 Seventh Avenue,
New York, NY 10001, USA
http://www.thieme.com

Some of the product names, patents, and registered designs referred to in this book are in fact registered trademarks or proprietary names even though specific reference to this fact is not always made in the text. Therefore, the appearance of a name without designation as proprietary is not to be construed as a representation by the publisher that it is in the public domain.

Cover design: Thieme Publishing Group
Typesetting by primustype Robert Hurler GmbH, Notzingen, Germany
Printed in China by Everbest Printing Co. Ltd.

ISBN 978-313-132452-8   1 2 3 4 5 6

*Dedicated to the memory of Jane Higdon (1958–2006),
scholar, athlete, and compassionate advocate of healthful eating
and exercise.*

Foreword

An Evidence-based Approach to Vitamins and Minerals: Health Benefits and Intake Recommendations by Dr. Jane Higdon and Dr. Victoria Drake provides a much needed source of authoritative information on the role of micronutrients in health promotion and in disease prevention and treatment. The book is especially important because of the potential health benefits of tuning up people's micronutrient metabolism, particularly those with inadequate diets, such as the many low-income and elderly people. A metabolic tune-up is likely to have enormous health benefits but is currently not being addressed adequately by the medical community.

Maximum health and life span require metabolic harmony. It is commonly thought that Americans' intake of the more than 40 essential micronutrients (vitamins, minerals, and other biochemicals that humans require) is adequate. Classic deficiency diseases such as scurvy, beriberi, pernicious anemia, and rickets are rare, but the evidence suggests that metabolic damage occurs at intake levels between the level causing acute micronutrient deficiency diseases and the recommended dietary allowances (RDAs). When one input in the metabolic network is inadequate, repercussions are felt on a large number of systems and can lead to degenerative disease. This may, for example, result in an increase in DNA damage (and possibly cancer), neuron decay (and possibly cognitive dysfunction), or mitochondrial decay (and possibly accelerated aging and degenerative diseases). The optimum amount of folate or zinc that is truly "required" is the amount that minimizes DNA damage and maximizes a healthy life span, which is higher than the amount to prevent acute disease. Vitamin and metabolite requirements of older people are likely to differ from those of younger people, but this issue has not been seriously examined. An optimal intake of micronutrients and metabolites will also vary with genetic constitution. A tune-up of micronutrient metabolism should give a marked increase in health at little cost. It is inexcusable that anyone in the world should have

an inadequate intake of a vitamin or mineral, at great cost to that person's health, when a year's supply of a daily multivitamin/multimineral pill as insurance against deficiencies costs less than a few packs of cigarettes. Low-income populations, in general, are the most likely to have poor diets and have the most to gain from multivitamin/multimineral supplementation. As Hippocrates said: "Leave your drugs in the chemist's pot if you can heal the patient with food."

Although many degenerative diseases will benefit from optimal nutrition, and optimal nutrition clearly involves more than adequate micronutrients, there are several important reasons for focusing on micronutrients and health, particularly DNA damage: (1) More than 20 years of efforts to improve the American diet have not been notably successful, though this work must continue. A parallel approach focusing on micronutrient intake is overdue and might be more successful, since it should be easier to convince people to take a multivitamin/multimineral pill as insurance against ill health than to change their diet significantly. (2) A multivitamin/multimineral pill is inexpensive, is recognized as safe, and supplies the range of vitamins and minerals that a person requires, though not the essential fatty acids. Fortification of food is another approach that is useful, but its implementation has been very slow, as with folic acid fortification. Moreover, fortification of food does not allow for differences between individuals. For example, menstruating women need more iron than men or postmenopausal women, who may be getting too much. That is why two types of vitamin pills are marketed, one with iron and one without. With better knowledge it seems likely that a broader variety of multivitamin/multimineral pills will be developed, reflecting such life-stage differences.

The above issues and many others discussed in this book highlight the need to educate the public about the crucial importance of optimal nutrition and the potential health benefits of something as simple and affordable as a daily multivitamin/multimineral supplement. The numerous advances in the science of nutrition and changing ideas about optimal intakes of micronutrients make *An Evidence-based Approach to Vitamins and Minerals: Health Benefits and Intake Recommendations* an excellent and timely resource. Dr. Higdon, who had a background in health care and nutrition science, and Dr. Drake, who has an expertise in toxicology and nutrition, have synthesized a large amount of recent scientific research on vitamins and nutritionally essential minerals into an organized volume that includes information on optimal micronutrient intakes to prevent and treat chronic diseases. The book also contains much needed and up-to-date information on safety and drug interactions of vitamins and minerals. The credibility of this book is enhanced by the fact that it is endorsed by the Linus Pauling Institute at Oregon State University and that each chapter has been critically reviewed by a recognized expert in the field. Tuning up the metabolism to maximize human health will require scientists, clinicians, and educators to abandon outdated paradigms of micronutrients merely preventing deficiency disease and to explore more meaningful ways to prevent chronic disease and achieve optimal health through optimal nutrition.

Bruce N. Ames, PhD
University of California, Berkeley
Children's Hospital Oakland Research Institute
Oakland, California

Preface to the Second Edition

I am honored to revise and update Dr. Jane Higdon's book, *An Evidence-based Approach to Vitamins and Minerals: Health Benefits and Intake Recommendations*. Since the first edition was published in 2003, there has been a dramatic expansion of the literature on the role of micronutrients in human health and disease. In this second edition, all 27 chapters have been revised to incorporate information from the relevant, more recently published peer-reviewed studies, especially studies with human subjects. This edition includes the latest recommendations by the Food and Nutrition Board (FNB) of the Institute of Medicine: the FNB established new dietary reference intakes for potassium and sodium in 2004 and revised their recommendations for calcium and vitamin D in 2010. Additionally, some of the Linus Pauling Institute (LPI) recommendations have been modified to reflect current knowledge in micronutrient research. The LPI recommendations are daily intake levels aimed at the promotion of optimum health and prevention of chronic disease in healthy individuals. A large literature indicates that inadequate or marginal intake of vitamins and nutritionally essential minerals may increase one's risk for a number of diseases, including cardiovascular diseases, certain cancers and neurodegenerative diseases, and osteoporosis. Micronutrient inadequacy can also impair immunity and thus increase susceptibility to communicable diseases like influenza. This book reviews the present knowledge on the roles of vitamins and minerals in disease prevention and disease treatment, in addition to providing basic information on biological function, deficiency, food sources, safety, and interactions with other micronutrients and drugs.

Acknowledgments

I wish to thank the faculty, staff, and students of the Linus Pauling Institute for their editorial advice and support in the revision of this book, especially Balz Frei, PhD, director and endowed chair; Stephen Lawson, administrative officer; and Barbara McVicar, assistant to the director. I am very appreciative to all of the distinguished scientists listed in the Editorial Advisory Board, who reviewed the contents of each chapter and provided helpful comments. I am particularly grateful to Donald M. Mock, MD, PhD, and Eva Obarzanek, PhD, for their valuable expertise in revising the chapters on biotin and salt, respectively. Finally, I deeply appreciate the skillful work by Dr. Higdon in writing the first edition of this book, which has been a popular resource for both health professionals and the public.

Victoria J. Drake, PhD
Manager, Micronutrient Information Center
Linus Pauling Institute
Oregon State University
Corvallis, Oregon

Preface to the First Edition

During my clinical training, I learned to approach micronutrient nutrition from the perspective of preventing or treating deficiency diseases, such as scurvy or iron-deficiency anemia. In clinical practice, I became increasingly interested in the potential for micronutrients to prevent and treat chronic diseases at intakes higher than those required to prevent deficiency. However, the standard medical and nutrition texts of the day rarely provided the kind of information I was looking for. Today, scientific and medical research on the roles of micronutrients in health and disease is expanding rapidly, as are, unfortunately, exaggerated health claims from numerous supplement manufacturers. Keeping up with the explosion of contradictory information regarding the safety and efficacy of dietary supplements has become an overwhelming task for consumers as well as health care and nutrition professionals. My goal in writing this book was to provide clinicians and consumers with a practical evidence-based reference to the rapidly expanding field of micronutrient nutrition.

While my own interest in nutrition and health led me to pursue doctoral work in nutrition and biochemistry, such a step should not be necessary for health care and nutrition professionals who want more information on the health implications of dietary and supplemental micronutrients. With the support of the Linus Pauling Institute at Oregon State University (LPI), I have synthesized and organized hundreds of experimental, clinical, and epidemiologic studies, providing an overview of the current scientific knowledge of the roles of vitamins and nutritionally important minerals in human health and disease. To ensure the accuracy of the information presented, I asked at least one recognized scientific expert in the field to review each chapter. The names and affiliations of these scientists are listed in the Editorial Advisory Board.

Throughout this book, I have tried to emphasize human research published in peer-reviewed journals. Where relevant, I have included the results of experimental studies in cell culture or animal models. Although randomized clinical trials provide the strongest evidence for the effect of micronutrient intake on disease outcomes in humans, it is not always ethical or practical to perform a double-blind, placebo-controlled trial. Observational studies can also provide useful information about micronutrient intake and disease outcomes. In reviewing the epidemiologic research, I have given more weight to the results of large prospective cohort studies, such as the Nurses Health Study, than retrospective case–control or cross-sectional studies. When available, I have included the results of systematic reviews and meta-analyses, which summarize information on the findings of many similar studies.

Nearly 35 years ago Linus Pauling, PhD, the only individual ever to win two unshared Nobel Prizes, concluded that micronutrients could play a significant role in enhancing human health and preventing chronic disease, not just deficiency disease. The basic premise that an optimum diet is the key to optimum health continues today as the foundation of the Linus Pauling Institute at Oregon State University. Scientists at the Linus Pauling Institute investigate the roles that micronutrients and other dietary constituents play in human aging and chronic diseases, particularly cancer, cardiovascular diseases, and neurodegenerative diseases. The goals of our research are to understand the molecular mechanisms behind the effects of nutrition on health and to determine how micronutrients and other dietary factors can be used in the prevention and treatment of diseases, thereby enhancing human health and well-being. The Linus Pauling Institute is also dedicated to training and supporting new researchers in the interdisciplinary science of nutrition and optimum health, as well as to educating the public about the science of optimum nutrition.

As you read this book, it will become apparent that the Linus Pauling Institute recommendations for certain micronutrients (e.g., vitamin C) differ considerably from those of Linus Pauling himself. Dr. Pauling, for whom the Linus Pauling Institute has great respect, based his own micronutrient recommendations largely on theoretical arguments. For example, in developing his recommendations for vitamin C intake, he used cross-species comparisons, evolutionary arguments, and the amount of vitamin C likely consumed in a raw plant food diet. At the Linus Pauling Institute, we base our micronutrient recommendations on current scientific evidence, much of which was unavailable to Dr. Pauling. The Linus Pauling Institute's recommendation for a vitamin C intake of at least 200 mg/day for generally healthy adults takes into account the currently available epidemiologic, biochemical, and clinical evidence. Similarly, the Linus Pauling Institute's intake recommendation for each micronutrient in this book is based on the current scientific research available, while, in many cases, acknowledging that the intake levels most likely to promote optimum health remain to be determined.

Acknowledgments

First and foremost, I wish to thank the faculty, staff, and students of the Linus Pauling Institute for providing me with the inspiration and the opportunity to write this book. Specifically, Balz Frei, PhD, the director, and Stephen Lawson, the chief administrative officer of the Linus Pauling Institute, provided valuable advice and editorial assistance throughout the project. Barbara McVicar also provided much needed technical assistance and support. I am very grateful for the support of Bruce N. Ames, PhD, who was enthusiastic about this project from the beginning. His research and his eloquent foreword have been invaluable in laying the groundwork for this book.

I would like to thank each of the distinguished scientists listed in the Editorial Advisory Board for taking the time to carefully review each chapter of this book and provide insightful and constructive comments. I am also grateful to Aram Chobanian, MD, for reviewing the information presented on salt. The artist, Pat Grimaldi of the Communication Media Center at Oregon State University, was both patient and skillful in creating the book's illustrations.

This project would not have been possible without the generous financial support of the donors to the Linus Pauling Institute, who deserve special thanks. Finally, although I did not know him personally, I would like to thank Dr. Linus Pauling for courageously stimulating scientific, medical, and popular interest in the roles played by micronutrients in promoting optimum health and preventing and treating disease.

Jane Higdon, PhD
Linus Pauling Institute
Oregon State University
Corvallis, Oregon

Editorial Advisory Board

Contents

How To Use This Book

Chapter Organization

Information on individual vitamins, organic (carbon-containing) compounds that are required by humans in small amounts from the diet to maintain normal physiological function, can be found in Chapters 1 through 13, in alphabetical order by vitamin. In addition to vitamins, a number of inorganic elements (minerals) are required in the human diet to support a wide range of biological functions. Information on nutritionally important minerals can be found in Chapters 14 through 27, in alphabetical order by mineral. For ease of use, the information in each chapter is organized in the following manner:

- **Function** Current scientific understanding of the function of the micronutrient with respect to maintaining health and preventing disease.
- **Deficiency** Risk factors, signs, symptoms, and physiological effects of frank deficiency of the micronutrient.
- **Disease Prevention** Where controlled research is available, information on the role(s) of the micronutrient in the prevention of disease.
- **Disease Treatment** Where controlled research is available, information on the role(s) of the micronutrient in the treatment of disease.
- **Sources** Information on dietary, supplemental, and other sources of the micronutrient. When available, this section includes a table of dietary sources.
- **Safety** Information on toxicity and adverse effects of the micronutrient, as well as micronutrient–drug interactions.
- **The Linus Pauling Institute Recommendation** A daily intake recommendation based on relevant scientific research and reflecting an intake level aimed at the prevention of chronic disease and the promotion of optimum health in generally healthy individuals. Recommendations for older adults (over the age of 50 years) are also addressed in this section.
- **References**
  In addition to the Linus Pauling Institute Recommendations, the Food and Nutrition Board (FNB) of the Institute of Medicine appoints committees of expert scientists to set Dietary Reference Intakes (DRIs), which are used to plan and evaluate diets of apparently healthy people. Three different DRIs appear regularly throughout this book:
  - The *Recommended Dietary Allowance* (RDA) is defined as the average daily dietary intake level of a specific nutrient sufficient to meet the requirement of nearly all (97%–98%) healthy individuals in a particular life-stage group. Because RDAs generally reflect intake levels designed to prevent deficiency, they are presented in the **Deficiency** section of each chapter.
  - An *Adequate Intake* (AI) is provided if there is insufficient evidence to determine an RDA. The AI is based on experimentally derived intake levels or observed average intake levels of apparently healthy people. For example, the AI of a nutrient for infants is generally based on the average daily intake of that nutrient supplied by human milk in healthy, full-term infants who are exclusively breast-fed. Because AIs reflect intake levels thought to prevent deficiency, they are also presented in the **Deficiency** section of each chapter.
  - The *Tolerable Upper Intake Level* (UL) is defined as the highest level of a nutrient determined to pose no risk of adverse effects for almost all individuals in the general population. The UL is discussed in the **Safety** section of each chapter.

Appendices

Several appendices have been included to facilitate the use of this book by clinicians as well as consumers.

- **Nutrient–Nutrient Interactions** A table summarizing the information on nutrient–nutrient interactions discussed in the book.
- **Drug–Nutrient Interactions** A table summarizing the information on nutrient–drug interactions discussed in the book.

- **Quick Reference to Diseases** A useful chart that allows the reader to locate micronutrient information by disease or health condition.
- **Glossary**
- **The Linus Pauling Institute Prescription for Health** A list summarizing the Linus Pauling Institute Recommendations for a healthy diet, lifestyle, and supplement use.

Table of Measures

In the metric system, a microgram (µg, mcg, or sometimes ug) is a unit of mass equal to one millionth (1/1 000 000) of a gram or one thousandth (1/1000) of a milligram. It is one of the smallest units of mass (or weight) commonly used. The abbreviation "µg" conforms to the International System of Units.

Weight	
Metric	**English (US)**
1 mg (1000 µg)	0.002 grain (0.000035 oz)
1 g (1000 mg)	0.04 oz
1 kg (1000 g)	35.27 oz (2.2 lb)
English (US)	**Metric**
1 grain	64.8 mg
1 oz	28.4 g
1 lb	453.6 g (0.45 kg)
Volume	
Metric	**English (US)**
1 mL	0.03 oz
1 L (1000 mL)	2.12 pt
1 L	1.06 qt
1 L	0.27 gal
English (US)	**Metric**
1 fl oz	30 mL
1 pt	470 mL
1 qt	950 mL
1 gal	3.79 L
Liquids	
Metric	**English (US)**
1 mL	⅕ tsp
5 mL	1 tsp
15 mL	1 tbsp
30 mL	⅛ cup
60 mL	¼ cup
100 mL (1 dL)	About ⅖ cup
120 mL	½ cup
240 mL	1 cup
480 mL	1 pt

Abbreviations:

dL	deciliter	µg	microgram
fl oz	fluid ounce	mL	milliliter
g	gram	oz	ounce
gal	gallon	pt	pint
kg	kilogram	qt	quart
L	liter	tbsp	tablespoon
lb	pound	tsp	teaspoon
mg	milligram		

1 Biotin

Biotin is a water-soluble vitamin that is generally classified as a B-complex vitamin. After the initial discovery of biotin, nearly 40 years of research were required to establish it as a vitamin.[1] Biotin is required by all organisms but can be synthesized only by bacteria, yeasts, molds, algae, and some plant species.[2]

Function

Biotin is attached at the active site of five mammalian enzymes known as carboxylases.[3] The attachment of biotin to another molecule, such as a protein, is known as *biotinylation*. Holocarboxylase synthetase (HCS) catalyzes the biotinylation of apocarboxylases (i.e., the catalytically inactive form of the enzyme) and of histones. Biotinidase catalyzes the release of biotin from histones and from the peptide products of carboxylase breakdown.

Enzyme Cofactor

Each carboxylase for which biotin acts as a cofactor catalyzes an essential metabolic reaction:
- *Acetyl-CoA carboxylase I and II* catalyze the binding of bicarbonate to acetyl-coenzyme A (CoA) to form malonyl-CoA, which is required for the synthesis of fatty acids. The former is crucial in cytosolic fatty acid synthesis, and the latter functions in regulating mitochondrial fatty acid oxidation.
- *Pyruvate carboxylase* is a critical enzyme in gluconeogenesis—the formation of glucose from sources other than carbohydrates, for example, amino acids.
- *Methylcrotonyl-CoA carboxylase* catalyzes an essential step in the catabolism of leucine, an essential amino acid.
- *Propionyl-CoA carboxylase* catalyzes essential steps in the metabolism of certain amino acids, cholesterol, and odd-chain fatty acids (fatty acids with an odd number of carbon molecules).[4]

Histone Biotinylation

Histones are proteins that bind to DNA and package it into compact structures to form nucleosomes—integral structural components of chromosomes. The compact packaging of DNA must be relaxed somewhat for DNA replication and transcription to occur. Modification of histones through the attachment of acetyl or methyl groups (acetylation or methylation) has been shown to affect the structure of histones, thereby affecting replication and transcription of DNA. Mounting evidence indicates that biotinylation of histones plays a role in regulating DNA replication and transcription as well as cellular proliferation and other cellular responses.[5–7]

Deficiency

Although overt biotin deficiency is very rare, the human requirement for dietary biotin has been demonstrated in two different situations: prolonged intravenous feeding (parenteral) without biotin supplementation and consumption of raw egg white for a prolonged period (many weeks to years). Avidin is an antimicrobial protein found in egg white that binds biotin and prevents its absorption. Cooking egg white denatures avidin, rendering it susceptible to digestion and therefore unable to prevent the absorption of dietary biotin.[8]

Three measures have been validated as indicators of biotin status: (1) high excretion of an organic acid (3-hydroxyisovaleric acid) that reflects decreased activity of the biotin-dependent enzyme, methylcrotonyl-CoA carboxylase; (2) reduced urinary excretion of biotin; and (3) propionyl-CoA carboxylase activity in peripheral blood lymphocytes.[4,9–11]

Signs and Symptoms

Signs of overt biotin deficiency include hair loss and a scaly red rash around the eyes, nose, mouth, and genital area. Neurological symptoms in adults have included depression, lethargy, hallucination, and numbness and tingling of the extremities. The characteristic facial rash, together with unusual facial fat distribution, has been termed the *biotin-deficient facies* by some investigators.[8] Individuals with hereditary disorders of biotin metabolism resulting in functional biotin deficiency often have similar physical findings as well as evidence of impaired immune system function and increased susceptibility to bacterial and fungal infections.[12]

Predisposing Conditions

There are several ways in which the hereditary disorder, biotinidase deficiency, leads to biotin deficiency. Intestinal absorption is decreased because a lack of biotinidase inhibits the release of biotin from dietary protein. Recycling of one's own biotin bound to protein is impaired, and urinary loss of biotin is increased because the kidneys more rapidly excrete biotin that is not bound to biotinidase.[5,8] Biotinidase deficiency uniformly responds to moderate biotin supplementation. Oral supplementation with as much as 5–10 mg biotin daily is sometimes required, although smaller doses are often sufficient. Some forms of HCS deficiency respond to biotin supplementation with large doses. HCS deficiency results in an enzyme that catalyzes the attachment of biotin to all four carboxylase enzymes. HCS deficiency results in decreased formation of all holocarboxylases at normal blood levels of biotin, so high-dose supplementation (40–100 mg biotin/day) is required. The inborn error, biotin transporter deficiency, also responds to high-dose biotin supplementation.[13] The prognosis of all three disorders is often, but not always, good if biotin therapy is introduced early (infancy or childhood) and continued for life.[12]

Aside from prolonged consumption of raw egg white or total intravenous nutritional support lacking biotin, other conditions may increase the risk of biotin depletion. The rapidly dividing cells of the developing fetus require biotin for histone biotinylation and synthesis of essential carboxylases; hence, the biotin requirement is likely increased during pregnancy. Research suggests that a substantial number of women develop marginal or subclinical biotin deficiency during normal pregnancy.[6,14] However, the recommended adequate intake does not change for pregnancy. In addition, some types of liver disease may decrease biotinidase activity and theoretically increase the requirement for biotin. A study of 62 children with chronic liver disease and 27 healthy control children found serum biotinidase activity to be abnormally low in those with severely impaired liver function due to cirrhosis.[15] However, this study did not provide evidence of biotin deficiency. Further, anticonvulsant medications, used to prevent seizures in individuals with epilepsy, increase the risk of biotin depletion.[16,17]

Adequate Intake

In 1998, the Food and Nutrition Board (FNB) of the Institute of Medicine felt that the existing scientific evidence was insufficient to calculate a recommended dietary amount (RDA) for biotin, so they set an adequate intake (AI) (**Table 1.1**). The AI for biotin assumes that current average intakes of biotin (35–60 µg/day) meet the dietary requirement.[1]

Table 1.1 Adequate intake (AI) for biotin

Life stage	Age	Males (µg/day)	Females (µg/day)
Infants	0–6 months	5	5
Infants	7–12 months	6	6
Children	1–3 years	8	8
Children	4–8 years	12	12
Children	9–13 years	20	20
Adolescents	14–18 years	25	25
Adults	≥19 years	30	30
Pregnancy	All ages	–	30
Breast-feeding	All ages	–	35

Disease Prevention

Birth Defects

Research indicates that biotin is broken down more rapidly during pregnancy and that biotin nutritional status declines during the course of pregnancy.[6] One study reported that biotin excretion dropped below the normal range during late pregnancy in 6 of 13 women, suggesting that their biotin status was abnormally low. Over half of pregnant women have abnormally high excretion of a metabolite (3-hydroxyisovaleric acid), thought to reflect decreased activity of a biotin-dependent enzyme. A study of 26 pregnant women found that biotin supplementation decreased the excretion of this metabolite compared with placebo, suggesting that marginal biotin deficiency may be relatively common in pregnancy.[14] In one study, the incidence of decreased lymphocyte propionyl-CoA carboxylase activity (a marker of biotin deficiency) in pregnancy was more than 75%.[18] Although the level of biotin depletion is not severe enough to cause diagnostic signs or symptoms, such observations are sources of concern because subclinical biotin deficiency has been shown to cause birth defects in several animal species.[16]

Currently, it is estimated that at least one-third of women develop marginal biotin deficiency during pregnancy.[8] Indirect evidence also suggests that marginal biotin deficiency causes birth defects in humans. On balance, the potential risk for teratogenesis (abnormal development of the embryo or fetus) from biotin deficiency makes it prudent to ensure adequate biotin intake throughout pregnancy. As pregnant women are advised to consume supplemental folic acid before and during pregnancy to prevent neural tube defects, it would be easy to consume supplemental biotin (at least 30 µg/day) in the form of a multivitamin that also contains at least 400 µg of folic acid. Toxicity at this level of biotin intake has never been reported.

Disease Treatment

Diabetes Mellitus

It has been known for many years that overt biotin deficiency impairs glucose utilization in rats.[19] In one human study, blood biotin levels were significantly lower in 43 patients with type 2 diabetes than in control individuals who did not have diabetes, and lower fasting blood glucose levels were associated with higher blood biotin levels. After 1 month of biotin supplementation (9000 µg/day), fasting blood glucose levels decreased by an average of 45%.[20] In contrast, a study in ten individuals with type 2 diabetes and seven controls without reported that biotin supplementation (15 000 µg/day) for 28 days did not decrease fasting blood glucose levels in either group.[21] A more recent, double-blind, placebo-controlled study by the same group of investigators found that the same biotin treatment protocol lowered plasma triglyceride levels in both diabetic and nondiabetic patients with hypertriglyceridemia.[22] In this study, biotin administration did not affect blood glucose concentrations in individuals who did or did not have diabetes. In addition, a few studies have shown that co-supplementation with biotin and chromium picolinate may be a beneficial adjunct therapy in patients with type 2 diabetes.[23-26] However, several studies have reported that administration of chromium picolinate alone improves glycemic control in individuals with diabetes.[27]

Reductions in blood glucose levels were found in seven individuals with type 1 diabetes after 1 week of supplementation with 16 000 µg biotin daily.[28] Several mechanisms could explain a possible blood glucose-lowering effect of biotin. As a cofactor of enzymes required for fatty acid synthesis, biotin may increase the utilization of glucose for fat synthesis. Biotin has been found to stimulate glucokinase, a liver enzyme that increases synthesis of glycogen, the storage form of glucose. Biotin has also been found to stimulate the secretion of insulin in the pancreas of rats, which has the effect of lowering blood glucose.[29] An effect on cellular glucose transporters (GLUTs) is currently under investigation. Currently, studies of the effect of supplemental biotin on blood glucose levels in humans are extremely limited, but they highlight the need for further research.

Brittle Fingernails

The finding that biotin supplements were effective in treating hoof abnormalities in horses and swine led to speculation that biotin supplements might also be helpful in strengthening brittle fingernails in humans. Three uncontrolled trials examining the effects of biotin supplementation (2.5 mg /day for up to 6 months) in women with brittle fingernails have been published.[29-31] In two of the trials, subjective evidence of clinical improvement was reported in 67%–91% of the participants available for follow-up at the end of the treatment period.[29,30] One trial that used scanning electron microscopy to assess fingernail thickness and splitting found that fingernail thickness increased by 25% and splitting decreased after biotin supplementation.[31] Although the results of these small uncontrolled trials suggest that biotin supplements may be helpful in strengthening brittle nails, larger placebo-controlled trials are needed to assess the efficacy of high-dose biotin supplementation for the treatment of brittle fingernails.

Hair Loss

Although hair loss is a symptom of severe biotin deficiency, there are no published scientific studies that support the claim that high-dose biotin supplements are effective in preventing or treating hair loss in men or women.

Sources

Food Sources

Biotin is found in many foods, but generally in lower amounts than other water-soluble vitamins. Egg yolk, liver, and yeast are rich sources of biotin. Large national nutritional surveys in the

Table 1.2 Food sources of biotin

Food	Serving	Biotin (µg)
Liver, cooked	3 ounces[a]	27–35
Egg, cooked	1 large	13–25
Yeast	1 packet (7 g)	1.4–14.0
Avocado	1 whole	2–6
Bread, whole-wheat	1 slice	0.02–6.0
Salmon, cooked	3 ounces[a]	4–5
Pork, cooked	3 ounces[a]	2–4
Cauliflower, raw	1 cup	0.2–4.0
Cheese, cheddar	1 ounce	0.4–2.0
Raspberries	1 cup	0.2–2.0

[a]A 3-ounce serving of meat or fish is about the size of a deck of cards.

United States were unable to estimate biotin intake due to the scarcity of data regarding biotin content of food. Smaller studies estimate average daily intakes of biotin to be from 40 µg/day to 60 µg/day in adults.[1] Table 1.2 lists some rich sources of biotin along with their content in micrograms.[32] However, a publication that employed chemical rather than microbial assays reported quite different contents for some common foods.[33]

Bacterial Synthesis

Most bacteria that normally colonize the small and large intestine (colon) synthesize biotin. Whether the biotin is released and absorbed by humans in meaningful amounts remains unknown. However, a specialized process for the uptake of biotin has been identified in cultured cells derived from the lining of the small bowel and colon,[34] suggesting that humans may be able to absorb biotin produced by enteric bacteria—a phenomenon documented in swine.

Safety

Toxicity

Biotin is not known to be toxic. Oral biotin supplementation has been well tolerated in doses up to 200 000 µg/day in people with hereditary disorders of biotin metabolism.[1] In people without disorders of biotin metabolism, doses of up to 5000 µg/day for 2 years were not associated with adverse effects.[35] However, there is one case report of life-threatening eosinophilic pleuropericardial effusion in an elderly woman who took a combination of 10 000 µg/day of biotin and 300 mg/day of pantothenic acid for 2 months.[36] Due to the lack of reports of adverse effects when the dietary reference intakes (DRIs) were established for biotin in 1998, the Institute of Medicine did not establish a tolerable upper intake level (UL) for biotin.[1]

Nutrient Interactions

Large doses of pantothenic acid (vitamin B_5) have the potential to compete with biotin for intestinal and cellular uptake due to their similar structures.[37] In addition, very high (pharmacologic) doses of lipoic acid have been found to decrease the activity of biotin-dependent carboxylases in rats, but such an effect has not been demonstrated in humans.[4,38]

Drug Interactions

Individuals on long-term anticonvulsant (anti-seizure) therapy reportedly have reduced blood levels of biotin as well as increased urinary excretion of organic acids that indicate decreased carboxylase activity.[39] The anticonvulsants primidone and carbamazepine inhibit biotin absorption in the small intestine. Chronic therapy with phenobarbital, phenytoin, or carbamazepine appears to increase urinary excretion of 3-hydroxyisovaleric acid. Use of the anticonvulsant valproic acid has been associated with decreased biotinidase activity in children.[17] Long-term treatment with sulfa drugs or other antibiotics may decrease bacterial synthesis of biotin, theoretically increasing the requirement for dietary biotin.

LPI Recommendation

Little is known about the amount of dietary biotin required to promote optimal health or prevent chronic disease. The Linus Pauling Institute supports the recommendation by the FNB of 30 µg biotin/day for adults. A varied diet should provide enough biotin for most people. However, following the Linus Pauling Institute recommendation to take a daily multivitamin/mineral supplement will generally provide an intake of at least 30 µg biotin/day.

Older Adults

Currently, there is no indication that older adults have an increased requirement for biotin. If dietary biotin intake is not sufficient, a daily multivitamin/mineral supplement will generally provide an intake of at least 30 µg biotin/day.

References

1. Food and Nutrition Board, Institute of Medicine. Biotin. In: Dietary Reference Intakes for Thiamin, Riboflavin, Niacin, Vitamin B$_6$, Vitamin B$_{12}$, Pantothenic Acid, Biotin, and Choline. Washington, DC: National Academy Press, 1998: 374–389
2. Mock DM. Biotin. In: Shils ME, Olson JA, Shike M, Ross AC, eds. Modern Nutrition in Health and Disease, 9th ed. Baltimore, MD: Lippincott Williams & Wilkins, 1999: 459–466
3. Chapman-Smith A, Cronan JE Jr. Molecular biology of biotin attachment to proteins. J Nutr 1999;129(2S, Suppl):477S–484S
4. Zempleni J, Mock DM. Biotin biochemistry and human requirements. J Nutr Biochem 1999;10(3):128–138
5. Hymes J, Wolf B. Human biotinidase isn't just for recycling biotin. J Nutr 1999;129(2S, Suppl):485S–489S
6. Zempleni J, Mock DM. Marginal biotin deficiency is teratogenic. Proc Soc Exp Biol Med 2000;223(1):14–21
7. Kothapalli N, Camporeale G, Kueh A, et al. Biological functions of biotinylated histones. J Nutr Biochem 2005;16(7):446–448
8. Mock DM. Biotin. In: Shils ME, Shike M, Ross AC, Caballero B, Cousins RJ, eds. Modern Nutrition in Health and Disease, 10th ed. Baltimore, MD: Lippincott Williams & Wilkins; 2006:498–506
9. Mock DM. Marginal biotin deficiency is teratogenic in mice and perhaps humans: a review of biotin deficiency during human pregnancy and effects of biotin deficiency on gene expression and enzyme activities in mouse dam and fetus. J Nutr Biochem 2005;16(7):435–437
10. Stratton SL, Bogusiewicz A, Mock MM, Mock NI, Wells AM, Mock DM. Lymphocyte propionyl-CoA carboxylase and its activation by biotin are sensitive indicators of marginal biotin deficiency in humans. Am J Clin Nutr 2006;84(2):384–388
11. Mock D, Henrich C, Carnell N, Mock N, Swift L. Lymphocyte propionyl-CoA carboxylase and accumulation of odd-chain fatty acid in plasma and erythrocytes are useful indicators of marginal biotin deficiency small star, filled. J Nutr Biochem 2002;13(8):462
12. Baumgartner ER, Suormala T. Inherited defects of biotin metabolism. Biofactors 1999;10(2-3):287–290
13. Mardach R, Zempleni J, Wolf B, et al. Biotin dependency due to a defect in biotin transport. J Clin Invest 2002;109(12):1617–1623
14. Mock DM, Quirk JG, Mock NI. Marginal biotin deficiency during normal pregnancy. Am J Clin Nutr 2002;75(2):295–299
15. Pabuçcuoğlu A, Aydoğdu S, Baş M. Serum biotinidase activity in children with chronic liver disease and its clinical significance. J Pediatr Gastroenterol Nutr 2002;34(1):59–62
16. Mock DM. Biotin status: which are valid indicators and how do we know? J Nutr 1999;129(2S, Suppl):498S–503S
17. Schulpis KH, Karikas GA, Tjamouranis J, Regoutas S, Tsakiris S. Low serum biotinidase activity in children with valproic acid monotherapy. Epilepsia 2001;42(10):1359–1362
18. Mock DM. Marginal biotin deficiency is common in normal human pregnancy and is highly teratogenic in mice. J Nutr 2009;139(1):154–157
19. Zhang H, Osada K, Sone H, Furukawa Y. Biotin administration improves the impaired glucose tolerance of streptozotocin-induced diabetic Wistar rats. J Nutr Sci Vitaminol (Tokyo) 1997;43(3):271–280
20. Maebashi M, Makino Y, Furukawa Y, Ohinata K, Kimura S, Sato T. Therapeutic evaluation of the effect of biotin on hyperglycemia in patients with non-insulin dependent diabetes mellitus. J Clin Biochem Nutr 1993;14:211–218
21. Báez-Saldaña A, Zendejas-Ruiz I, Revilla-Monsalve C, et al. Effects of biotin on pyruvate carboxylase, acetyl-CoA carboxylase, propionyl-CoA carboxylase, and markers for glucose and lipid homeostasis in type 2

diabetic patients and nondiabetic subjects. Am J Clin Nutr 2004;79(2):238–243

22. Revilla-Monsalve C, Zendejas-Ruiz I, Islas-Andrade S, et al. Biotin supplementation reduces plasma triacylglycerol and VLDL in type 2 diabetic patients and in nondiabetic subjects with hypertriglyceridemia. Biomed Pharmacother 2006;60(4):182–185

23. Geohas J, Daly A, Juturu V, Finch M, Komorowski JR. Chromium picolinate and biotin combination reduces atherogenic index of plasma in patients with type 2 diabetes mellitus: a placebo-controlled, double-blinded, randomized clinical trial. Am J Med Sci 2007;333(3):145–153

24. Albarracin C, Fuqua B, Geohas J, Juturu V, Finch MR, Komorowski JR. Combination of chromium and biotin improves coronary risk factors in hypercholesterolemic type 2 diabetes mellitus: a placebo-controlled, double-blind randomized clinical trial. J Cardiometab Syndr 2007;2(2):91–97

25. Singer GM, Geohas J. The effect of chromium picolinate and biotin supplementation on glycemic control in poorly controlled patients with type 2 diabetes mellitus: a placebo-controlled, double-blinded, randomized trial. Diabetes Technol Ther 2006;8(6):636–643

26. Albarracin CA, Fuqua BC, Evans JL, Goldfine ID. Chromium picolinate and biotin combination improves glucose metabolism in treated, uncontrolled overweight to obese patients with type 2 diabetes. Diabetes Metab Res Rev 2008;24(1):41–51

27. Broadhurst CL, Domenico P. Clinical studies on chromium picolinate supplementation in diabetes mellitus—a review. Diabetes Technol Ther 2006;8(6):677–687

28. Coggeshall JC, Heggers JP, Robson MC, Baker H. Biotin status and plasma glucose levels in diabetics. Ann N Y Acad Sci 1985;447:389–392

29. Romero-Navarro G, Cabrera-Valladares G, German MS, et al. Biotin regulation of pancreatic glucokinase and insulin in primary cultured rat islets and in biotin-deficient rats. Endocrinology 1999;140(10):4595–4600

30. Floersheim GL. [Treatment of brittle fingernails with biotin]. Z Hautkr 1989;64(1):41–48

31. Hochman LG, Scher RK, Meyerson MS. Brittle nails: response to daily biotin supplementation. Cutis 1993;51(4):303–305

32. Briggs DR, Wahlqvist ML. Food Facts: The Complete No-Fads-Plain-Facts Guide to Healthy Eating. Victoria, Australia: Penguin Books; 1988

33. Staggs CG, Sealey WM, McCabe BJ, Teague AM, Mock DM. Determination of the biotin content of select foods using accurate and sensitive HPLC/avidin binding. J Food Compost Anal 2004;17(6):767–776

34. Said HM, Ortiz A, McCloud E, Dyer D, Moyer MP, Rubin S. Biotin uptake by human colonic epithelial NCM460 cells: a carrier-mediated process shared with pantothenic acid. Am J Physiol 1998;275(5 Pt 1):C1365–C1371

35. Koutsikos D, Agroyannis B, Tzanatos-Exarchou H. Biotin for diabetic peripheral neuropathy. Biomed Pharmacother 1990;44(10):511–514

36. Debourdeau PM, Djezzar S, Estival JL, Zammit CM, Richard RC, Castot AC. Life-threatening eosinophilic pleuropericardial effusion related to vitamins B5 and H. Ann Pharmacother 2001;35(4):424–426

37. Zempleni J, Mock DM. Human peripheral blood mononuclear cells: Inhibition of biotin transport by reversible competition with pantothenic acid is quantitatively minor. J Nutr Biochem 1999;10(7):427–432

38. Flodin N. Pharmacology of Micronutrients. New York: Alan R. Liss, Inc.; 1988

39. Camporeale G, Zempleni J. Biotin. In: Bowman BA, Russell RM, eds. Present Knowledge in Nutrition, 9th ed, Volume 1. Washington, DC: ILSI Press; 2006:314–326

2 Folic Acid

The terms *folic acid* and *folate* are often used interchangeably for this water-soluble B-complex vitamin. Folic acid, the more stable form, occurs rarely in foods or the human body but is the form most often used in vitamin supplements and fortified foods. Naturally occurring folates exist in many chemical forms. They are found in foods as well as in metabolically active forms in the human body.[1] In the following discussion, forms found in food or the body are referred to as *folates*, whereas the form found in supplements or fortified foods is referred to as *folic acid*.

Function

One-carbon Metabolism

The only function of folate coenzymes in the body appears to be in mediating the transfer of one-carbon units.[2] Folate coenzymes act as acceptors and donors of one-carbon units in a variety of reactions critical to the metabolism of nucleic acids and amino acids.[3]

Nucleic acid metabolism. Folate coenzymes play a vital role in DNA metabolism through two different pathways (**Fig. 2.1**):
1. The synthesis of DNA from its precursors (thymidine and purines) is dependent on folate coenzymes.
2. A folate coenzyme is required for the synthesis of methionine, and methionine is required for the synthesis of *S*-adenosylmethionine (SAM).

SAM is a methyl group (one-carbon unit) donor used in many biological methylation reactions, including the methylation of a number of sites within DNA and RNA. Methylation of DNA may be important in cancer prevention.

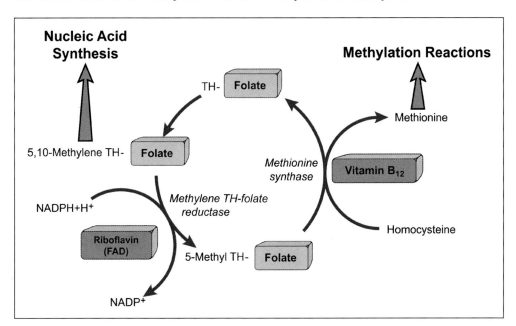

Fig. 2.1 Folate and nucleic acid metabolism: 5,10-methylene tetrahydrofolate (THF) is required for the synthesis of nucleic acids, and 5-methyl THF is required for the formation of methionine from homocysteine. Methionine, in the form of *S*-adenosylmethionine, is required for many biological methylation reactions, including DNA methylation. Methylene TH-folate reductase is a flavin-dependent enzyme required to catalyze the reduction of 5,10-methylene THF to 5-methyl THF.

Amino acid metabolism. Folate coenzymes are required for the metabolism of several important amino acids. The synthesis of methionine from homocysteine requires a folate coenzyme as well as a vitamin B_{12}-dependent enzyme. Thus, folate deficiency can result in decreased synthesis of methionine and a build-up of homocysteine. Increased levels of homocysteine may be a risk factor for heart disease as well as several other chronic diseases.

Nutrient Interactions

The metabolism of homocysteine, an intermediate in the metabolism of sulfur-containing amino acids, provides an example of the interrelationships of nutrients necessary for optimal physiological function and health. Healthy individuals use two different pathways to metabolize homocysteine (**Fig. 2.2**). One pathway (methionine synthase) synthesizes methionine from homocysteine and depends on a folate coenzyme and a vitamin B_{12}-dependent enzyme. The other pathway converts homocysteine to another amino acid, cysteine, and requires two vitamin B_6-dependent enzymes. Thus, the amount of homocysteine in the blood is regulated by three vitamins: folate, vitamin B_{12}, and vitamin B_6.[4]

Deficiency

Causes

Folate deficiency is most often caused by a dietary insufficiency; however, it can occur in a number of other situations, for example, alcoholism is associated with low dietary intake and diminished absorption of folate, which can lead to

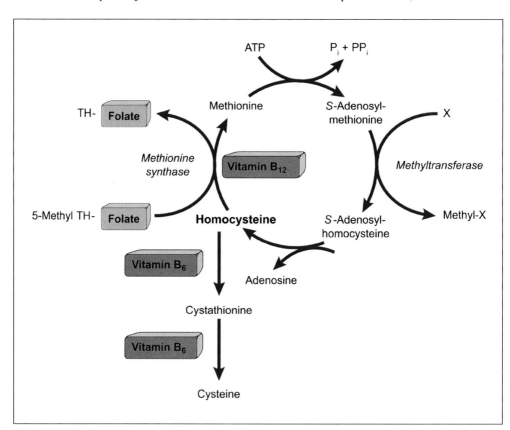

Fig. 2.2 Homocysteine metabolism: S-adenosylhomocysteine is formed during S-adenosylmethionine-dependent methylation reactions, and the hydrolysis of S-adenosylhomocysteine results in homocysteine. Homocysteine may be remethylated to form methionine by a folate-dependent reaction that is catalyzed by methionine synthase, a vitamin B_{12}-dependent enzyme. Alternately, homocysteine may be metabolized to cysteine in reactions catalyzed by two vitamin B_6-dependent enzymes.

folate deficiency. In addition, certain conditions such as pregnancy or cancer result in increased rates of cell division and metabolism, causing an increase in the body's demand for folate.[5] Several medications may also contribute to deficiency (see "Drug Interactions," p. 14).

Symptoms

Individuals in the early stages of folate deficiency may not show obvious symptoms, but their blood levels of homocysteine may increase. Rapidly dividing cells are most vulnerable to the effects of folate deficiency, so when the folate supply to the rapidly dividing cells of the bone marrow is inadequate, blood cell division becomes abnormal, resulting in fewer but larger red blood cells. This type of anemia is called *megaloblastic* or *macrocytic* anemia, referring to the enlarged, immature red blood cells. Neutrophils, a type of white blood cell, become hypersegmented, a change that can be found by examining a blood sample microscopically. As normal red blood cells have a lifetime in the circulation of approximately 4 months, it can take months for folate-deficient individuals to develop the characteristic megaloblastic anemia. Progression of such an anemia leads to decreased oxygen-carrying capacity of the blood and may ultimately result in symptoms of fatigue, weakness, and shortness of breath.[1] It is important to point out that megaloblastic anemia resulting from folate deficiency is identical to the megaloblastic anemia resulting from vitamin B_{12} deficiency, and further clinical testing is required to diagnose the true cause of megaloblastic anemia.

Recommended Dietary Allowance

Traditionally, the dietary folate requirement was defined as the amount needed to prevent a deficiency severe enough to cause symptoms such as anemia. The most recent recommended dietary allowance (RDA) (**Table 2.1**) was based primarily on the adequacy of red blood cell folate concentrations at different levels of folate intake, as judged by the absence of abnormal hematological indicators. Red cell folate has been shown to correlate with liver folate stores. Maintenance of normal blood homocysteine levels, an indicator of one-carbon metabolism, was considered only as an ancillary indicator of adequate folate intake. As pregnancy is associated with a significant increase in cell division and other metabolic processes that require folate coenzymes, the RDA for pregnant women is considerably higher than for women who are not pregnant.[3] However, the prevention of neural tube defects (NTDs) was not considered when setting the RDA for pregnant women. Rather, reducing the risk of NTDs was considered in a separate recommendation for women capable of becoming pregnant, because the crucial events in neural tube development occur before many women are aware that they are pregnant.[6]

Dietary Folate Equivalents

When the Food and Nutrition Board (FNB) of the Institute of Medicine set the new dietary recommendation for folate, they introduced a new unit, the dietary folate equivalent (DFE):

Table 2.1 Recommended dietary allowance for folate in DFEs

Life stage	Age	Males (µg/day)	Females (µg/day)
Infants	0–6 months	65 (AI)	65 (AI)
Infants	7–12 months	80 (AI)	80 (AI)
Children	1–3 years	150	150
Children	4–8 years	200	200
Children	9–13 years	300	300
Adolescents	14–18 years	400	400
Adults	≥ 19 years	400	400
Pregnancy	All ages	–	600
Breast-feeding	All ages	–	500

AI, adequate intake; DFE, dietary folate equivalent.

- 1 μg of food folate provides 1 μg DFE.
- 1 μg folic acid taken with meals or as fortified food provides 1.7 μg DFE.
- 1 μg folic acid (supplement) taken on an empty stomach provides 2 μg DFE.

Use of the DFE reflects the higher bioavailability of the synthetic folic acid in supplements and fortified foods compared with that of naturally occurring food folates,[6] for example, a serving of food containing 60 μg folate would provide 60 μg DFE, whereas a serving of pasta fortified with 60 μg folic acid would provide $1.7 \times 60 = 102$ μg DFE due to the higher bioavailability of folic acid. A folic acid supplement of 400 μg taken on an empty stomach would provide 800 μg DFE.

Genetic Variation in Folate Requirements

A common polymorphism or variation in the gene for the enzyme methylene tetrahydrofolate reductase (MTHFR), known as the C 677 T *MTHFR* polymorphism, results in a less stable enzyme.[7] Depending on the population, 50% of individuals may have inherited one copy (C/T), and 5%–25% may have inherited two copies (T/T) of the abnormal *MTHFR* gene. *MTHFR* plays an important role in maintaining the specific folate coenzyme required to form methionine from homocysteine (see **Fig. 2.1**). When folate intake is low, individuals who are homozygous (T/T) for the abnormal gene have lower levels of MTHFR and thus higher levels of homocysteine in their blood.[8] Improved folate nutritional status appears to stabilize MTHFR, resulting in improved enzyme levels and lower homocysteine levels. An important unanswered question about folate is whether the current RDA is enough to normalize MTHFR levels in individuals who are homozygous for the C 677 T polymorphism, or whether those individuals have a higher folate requirement than the RDA.[9]

Disease Prevention

Pregnancy Complications

Neural tube defects. Fetal growth and development are characterized by widespread cell division. Adequate folate is critical for DNA and RNA synthesis. NTDs result in either anencephaly or spina bifida, both of which are devastating and sometimes fatal birth defects. The defects occur between days 21 and 27 after conception, a time when many women do not realize that they are pregnant.[10] The risk of NTDs in the United States before fortification of foods with folic acid was estimated to be 1 per 1000 pregnancies.[1] Results of randomized trials have demonstrated 60%–100% reductions in NTD cases when women consumed folic acid supplements in addition to a varied diet during the periconceptional period (about 1 month before and 1 month after conception). The results of these and other studies prompted the US Public Health Service to recommend that all women capable of becoming pregnant consume 400 μg folic acid daily to prevent NTDs. The recommendation was made to all women of childbearing age because adequate folic acid must be available very early in pregnancy and many pregnancies in the United States are unplanned. Despite the effectiveness of folic acid supplementation, it appears that fewer than half of women who become pregnant follow the recommendation.[11] To decrease the incidence of NTDs, the US Food and Drug Administration (FDA) implemented legislation in 1998 requiring the fortification of all enriched grain products with folic acid. The required level of folic acid fortification in the United States was estimated to provide 100 μg additional folic acid in the average person's diet, though it probably provides even more due to overuse of folic acid by food manufacturers.[9]

The Centers for Disease Control and Prevention reported that the frequency of NTDs in the United States has decreased by 26% since the mandate.[12] However, studies in Canada, where fortification is nearly identical to that in the United States (1.5 and 1.4 mg folic acid/kg grain, respectively), have reported greater reductions in the incidence of NTDs. In fact, it was recently proposed that the fortification legislation has prevented approximately 50% of NTDs in Canada and the United States, but that improvements in the latter have been largely underestimated.[13]

Other pregnancy complications. Adequate folate status may also prevent the occurrence of other types of birth defects, including certain heart defects and limb malformations. However, the support for these findings is not as consistent or clear as support for NTD prevention.[10] In addition, low levels of dietary folate during pregnancy have been associated with increased risks of premature delivery and low infant birth weights. More recently, elevated blood homocysteine levels, considered an indicator of functional folate deficiency, have been associated with increased incidence of miscarriage as well as pregnancy complications such as pre-eclampsia and placental abruption.[14] Thus, it is reasonable to maintain folic acid supplementation throughout pregnancy, even after closure of the neural tube in order to decrease the risk of other problems during pregnancy.

Cardiovascular Diseases

Homocysteine and cardiovascular diseases. The results of more than 80 studies indicate that even moderately elevated levels of homocysteine in the blood increase the risk of cardiovascular diseases.[4] An analysis of the observational studies on blood homocysteine and vascular disease indicated that a prolonged decrease in plasma homocysteine level of only 1 μmol/L resulted in about a 10% risk reduction.[15] The mechanism by which homocysteine increases the risk of vascular disease remains the subject of a great deal of research, but it may involve adverse effects of homocysteine on blood clotting, arterial vasodilation, and thickening of arterial walls.[16] Although increased homocysteine levels in the blood have been consistently associated with increased risk of cardiovascular diseases, it is not yet clear whether lowering homocysteine levels will reduce cardiovascular disease risk. Consequently, the American Heart Association (AHA) recommends screening for elevated total homocysteine levels only in "high-risk" individuals, for example, those with a personal or family history of premature cardiovascular disease, malnutrition or malabsorption syndromes, hypothyroidism, kidney failure, lupus, or individuals taking certain medications (nicotinic acid, theophylline, bile acid-binding resins, methotrexate, and L-dopa). Most research indicates that a plasma homocysteine level of less than 10 μmol/L is associated with a lower risk of cardiovascular disease and is a reasonable treatment goal for individuals at high risk.[17]

Folate and homocysteine. Folate-rich diets have been associated with decreased risk of cardiovascular disease. A study that followed 1980 Finnish men for 10 years found that those who consumed the most dietary folate had a 55% lower risk of an acute coronary event when compared with those who consumed the least dietary folate.[18] Of the three vitamins that regulate homocysteine levels, folic acid has been shown to have the greatest effect in lowering basal levels of homocysteine in the blood when there is no coexisting deficiency of vitamin B_{12} or vitamin B_6. Increasing folate intake through folate-rich foods or supplements has been found to lower homocysteine levels. Moreover, blood homocysteine levels have declined since the FDA mandated folic acid fortification of the grain supply.[9] A recent meta-analysis of 25 randomized controlled trials found that supplementation with 0.8 mg folic acid daily maximally reduced plasma homocysteine concentrations; daily doses of 0.2 and 0.4 mg folic acid were associated with 60% and 90% reductions, respectively, in plasma homocysteine.[19] A supplement regimen of 400 μg folic acid, 2 mg vitamin B_6, and 6 μg vitamin B_{12} has been advocated by the AHA if an initial trial of a folate-rich diet is not successful in adequately lowering homocysteine levels.[17]

Although increased folic acid intake has been found to decrease homocysteine levels, it is currently not clear whether increasing folic acid intake results in decreased risk of cardiovascular diseases. Several randomized, placebo-controlled trials have been conducted or are ongoing to determine whether homocysteine lowering through folic acid and other B-vitamin supplementation reduces the incidence of cardiovascular diseases. A preliminary meta-analysis of data from four of the ongoing trials, including about 14 000 participants, showed that B-vitamin supplementation had no significant effect on risk of coronary heart disease or stroke.[20] Similarly, another meta-analysis of 12 randomized controlled trials, including data from 16958 individuals with pre-existing cardiovascular or renal disease, found that folic acid supplementation had no effect on coronary heart disease, stroke, or all-cause mortality despite 13%–52% reductions in plasma homocysteine concentrations.[21] Consequently, the AHA removed its recommendation for using folic acid to prevent cardiovascular diseases in high-risk women.[22] Completion of the ongoing clinical trials should provide a more definitive answer on whether folic acid is beneficial for the prevention or treatment of heart disease or stroke.

Cancer

Cancer is thought to arise from DNA damage in excess of ongoing DNA repair and/or the inappropriate expression of critical genes. As a result of the important roles played by folate in DNA and RNA synthesis and methylation, it is possible for folate intake to affect both DNA repair and gene expression. The consumption of at least five servings of fruit and vegetables daily has been consistently associated with a decreased incidence of cancer. Fruit and vegetables are excellent sources of folate, which may play a role in their anti-carcinogenic effect. Observational studies have found diminished folate status to be associated with cancers of the cervix, colon and rectum, lung, esophagus, brain, pancreas, and breast. Intervention trials of folic acid supplementation in humans have been conducted mainly with respect to cervical and colorectal (colon and rectum) cancer. Although the results in cervical cancer have been inconsistent,[2] randomized intervention trials regarding colorectal cancer have been more promising.[23,24]

Colorectal cancer. A recent meta-analysis of seven cohort and nine case–control studies found that folate from food was inversely associated with colorectal cancer risk; however, total folate from food and folic acid supplements was not associated with colorectal cancer risk.[25] It is important to note that the case–control studies examined in this meta-analysis were highly heterogeneous, and that the authors stated that dietary fiber or other vitamins could have confounded their results. Overall, the role of folate in the possible prevention of colorectal cancer provides an example of the complexity of the interactions between genetics and nutrition. In general, observational studies have found that relatively low folate intake and high alcohol intake are associated with increased incidence of colorectal cancer.[1,26,27] Alcohol interferes with the absorption and metabolism of folate.[5] In a prospective study of more than 45 000 male health professionals, current intake of more than two alcoholic drinks per day doubled the risk of colon cancer. The combination of high alcohol and low folate intake yielded an even greater risk of colon cancer; however, increased alcohol intake in individuals who consumed 650 µg folate or more per day was not associated with an increased risk of colon cancer.[28]

In some studies, individuals who are homozygous for the C 677 T *MTHFR* polymorphism (T/T) have been found to be at decreased risk for colon cancer when folate intake is adequate. However, when folate intake is low and/or alcohol intake is high, individuals with the T/T genotype have been found to be at increased risk of colorectal cancer.[29,30]

Although dietary folate may protect against colorectal cancer, high doses of supplemental folic acid may actually accelerate tumor growth in cancer patients. A recent chemopreventive trial in patients with a history of colorectal adenoma associated supplementation of 1 mg/day of folic acid (more than twice the RDA) with a statistical trend for advanced colorectal lesions, as well as with a significantly increased risk (more than twofold) for the presence of three or more colorectal adenomas.[31] In this study, folic acid supplementation was also associated with an increased risk for cancers at other sites, primarily the prostate. Human observational studies as well as animal studies on high-dose folate and cancer have reported mixed results. Thus, more research is needed to determine the role of high-dose folate in cancer progression.

Breast cancer. Studies investigating whether folate intake affects breast cancer risk have reported mixed results.[32] The results of two prospective studies suggest that increased folate intake may reduce the risk of breast cancer in women who regularly consume alcohol,[33-35] and moderate alcohol intake has been associated with increased risk of breast cancer in women in several studies. Interestingly, a very large prospective study in more than 88 000 nurses reported that folic acid intake was not associated with breast cancer in women who consumed less than one alcoholic drink per day. However, in women consuming at least one alcoholic drink per day, folic acid intake of at least 600 µg daily resulted in about half the risk of breast cancer compared with women who consumed less than 300 µg folic acid daily.[35]

Alzheimer Disease and Cognitive Impairment

The role of folate in nucleic acid synthesis and methylation reactions is essential for normal brain function. Over the past decade several investigators have described associations between decreased folate levels and cognitive impairment in elderly people.[36] A large cross-sectional study in elderly Canadians found that those individuals with low serum folate levels were more likely to have dementia, be institutionalized, and be depressed. However, these findings could reflect the poorer nutritional status of institutionalized elderly people and individuals with dementia. In the same study, low serum folate levels were associated with an increased likelihood of short-term memory problems in elderly individuals who had no signs of dementia.[37] A study in 30 elderly nuns, who lived in the same convent, ate the same diet, and had similar lifestyles, reported a strong association between decreased blood folate levels and the severity of brain atrophy related to Alzheimer disease.[38] More recent studies have reported conflicting results as to whether folate status impacts Alzheimer disease risk. One study in elderly people of predominantly Hispanic and African–American ethnicity with a high prevalence of vascular risk factors reported that a higher folate intake, from diet and folic acid supplements, was associated with a decreased risk for Alzheimer disease.[39]

In contrast, a prospective study in elderly individuals reported that dietary folate is not associated with Alzheimer disease,[40] whereas another prospective study reported that a high folate intake, from foods and folic acid supplements, was associated with increased rates of cognitive decline in elderly people.[41] Moderately increased homocysteine levels, as well as decreased folate and vitamin B_{12} levels, have been associated with Alzheimer disease and vascular dementia. One study in 370 elderly men and women, who were followed over 3 years, associated low serum levels of vitamin B_{12} ($\leq$150 pmol/L) or folate ($\leq$10 nmol/L) with a doubling of the risk of developing Alzheimer disease.[42] In a sample of 1092 men and women without dementia followed for an average of 10 years, those with higher plasma homocysteine levels at baseline had a significantly higher risk of developing Alzheimer disease and other types of dementia.[43] Those with plasma homocysteine levels > 14 μmol/L had nearly twice the risk of developing Alzheimer disease.

Disease Treatment

Currently, there is insufficient evidence to support the use of supplemental folic acid for the treatment of diseases or health conditions other than folate deficiency. The use of folic acid supplements to treat elevated plasma homocysteine levels (hyperhomocysteinemia) is discussed under "Cardiovascular Diseases," p. 11.

Table 2.2 Food sources of folate

Food	Serving	Folate (μg DFE)
Fortified breakfast cereal	1 cup	200–400[a]
White rice, cooked	1 cup	221[a]
White spaghetti, cooked	1 cup	196[a]
Lentils, cooked	½ cup	179
Garbanzo beans, cooked	½ cup	14
Asparagus, cooked	½ cup (about 6 spears)	134
Spinach, cooked	½ cup	132
Orange juice from concentrate	6 ounces	83
Lima beans, cooked	½ cup	78
White bread	1 slice	35[a]

[a]Fortified with folic acid (1.4 mg folic acid/kg).
DFE, dietary folate equivalent.

Sources

Food Sources

Green leafy vegetables (foliage) are rich sources of folate and provide the basis for its name. Citrus fruit juices, legumes, and fortified cereals are also excellent sources of folate.[1] A number of folate-rich foods are listed in **Table 2.2** along with their folate content. To help prevent NTDs, the FDA required the addition of 1.4 mg folic acid/kg grain to be added to refined grain products, which are already enriched with niacin, thiamin, riboflavin, and iron, as of January 1, 1998. The addition of nutrients to foods in order to prevent a nutritional deficiency or restore nutrients lost in processing is known as *fortification*. It has been estimated that this level of fortification increases dietary intake by an average of 100 µg folic acid/day.[10]

Supplements

The principal form of supplementary folate is folic acid, which is available in single ingredient and combination products such as B-complex vitamins and multivitamins. Doses of 1000 µg (1 mg) or more require a prescription.[44]

Safety

Toxicity

No adverse effects have been associated with the consumption of excess folate from foods. Concerns about safety are limited to synthetic folic acid intake. Deficiency of vitamin B_{12}, although often undiagnosed, may affect a significant number of people, especially older adults. One symptom of vitamin B_{12} deficiency is megaloblastic

Table 2.3 Tolerable upper intake level (UL) for folic acid

Life stage	Age	UL (µg/day)
Infants	0–12 months	Not possible to establish[a]
Children	1–3 years	300
Children	4–8 years	400
Children	9–13 years	600
Adolescents	14–18 years	800
Adults	≥ 19 years	1000

[a] Source of intake should be from food and formula only.

anemia, which is indistinguishable from that associated with folate deficiency. Large doses of folic acid given to an individual with an undiagnosed vitamin B_{12} deficiency could correct megaloblastic anemia without correcting the underlying vitamin B_{12} deficiency, leaving the individual at risk of developing irreversible neurological damage. Such cases of neurological progression in vitamin B_{12} deficiency have been mostly seen at folic acid doses of 5000 µg (5 mg) and above. To be very sure of preventing irreversible neurological damage in vitamin B_{12}-deficient individuals, the FNB advises that all adults limit their intake of folic acid (supplements and fortification) to 1000 µg (**Table 2.3**). The board also noted that vitamin B_{12} deficiency is very rare in women in their childbearing years, making the consumption of folic acid at or above 1000 µg/day unlikely to cause problems;[1] however, there are limited data on the effects of large doses.

Drug Interactions

When nonsteroidal anti-inflammatory drugs (NSAIDs), such as aspirin or ibuprofen, are taken in very large therapeutic dosages (i.e., to treat severe arthritis), they may interfere with folate metabolism. In contrast, routine low-dose use of NSAIDs has not been found to adversely affect folate status. The anticonvulsant, phenytoin, has been shown to inhibit the intestinal absorption of folate, and several studies have associated decreased folate status with long-term use of the anticonvulsants, phenytoin, phenobarbital, and primidone.[45] However, few studies controlled for differences in dietary folate intake between anticonvulsant users and nonusers. Also, taking folic acid at the same time as the cholesterol-lowering agents, cholestyramine and colestipol, may decrease the absorption of folic acid.[44]

Methotrexate is a folic acid antagonist used to treat a number of diseases, including rheumatoid arthritis and psoriasis. Some of the side effects of methotrexate are similar to those of severe folate deficiency, and increased dietary folate or supplemental folic acid may decrease side effects without reducing the efficacy of methotrexate. A number of other medications have been shown to have antifolate activity, including trimethoprim (an antibiotic), pyrimethamine (an antimalarial), triamterene (a blood pressure medication), and sulfasalazine (a treatment for ulcerative colitis). Early studies of oral contraceptives (birth control pills) containing high doses of estrogen indicated adverse effects on folate status; however, this finding has not been supported by more recent studies on low-dose oral contraceptives that controlled for dietary folate.[1]

LPI Recommendation

The available scientific evidence shows that adequate folate intake prevents neural tube defects and other poor outcomes of pregnancy, is helpful in lowering the risk of some forms of cancer, especially in genetically susceptible individuals, and may lower the risk of cardiovascular diseases. The Linus Pauling Institute recommends that adults take a 400 µg supplement of folic acid daily, in addition to folate and folic acid consumed in the diet. A daily multivitamin/mineral supplement, containing 100% of the daily value (DV) for folic acid provides 400 µg folic acid. Even with a larger than average intake of folic acid from fortified foods, it is unlikely that an individual's daily folic acid intake would regularly exceed the tolerable upper intake level of 1000 µg/day established by the FNB.

Older Adults

The recommendation for 400 µg/day of supplemental folic acid as part of a daily multivitamin/multimineral supplement, in addition to a folate-rich diet, is especially important for older adults because blood homocysteine levels tend to increase with age.

Women Capable of Becoming Pregnant

As the crucial events in neural tube development occur before many women are aware that they are pregnant, women who are capable of becoming pregnant should consume 400 µg/day folic acid from supplements or fortified food, in addition to dietary sources to prevent NTDs.

References

1. Food and Nutrition Board, Institute of Medicine. Folate. In: Dietary Reference Intakes for Thiamin, Riboflavin, Niacin, Vitamin B_6, Folate, Vitamin B_{12}, Pantothenic Acid, Biotin, and Choline. Washington, DC: National Academy Press, 1998:196–305
2. Choi SW, Mason JB. Folate and carcinogenesis: an integrated scheme. J Nutr 2000;130(2):129–132
3. Bailey LB, Gregory JF III. Folate metabolism and requirements. J Nutr 1999;129(4):779–782
4. Gerhard GT, Duell PB. Homocysteine and atherosclerosis. Curr Opin Lipidol 1999;10(5):417–428
5. Herbert V. Folic acid. In: Shils M, Olson JA, Shike M, Ross AC, eds. Modern Nutrition in Health and Disease, 9th ed. Baltimore, MD: Lippincott Williams & Wilkins; 1999:433–446
6. Bailey LB. Dietary reference intakes for folate: the debut of dietary folate equivalents. Nutr Rev 1998;56(10):294–299
7. Bailey LB, Gregory JF III. Polymorphisms of methylenetetrahydrofolate reductase and other enzymes: metabolic significance, risks and impact on folate requirement. J Nutr 1999;129(5):919–922
8. Kauwell GP, Wilsky CE, Cerda JJ, et al. Methylenetetrahydrofolate reductase mutation (677C−>T) negatively influences plasma homocysteine response to marginal folate intake in elderly women. Metabolism 2000;49(11):1440–1443
9. Shane B. Folic acid, vitamin B-12, and vitamin B-6. In: Stipanuk M, ed. Biochemical and Physiological Aspects of Human Nutrition. Philadelphia, PA: WB Saunders Co.; 2000:483–518
10. Eskes TK. Open or closed? A world of difference: a history of homocysteine research. Nutr Rev 1998; 56(8):236–244
11. McNulty H, Cuskelly GJ, Ward M. Response of red blood cell folate to intervention: implications for folate recommendations for the prevention of neural tube defects. Am J Clin Nutr 2000; 71(5, Suppl):1308S–1311S
12. Centers for Disease Control and Prevention (CDC). Spina bifida and anencephaly before and after folic acid mandate–United States, 1995–1996 and 1999–2000. MMWR Morb Mortal Wkly Rep 2004; 53(17):362–365
13. Mills JL, Signore C. Neural tube defect rates before and after food fortification with folic acid. Birth Defects Res A Clin Mol Teratol 2004;70(11):844–845
14. Scholl TO, Johnson WG. Folic acid: influence on the outcome of pregnancy. Am J Clin Nutr 2000; 71(5, Suppl)1295S–1303S
15. Boushey CJ, Beresford SA, Omenn GS, Motulsky AG. A quantitative assessment of plasma homocysteine as a risk factor for vascular disease. Probable benefits of increasing folic acid intakes. JAMA 1995; 274(13):1049–1057
16. Seshadri N, Robinson K. Homocysteine, B vitamins, and coronary artery disease. Med Clin North Am 2000;84(1):215–237
17. Malinow MR, Bostom AG, Krauss RM. Homocyst(e)ine, diet, and cardiovascular diseases: a statement for healthcare professionals from the Nutrition Committee, American Heart Association. Circulation 1999;99(1):178–182
18. Voutilainen S, Rissanen TH, Virtanen J, Lakka TA, Salonen JT; Kuopio Ischemic Heart Disease Risk Factor Study. Low dietary folate intake is associated with an excess incidence of acute coronary events: The Kuopio Ischemic Heart Disease Risk Factor Study. Circulation 2001;103(22):2674–2680
19. Homocysteine Lowering Trialists' Collaboration. Dose-dependent effects of folic acid on blood concentrations of homocysteine: a meta-analysis of the randomized trials. Am J Clin Nutr 2005;82(4):806–812
20. Clarke R, Lewington S, Sherliker P, Armitage J. Effects of B-vitamins on plasma homocysteine concentrations and on risk of cardiovascular disease and dementia. Curr Opin Clin Nutr Metab Care 2007; 10(1):32–39
21. Bazzano LA, Reynolds K, Holder KN, He J. Effect of folic acid supplementation on risk of cardiovascular diseases: a meta-analysis of randomized controlled trials. JAMA 2006;296(22):2720–2726
22. Updated guidelines advise focusing on women's lifetime heart risk. Update gives definitive answers on HRT, aspirin, supplements [website]. Available at: http://www.goredforwomen.org/press_release.aspx?release_id=918. Accessed 4 Jan 2011

23. Kim YI, Baik HW, Fawaz K, et al. Effects of folate supplementation on two provisional molecular markers of colon cancer: a prospective, randomized trial. Am J Gastroenterol 2001;96(1):184–195
24. Cravo ML, Pinto AG, Chaves P, et al. Effect of folate supplementation on DNA methylation of rectal mucosa in patients with colonic adenomas: correlation with nutrient intake. Clin Nutr 1998;17(2):45–49
25. Sanjoaquin MA, Allen N, Couto E, Roddam AW, Key TJ. Folate intake and colorectal cancer risk: a meta-analytical approach. Int J Cancer 2005;113(5):825–828
26. Su LJ, Arab L. Nutritional status of folate and colon cancer risk: evidence from NHANES I epidemiologic follow-up study. Ann Epidemiol 2001;11(1):65–72
27. Terry P, Jain M, Miller AB, Howe GR, Rohan TE. Dietary intake of folic acid and colorectal cancer risk in a cohort of women. Int J Cancer 2002;97(6):864–867
28. Giovannucci E, Rimm EB, Ascherio A, Stampfer MJ, Colditz GA, Willett WC. Alcohol, low-methionine—low-folate diets, and risk of colon cancer in men. J Natl Cancer Inst 1995;87(4):265–273
29. Slattery ML, Potter JD, Samowitz W, Schaffer D, Leppert M. Methylenetetrahydrofolate reductase, diet, and risk of colon cancer. Cancer Epidemiol Biomarkers Prev 1999;8(6):513–518
30. Ma J, Stampfer MJ, Giovannucci E, et al. Methylenetetrahydrofolate reductase polymorphism, dietary interactions, and risk of colorectal cancer. Cancer Res 1997;57(6):1098–1102
31. Cole BF, Baron JA, Sandler RS, et al; Polyp Prevention Study Group. Folic acid for the prevention of colorectal adenomas: a randomized clinical trial. JAMA 2007;297(21):2351–2359
32. Kim YI. Does a high folate intake increase the risk of breast cancer? Nutr Rev 2006;64(10 Pt 1):468–475
33. Rohan TE, Jain MG, Howe GR, Miller AB. Dietary folate consumption and breast cancer risk. J Natl Cancer Inst 2000;92(3):266–269
34. Sellers TA, Kushi LH, Cerhan JR, et al. Dietary folate intake, alcohol, and risk of breast cancer in a prospective study of postmenopausal women. Epidemiology 2001;12(4):420–428
35. Zhang S, Hunter DJ, Hankinson SE, et al. A prospective study of folate intake and the risk of breast cancer. JAMA 1999;281(17):1632–1637
36. Weir DG, Molloy AM. Microvascular disease and dementia in the elderly: are they related to hyperhomocysteinemia? Am J Clin Nutr 2000;71(4):859–860
37. Ebly EM, Schaefer JP, Campbell NR, Hogan DB. Folate status, vascular disease and cognition in elderly Canadians. Age Ageing 1998;27(4):485–491
38. Snowdon DA, Tully CL, Smith CD, Riley KP, Markesbery WR. Serum folate and the severity of atrophy of the neocortex in Alzheimer disease: findings from the Nun study. Am J Clin Nutr 2000;71(4):993–998
39. Luchsinger JA, Tang MX, Miller J, Green R, Mayeux R. Relation of higher folate intake to lower risk of Alzheimer disease in the elderly. Arch Neurol 2007;64(1):86–92
40. Morris MC, Evans DA, Schneider JA, Tangney CC, Bienias JL, Aggarwal NT. Dietary folate and vitamins B-12 and B-6 not associated with incident Alzheimer's disease. J Alzheimers Dis 2006;9(4):435–443
41. Morris MC, Evans DA, Bienias JL, et al. Dietary folate and vitamin B12 intake and cognitive decline among community-dwelling older persons. Arch Neurol 2005;62(4):641–645
42. Wang HX, Wahlin A, Basun H, Fastbom J, Winblad B, Fratiglioni L. Vitamin B(12) and folate in relation to the development of Alzheimer's disease. Neurology 2001;56(9):1188–1194
43. Seshadri S, Beiser A, Selhub J, et al. Plasma homocysteine as a risk factor for dementia and Alzheimer's disease. N Engl J Med 2002;346(7):476–483
44. Hendler SS, Rorvik DR, eds. PDR for Nutritional Supplements. Montvale: Medical Economics Company, Inc; 2001
45. Apeland T, Mansoor MA, Strandjord RE. Antiepileptic drugs as independent predictors of plasma total homocysteine levels. Epilepsy Res 2001;47(1-2):27–35

3 Niacin

Niacin is a water-soluble vitamin, which is also known as nicotinic acid or vitamin B_3. Nicotinamide is the derivative of niacin; it is used by the body to form the coenzymes nicotinamide adenine dinucleotide (NAD) and nicotinamide adenine dinucleotide phosphate (NADP). The chemical structures of the various forms of niacin are shown in **Fig. 3.1**. None of the forms is related to the nicotine found in tobacco, although their names are similar.[1]

Function

Oxidation–Reduction (Redox) Reactions

Living organisms derive most of their energy from oxidation–reduction (redox) reactions, which are processes involving the transfer of electrons. As many as 200 enzymes require the niacin coenzymes, NAD and NADP, mainly to accept or donate electrons for redox reactions. NAD functions most often in energy-producing reactions involving the degradation (catabolism) of carbohydrates, fats, proteins, and alcohol. NADP functions more often in biosynthetic (anabolic) reactions, such as in the synthesis of all macromolecules, including fatty acids and cholesterol.[1,2]

Non-redox Reactions

The niacin coenzyme, NAD, is the substrate (reactant) for two classes of enzymes (mono-ADP-ribosyltransferases and poly-ADP-ribose polymerases) that separate the niacin moiety from NAD and transfer ADP-ribose to proteins (**Fig. 3.2**). Mono-ADP-ribosyltransferases were first discovered in certain bacteria, in which they were found to produce toxins, such as cholera and diphtheria. These enzymes and their products, ADP-ribosylated proteins, have also been found in the cells of mammals and are thought to play a role in cell signaling by affecting G-protein activity.[3] G-proteins are proteins that bind guanosine-5′-triphosphate (GTP) and act as intermediaries in a number of cell-signaling pathways. Poly-ADP-ribose polymerases (PARPs) are enzymes that catalyze the transfer of many ADP-ribose units from NAD to acceptor proteins. PARPs appear to function in DNA repair and stress responses, cell signaling, transcription, regulation, apoptosis, chromatin structure, and cell differentiation, suggesting a possible role for NAD in cancer prevention.[2] At least five different PARPs have been identified and, although their functions are not yet well understood, their existence indicates a potential for considerable consumption of NAD.[4] A third class of enzymes (ADP-ribosyl cyclases) catalyzes the formation of cyclic ADP-ribose, a molecule that works within cells to

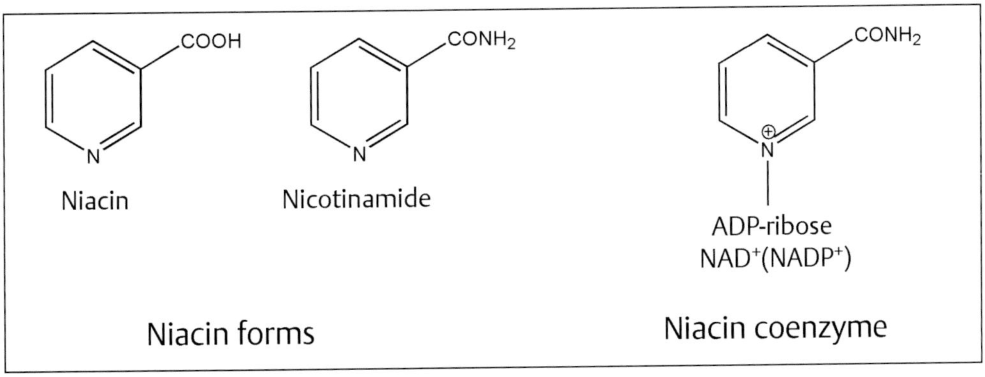

Fig. 3.1 Chemical structures of niacin and related compounds.

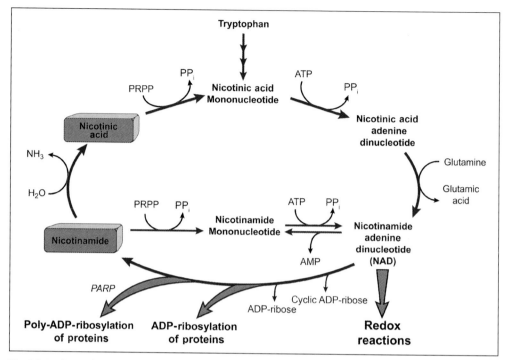

Fig. 3.2 Synthesis of nicotinamide adenine dinucleotide (NAD). NAD is required for numerous redox reactions. It is also consumed in ADP-ribosylation reactions. AMP, adenosine monophosphate; ADP, adenosine diphosphate; ATP, adenosine triphosphate; PARP, poly-ADP-ribose polymerase; PP$_i$, inorganic pyrophosphate; PRPP, phosphoribosyl pyrophosphate.

provoke the release of calcium ions from internal storage sites and probably also plays a role in cell signaling.[1]

Deficiency

Pellagra

The late stage of severe niacin deficiency is known as pellagra. Early records of pellagra followed the widespread cultivation of corn in Europe in the 1700s.[1] The disease was generally associated with poorer social classes whose chief dietary staple consisted of cereals such as corn or sorghum. Pellagra was also common in the southern United States during the early 1900s where income was low and corn products were a major dietary staple.[5] Interestingly, pellagra was not known in Mexico, where also corn was an important dietary staple and much of the population was poor. In fact, corn contains appreciable amounts of niacin, but it is present in a bound

form that is not nutritionally available to humans. The traditional preparation of corn tortillas in Mexico involves soaking the corn in a lime (calcium oxide) solution, before cooking. Heating the corn in an alkaline solution results in the release of bound niacin, increasing its bioavailability.[6]

The most common symptoms of niacin deficiency involve the skin, digestive system, and nervous system.[2] The symptoms of pellagra were commonly referred to as the four Ds: dermatitis, diarrhea, dementia, and death. In the skin, a thick, scaly, darkly pigmented rash develops symmetrically in areas exposed to sunlight. In fact, the word "pellagra" comes from the Italian phrase for rough or raw skin. Symptoms related to the digestive system include a bright red tongue, vomiting, and diarrhea. Neurological symptoms include headache, apathy, fatigue, depression, disorientation, and memory loss. If untreated, pellagra is ultimately fatal.[3]

Nutrient Interactions

Tryptophan and niacin. In addition to its synthesis from dietary niacin, NAD may also be synthesized in the liver from the dietary amino acid, tryptophan. The relative ability to make this conversion varies greatly from mice to humans. The synthesis of niacin from tryptophan also depends on enzymes that require vitamin B_6 and riboflavin as well as an enzyme containing heme (iron). On average, 1 mg niacin can be synthesized from the ingestion of 60 mg tryptophan. Thus, 60 mg tryptophan is considered to be 1 mg of niacin equivalents (NE). However, studies of pellagra in the southern United States during the early twentieth century indicated that the diets of many individuals who had pellagra contained enough NE to prevent pellagra,[3] challenging the idea that 60 mg dietary tryptophan is equivalent to 1 mg niacin. In particular, one study in young men found that the tryptophan content of the diet had no effect on the decrease in red blood cell niacin content that resulted from low dietary niacin.[7]

Causes of niacin deficiency. Niacin deficiency or pellagra may result from inadequate dietary intake of niacin and/or tryptophan. As mentioned above, other nutrient deficiencies may also contribute to the development of niacin deficiency; for example, patients with Hartnup disease, a hereditary disorder resulting in defective tryptophan absorption, have developed pellagra.[2] Carcinoid syndrome, a condition of increased secretion of serotonin and other catecholamines by carcinoid tumors, may also result in pellagra due to increased utilization of dietary tryptophan for serotonin rather than niacin synthesis. Further, prolonged treatment with the anti-tuberculosis drug, isoniazid, has resulted in niacin deficiency.[8]

Recommended Dietary Allowance

The recommended dietary allowance (RDA) for niacin, revised in 1998, was based on the prevention of deficiency (**Table 3.1**). Pellagra can be prevented by about 11 mg NE/day, but 12–16 mg/day has been found to normalize the urinary excretion of niacin metabolites (breakdown products) in healthy young adults. As pellagra represents severe deficiency, the Food and Nutrition Board (FNB) of the Institute of Medicine chose to use the excretion of niacin metabolites as an indicator of niacin nutritional status rather than symptoms of pellagra.[8] However, some researchers feel that cellular NAD and NADP content may be more relevant indicators of niacin nutritional status.[7,9,10]

Disease Prevention

Cancer

Studies of cultured cells (in vitro) provide evidence that NAD content influences the cellular response to DNA damage, an important risk factor in cancer development. Cellular NAD is con-

Table 3.1 Recommended dietary allowance for niacin

Life stage	Age	Males (mg NE[a]/day)	Females (mg NE/day)
Infants	0–6 months	2 (AI)[b]	2 (AI)[b]
Infants	7–12 months	4 (AI)	4 (AI)
Children	1–3 years	6	6
Children	4–8 years	8	8
Children	9–13 years	12	12
Adolescents	14–18 years	16	14
Adults	≥19 years	16	14
Pregnancy	All ages	–	18
Breast-feeding	All ages	–	17

AI, adequate intake; NE, niacin equivalent.
[a] 1 mg NE = 60 mg tryptophan = 1 mg niacin.
[b] 2 mg preformed niacin/day.

sumed in the synthesis of ADP-ribose polymers, which play a role in DNA repair, and cyclic ADP-ribose may also mediate cell-signaling pathways important in cancer prevention.[11] In addition, cellular depletion of NAD has been found to decrease levels of the tumor-suppressor protein, p53, in human breast, skin, and lung cells.[10] Neither the cellular NAD content nor the dietary intake of NAD precursors (niacin and tryptophan) necessary for optimizing protective responses after DNA damage has been determined, but both are likely to be higher than that required for the prevention of pellagra. Niacin deficiency was found to decrease bone marrow NAD and poly-ADP-ribose levels and increase the risk of chemically induced leukemia.[12] Moreover, one study reported that niacin supplementation decreased the risk of ultraviolet light-induced skin cancers in mice.[13] However, little is known about cellular NAD levels and the prevention of DNA damage or cancer in humans. One study in two healthy individuals involved elevating NAD levels in blood lymphocytes by supplementation with 100 mg nicotinic acid/day for 8 weeks. Compared with nonsupplemented individuals, the supplemented individuals had reduced DNA strand breaks in lymphocytes exposed to free radicals in a test tube assay.[14] More recently, nicotinic acid supplementation of up to 100 mg/day in 21 healthy smokers failed to provide any evidence of a decrease in cigarette smoke-induced genetic damage in blood lymphocytes compared with placebo.[15]

Generally, relationships between dietary factors and cancer are established first in epidemiological studies and followed up by basic cancer research at the cellular level. In the case of niacin, research on biochemical and cellular aspects of DNA repair has stimulated an interest in the relationship between niacin intake and cancer risk in human populations.[16] A large case–control study found increased consumption of niacin, along with antioxidant nutrients, to be associated with decreased incidence of oral (mouth), pharyngeal (throat), and esophageal cancers in northern Italy and Switzerland.[17,18] An increase in niacin intake of 6.2 mg was associated with about a 40% decrease in cases of cancers of the mouth and throat, whereas a 5.2 mg increase in niacin intake was associated with a similar decrease in cases of esophageal cancer.

Type 1 Diabetes Mellitus

Type 1 diabetes mellitus, formerly called insulin-dependent diabetes mellitus in children, is known to result from the autoimmune destruction of insulin-secreting β cells in the pancreas. Before the onset of symptomatic diabetes, specific antibodies, including islet cell antibodies (ICAs), can be detected in the blood of high-risk individuals. The ability to detect individuals at high risk for the development of type 1 diabetes led to the enrollment of high-risk siblings of children with type 1 diabetes into trials designed to prevent its onset. Evidence from in vitro and animal research indicates that high levels of nicotinamide protect β cells from damage by toxic chemicals, inflammatory white blood cells, and reactive oxygen species. Pharmacological doses of nicotinamide (up to 3 g/day) were first used to protect β cells in patients shortly after the onset of type 1 diabetes. An analysis of ten published trials (five placebo controlled) found evidence of improved β-cell function after 1 year of treatment with nicotinamide, but the analysis failed to find any clinical evidence of improved glycemic (blood glucose) control.[19]

High doses of nicotinamide have been found to decrease insulin sensitivity in high-risk relatives of patients with type 1 diabetes,[20] which might explain the finding of improved β-cell function without concomitant improvement in glycemic control. Several pilot studies for the prevention of type 1 diabetes in ICA-positive relatives of patients with type 1 diabetes yielded conflicting results, whereas a large randomized trial in schoolchildren that was not placebo controlled found a significantly lower incidence of type 1 diabetes in the nicotinamide-treated group. A large, multicenter, randomized controlled trial of nicotinamide in ICA-positive siblings of patients with diabetes aged between 3 and 12 years recently failed to find a difference in the incidence of type 1 diabetes after 3 years.[19] Another large multicenter trial of nicotinamide in high-risk relatives of patients with type 1 diabetes is currently in progress.[21] Unlike nicotinamide, nicotinic acid has not been found to be effective in the prevention of type 1 diabetes.

Disease Treatment

High Cholesterol and Cardiovascular Disease

Pharmacological doses of nicotinic acid, but not nicotinamide, have been known to reduce serum cholesterol since 1955.[22] Today, niacin is commonly prescribed with other lipid-lowering medications. However, one randomized, placebo-controlled, multicenter trial examined the effect of nicotinic acid therapy (3 g/day), alone, on outcomes of cardiovascular disease. Specifically, the Coronary Drug Project (CDP) followed more than 8000 men with a previous myocardial infarction (heart attack) for 6 years.[23] Compared with the placebo group, the group that took 3 g/day of nicotinic acid experienced an average 10% reduction in total blood cholesterol, a 26% decrease in triglycerides, a 27% reduction in recurrent nonfatal myocardial infarction, and a 26% reduction in cerebrovascular events (stroke + transient ischemic attacks). Although nicotinic acid therapy did not decrease total deaths or deaths from cardiovascular disease during the 6-year study period, post-trial follow-up 9 years later revealed a 10% reduction in total deaths with nicotinic acid treatment. Four out of five major cardiovascular outcome trials found nicotinic acid in combination with other therapies to be of statistically significant benefit in men and women.[24] Nicotinic acid therapy markedly increases high-density lipoprotein (HDL)-cholesterol levels, decreases serum Lp(a) (lipoprotein-a) concentrations, and shifts small, dense low-density lipoprotein (LDL) particles to large, buoyant LDL particles; all of these changes in the blood lipid profile are considered cardioprotective.

As a result of the adverse side effects associated with high doses of nicotinic acid (see under "Safety," p. 22), it has most recently been used in combination with other lipid-lowering medications in slightly lower doses.[22] A recent randomized controlled trial found that a combination of nicotinic acid (2–3 g/day) and a cholesterol-lowering drug (simvastatin) resulted in greater benefits on serum HDL levels and cardiovascular events, such as heart attack and stroke, than placebo in patients with coronary artery disease and low HDL levels.[25] However, an antioxidant combination (vitamin E, vitamin C, selenium, and β-carotene) appeared to blunt the beneficial effects of niacin plus simvastatin.[26] The effects of niacin are dose dependent.[27] A placebo-controlled study in 39 patients taking statins (cerivastatin, atorvastatin, or simvastatin) found that a very low dose of niacin, 100 mg daily, increased HDL-cholesterol by only 2.1 mg/dL, and the combination had no effect on LDL-cholesterol, total cholesterol, or triglyceride levels.[28] Doses of niacin higher than 1 g/day are typically used to treat hyperlipidemia. A few case reports have raised concerns that concurrent use of niacin and statins may result in myopathy; however, clinical trials have not confirmed such adverse effects.[25,29]

Although it is a nutrient, at the pharmacological dose required for cholesterol-lowering effects, the use of nicotinic acid should be approached as if it were a drug. Individuals should only undertake cholesterol-lowering therapy with nicotinic acid under the supervision of a qualified health-care provider in order to minimize potentially adverse effects and maximize therapeutic benefits.

Human Immunodeficiency Virus

It has been hypothesized that infection with human immunodeficiency virus (HIV), the virus that causes acquired immune deficiency syndrome (AIDS), increases the risk of niacin deficiency. Interferon-γ (IF-γ) is a cytokine produced by cells of the immune system in response to infection. IF-γ levels are elevated in individuals infected with HIV, and higher IF-γ levels have been associated with poorer prognoses. By stimulating the enzyme, indoleamine-2,3-dioxygenase (IDO), IF-γ increases the breakdown of tryptophan, a niacin precursor, thus supporting the idea that HIV infection increases the risk of niacin deficiency.[30] In a very small, uncontrolled study, treatment of four HIV-positive individuals with 1000–1500 mg/day of nicotinamide for 2 months resulted in 40% increases in plasma tryptophan levels.[31] An observational study of 281 HIV-positive men found that higher levels of niacin intake were associated with decreased progression rate to AIDS and improved survival.[32]

Sources

Food Sources

Good sources of niacin include yeast, meat, poultry, red fishes (e.g., tuna, salmon), cereals (especially fortified cereals), legumes, and seeds. Milk, green leafy vegetables, coffee, and tea also provide some niacin.[3] In plants, especially mature cereal grains such as corn and wheat, niacin may be bound to sugar molecules in the form of glycosides, which significantly decrease niacin bioavailability.[6]

In the United States, the average dietary intake of niacin is about 30 mg/day for young men and 20 mg/day for young women. In a sample of adults aged over 60, men and women were found to have an average dietary intake of 21 and 17 mg/day, respectively.[8] Some foods with substantial amounts of niacin are listed in **Table 3.2** along with their niacin content. Food composition tables generally list niacin content without including NE from tryptophan, or any adjustment for niacin bioavailability.

Supplements

Niacin supplements are available as nicotinamide or nicotinic acid. Nicotinamide is the form of niacin typically used in nutritional supplements and in food fortification. Nicotinic acid is available over the counter and with a prescription as a cholesterol-lowering agent.[33] The nomenclature for nicotinic acid formulations can be confusing. Nicotinic acid is available over the counter in an "immediate-release" (crystalline) and "slow-release" or "timed-release" form. A shorter-acting timed-release preparation referred to as "intermediate-release" or "extended-release" nicotinic acid is available by prescription.[34,35] Due to the potential for side effects, medical supervision is recommended for the use of nicotinic acid as a cholesterol-lowering agent.

Safety

Toxicity

Niacin from foods is not known to cause adverse effects. Although one study noted adverse effects after consumption of bagels with 60 times the normal amount of niacin fortification, most adverse effects have been reported with pharmacological preparations of niacin.[8]

Nicotinic acid. Common side effects of nicotinic acid include flushing, itching, and gastrointestinal disturbances such as nausea and vomiting. Hepatotoxicity (liver cell damage), including elevated liver enzymes and jaundice, has been observed at intakes as low as 750 mg nicotinic acid/day for less than 3 months.[34,35] Hepatitis has been

Table 3.2 Food sources of niacin

Food	Serving	Niacin (mg)
Cereal, fortified	1 cup	20–27
Tuna, light, packed in water	3 ounces[a]	11.3
Salmon, chinook	3 ounces,[a] cooked	8.5
Chicken, light meat	3 ounces,[a] cooked without skin	7.3
Turkey, light meat	3 ounces,[a] cooked without skin	5.8
Cereal, unfortified	1 cup	5–7
Peanuts	1 ounce, dry roasted	3.8
Beef, lean	3 ounces, cooked	3.1
Pasta, enriched	1 cup, cooked	2.3
Lentils	1 cup, cooked	2.1
Lima beans	1 cup, cooked	1.8
Bread, whole-wheat	1 slice	1.3
Coffee, brewed	1 cup	0.5

[a]A 3-ounce serving of meat or fish is about the size of a deck of cards.

observed with timed-release nicotinic acid at dosages as small as 500 mg/day for 2 months, although almost all reports of severe hepatitis have been associated with the timed-release form of nicotinic acid at doses of 3–9 g/day used to treat high cholesterol for months or years.[8] Immediate-release (crystalline) nicotinic acid appears to be less toxic to the liver than extended-release forms. Immediate-release nicotinic acid is often used at higher doses than timed-release forms, and severe liver toxicity has occurred in individuals who substituted timed-release niacin for immediate-release niacin at equivalent doses.[33]

Skin rashes and dry skin have been noted with nicotinic acid supplementation. Transient episodes of low blood pressure (hypotension) and headache have also been reported. Large doses of nicotinic acid have been observed to impair glucose tolerance, likely due to decreased insulin sensitivity. Impaired glucose tolerance in susceptible (pre-diabetic) individuals could result in elevated blood glucose levels and clinical diabetes. Elevated blood levels of uric acid, occasionally resulting in attacks of gout in susceptible individuals, have also been observed with high-dose nicotinic acid therapy.[34] Nicotinic acid at doses of 1.5–5.0 g/day has resulted in a few case reports of blurred vision and other eye problems, which have generally been reversible on discontinuation. People with abnormal liver function or a history of liver disease, diabetes, active peptic ulcer disease, gout, cardiac arrhythmias, inflammatory bowel disease, migraine headaches, and alcoholism may be more susceptible to the adverse effects of excess nicotinic acid intake than the general population.[8]

Nicotinamide. Nicotinamide is generally better tolerated than nicotinic acid. It does not usually cause flushing. However, nausea, vomiting, and signs of liver toxicity (elevated liver enzymes, jaundice) have been observed at doses of 3 g/day.[33] Nicotinamide has resulted in decreased insulin sensitivity at doses of 2 g/day in adults at high risk for type 1 diabetes.[20]

The tolerable upper intake level. Flushing of the skin, primarily on the face, arms, and chest, is a common side effect of nicotinic acid and may occur initially at doses as low as 30 mg/day. Although flushing from nicotinamide is rare, the FNB set the tolerable upper intake level (UL) for

Table 3.3 Tolerable upper intake level (UL) for niacin

Life stage	Age	UL (mg/day)
Infants	0–12 months	Not possible to establish[a]
Children	1–3 years	10
Children	4–8 years	15
Children	9–13 years	20
Adolescents	14–18 years	30
Adults	≥19 years	35

[a]Source of intake should be from food and formula only.

niacin (nicotinic acid and nicotinamide) at 35 mg/day to avoid the adverse effect of flushing (**Table 3.3**). The UL applies to the general population and is not meant to apply to individuals who are being treated with a nutrient under medical supervision, as should be the case with high-dose nicotinic acid for elevated blood cholesterol levels.[8]

Drug Interactions

Coadministration of nicotinic acid with lovastatin (another cholesterol-lowering medication) may have resulted in rhabdomyolysis in a small number of case reports.[33] Rhabdomyolysis is a relatively uncommon condition in which muscle cells are broken down, releasing muscle enzymes and electrolytes into the blood, and sometimes resulting in kidney failure. A three-year randomized controlled trial in 160 patients with documented coronary heart disease (CHD) and low HDL levels found that a combination of simvastatin and niacin increased HDL2 levels, inhibited the progression of coronary artery stenosis (narrowing), and decreased the frequency of cardiovascular events such as myocardial infarction and stroke.[25] However, concurrent therapy with antioxidants (1000 mg/day vitamin C, 800 IU/day α-tocopherol, 100 µg/day selenium, and 25 mg/day β-carotene) diminished the protective effects of the simvastatin–niacin combination. Although the mechanism for these effects is not known, some scientists have questioned the benefit of concurrent antioxidant therapy in patients on lipid-lowering agents.[36]

Several other medications may interact with niacin therapy or with absorption and metabolism of the vitamin. Sulfinpyrazone is a medication for the treatment of gout that promotes excretion of uric acid from the blood into urine. Nicotinic acid may inhibit this "uricosuric" effect of sulfinpyrazone.[33] Long-term administration of the cancer chemotherapy agent, 5-fluorouracil (5-FU), has been reported to cause symptoms of pellagra, and thus niacin supplementation may be needed. Niacin supplementation is also recommended during long-term treatment of tuberculosis with isoniazid, a niacin antagonist, because such treatment has resulted in pellagra-like symptoms.[37] Further, estrogen and estrogen-containing oral contraceptives increase the efficiency of niacin synthesis from tryptophan, resulting in a decreased dietary requirement for niacin.[2]

LPI Recommendation

The optimum intake of niacin for health promotion and chronic disease prevention is not yet known. The RDA (16 mg NE/day for men and 14 mg NE/day for women) is easily obtainable in a varied diet and should prevent deficiency in most people. Following the Linus Pauling Institute recommendation to take a daily multivitamin/mineral supplement, containing 100% of the daily value for niacin, will provide at least 20 mg niacin daily.

Older Adults

Dietary surveys indicate that 15%–25% of older adults do not consume enough niacin in their diets to meet the RDA (16 mg NE/day for men and 14 mg NE/day for women), and that dietary intake of niacin decreases between the ages of 60 and 90 years. Thus, it is advisable for older adults to supplement their dietary intake with a multivitamin/multimineral supplement, which will generally provide at least 20 mg niacin daily.

References

1. Brody T. Nutritional Biochemistry, 2nd ed. San Diego, CA: Academic Press; 1999
2. Cervantes-Laurean D, McElvaney NG, Moss J. Niacin. In: Shils M, Olson JA, Shike M, Ross AC, eds. Modern Nutrition in Health and Disease, 9th ed. Baltimore, MA: Lippincott Williams & Wilkins; 1999:401–411
3. Jacob R, Swenseid M. Niacin. In: Ziegler EE, Filer LJ, eds. Present Knowledge in Nutrition, 7th ed. Washington, DC: ILSI Press, 1996:185–190
4. Jacobson MK, Jacobson EL. Discovering new ADP-ribose polymer cycles: protecting the genome and more. Trends Biochem Sci 1999;24(11):415–417
5. Park YK, Sempos CT, Barton CN, Vanderveen JE, Yetley EA. Effectiveness of food fortification in the United States: the case of pellagra. Am J Public Health 2000;90(5):727–738
6. Gregory JF III. Nutritional properties and significance of vitamin glycosides. Annu Rev Nutr 1998;18:277–296
7. Fu CS, Swendseid ME, Jacob RA, McKee RW. Biochemical markers for assessment of niacin status in young men: levels of erythrocyte niacin coenzymes and plasma tryptophan. J Nutr 1989;119(12):1949–1955
8. Food and Nutrition Board, Institute of Medicine. Niacin. In: Dietary Reference Intakes for Thiamin, Riboflavin, Niacin, Vitamin B_6, Vitamin B_{12}, Pantothenic Acid, Biotin, and Choline. Washington, DC: National Academy Press; 1998:123–149
9. Jacobson EL, Jacobson MK. Tissue NAD as a biochemical measure of niacin status in humans. Methods Enzymol 1997;280:221–230
10. Jacobson EL, Shieh WM, Huang AC. Mapping the role of NAD metabolism in prevention and treatment of carcinogenesis. Mol Cell Biochem 1999;193(1-2):69–74
11. Hageman GJ, Stierum RH. Niacin, poly(ADP-ribose) polymerase-1 and genomic stability. Mutat Res 2001;475(1-2):45–56
12. Boyonoski AC, Spronck JC, Gallacher LM, et al. Niacin deficiency decreases bone marrow poly(ADP-ribose) and the latency of ethylnitrosourea-induced carcinogenesis in rats. J Nutr 2002;132(1):108–114
13. Gensler HL, Williams T, Huang AC, Jacobson EL. Oral niacin prevents photocarcinogenesis and photoimmunosuppression in mice. Nutr Cancer 1999; 34(1):36–41
14. Weitberg AB. Effect of nicotinic acid supplementation in vivo on oxygen radical-induced genetic damage in human lymphocytes. Mutat Res 1989;216(4):197–201
15. Hageman GJ, Stierum RH, van Herwijnen MH, van der Veer MS, Kleinjans JC. Nicotinic acid supplementation: effects on niacin status, cytogenetic damage, and poly(ADP-ribosylation) in lymphocytes of smokers. Nutr Cancer 1998;32(2):113–120
16. Jacobson EL. Niacin deficiency and cancer in women. J Am Coll Nutr 1993;12(4):412–416
17. Negri E, Franceschi S, Bosetti C, et al. Selected micronutrients and oral and pharyngeal cancer. Int J Cancer 2000;86(1):122–127
18. Franceschi S, Bidoli E, Negri E, et al. Role of macronutrients, vitamins and minerals in the aetiology of squamous-cell carcinoma of the oesophagus. Int J Cancer 2000;86(5):626–631
19. Lampeter EF, Klinghammer A, Scherbaum WA, et al; DENIS Group. The Deutsche Nicotinamide Intervention Study: an attempt to prevent type 1 diabetes. Diabetes 1998;47(6):980–984
20. Greenbaum CJ, Kahn SE, Palmer JP. Nicotinamide's effects on glucose metabolism in subjects at risk for IDDM. Diabetes 1996;45(11):1631–1634
21. Schatz DA, Bingley PJ. Update on major trials for the prevention of type 1 diabetes mellitus: the American Diabetes Prevention Trial (DPT-1) and the European Nicotinamide Diabetes Intervention Trial (ENDIT). J Pediatr Endocrinol Metab 2001;14(Suppl 1):619–622
22. Knopp RH. Drug treatment of lipid disorders. N Engl J Med 1999;341(7):498–511
23. Canner PL, Berge KG, Wenger NK, et al. Fifteen year mortality in Coronary Drug Project patients: long-term benefit with niacin. J Am Coll Cardiol 1986;8(6):1245–1255

24. Guyton JR, Capuzzi DM. Treatment of hyperlipidemia with combined niacin-statin regimens. Am J Cardiol 1998;82(12A):82U–84U; discussion 85U–86U

25. Brown BG, Zhao XQ, Chait A, et al. Simvastatin and niacin, antioxidant vitamins, or the combination for the prevention of coronary disease. N Engl J Med 2001;345(22):1583–1592

26. Cheung MC, Zhao XQ, Chait A, Albers JJ, Brown BG. Antioxidant supplements block the response of HDL to simvastatin-niacin therapy in patients with coronary artery disease and low HDL. Arterioscler Thromb Vasc Biol 2001;21(8):1320–1326

27. McKenney J. New perspectives on the use of niacin in the treatment of lipid disorders. Arch Intern Med 2004;164(7):697–705

28. Wink J, Giacoppe G, King J. Effect of very-low-dose niacin on high-density lipoprotein in patients undergoing long-term statin therapy. Am Heart J 2002;143(3):514–518

29. Kashyap ML, McGovern ME, Berra K, et al. Long-term safety and efficacy of a once-daily niacin/lovastatin formulation for patients with dyslipidemia. Am J Cardiol 2002;89(6):672–678

30. Brown RR, Ozaki Y, Datta SP, Borden EC, Sondel PM, Malone DG. Implications of interferon-induced tryptophan catabolism in cancer, auto-immune diseases and AIDS. Adv Exp Med Biol 1991;294:425–435

31. Murray MF, Langan M, MacGregor RR. Increased plasma tryptophan in HIV-infected patients treated with pharmacologic doses of nicotinamide. Nutrition 2001;17(7-8):654–656

32. Tang AM, Graham NM, Saah AJ. Effects of micronutrient intake on survival in human immunodeficiency virus type 1 infection. Am J Epidemiol 1996; 143(12):1244–1256

33. Hendler SS, Rorvik DR, eds. PDR for Nutritional Supplements. Montvale: Medical Economics Co., Inc.; 2001

34. Vitamins. Drug Facts and Comparisons. 54th ed. St. Louis, Facts and Comparisons; 2000:16.

35. Knopp RH. Evaluating niacin in its various forms. Am J Cardiol 2000;86(12A):51 L–56 L

36. Brown BG, Cheung MC, Lee AC, Zhao XQ, Chait A. Antioxidant vitamins and lipid therapy: end of a long romance? Arterioscler Thromb Vasc Biol 2002; 22(10):1535–1546

37. Flodin N. Pharmacology of Micronutrients. New York: Alan R. Liss, Inc., 1988

4   Pantothenic Acid

Pantothenic acid, also known as vitamin B_5, is essential to all forms of life.[1] It is found throughout living cells in the form of coenzyme A (CoA), a vital coenzyme in numerous chemical reactions.[2]

Function

Coenzyme A

Pantothenic acid is a component of CoA, an essential coenzyme in a variety of reactions that sustain life. CoA is required for chemical reactions that generate energy from food (fat, carbohydrates, and proteins). The synthesis of essential fats, cholesterol, and steroid hormones requires CoA, as does the synthesis of the neurotransmitter acetylcholine, and the hormone melatonin. Heme, a component of hemoglobin, requires a CoA-containing compound for its synthesis. Metabolism of a number of drugs and toxins by the liver requires CoA.[3]

Coenzyme A was named for its role in acetylation reactions. Most acetylated proteins in the body have been modified by the addition of an acetate group donated by CoA. Protein acetylation affects the three-dimensional structure of proteins, potentially altering their function; for example, acetylation reactions can alter the activity of peptide hormones. Protein acetylation appears to play a role in cell division and DNA replication, and also affects gene expression by facilitating the transcription of mRNA. In addition, a number of proteins are modified by the attachment of long-chain fatty acids donated by CoA. These modifications are known as protein acylation and appear to play a central role in cell signaling.[4]

Acyl-carrier Protein

The acyl-carrier protein requires pantothenic acid in the form of 4′-phosphopantetheine for its activity as an enzyme.[4,5] Both CoA and the acyl-carrier protein are required for the synthesis of fatty acids. Fatty acids are a component of some lipids, which are fat molecules essential for normal physiological function. Among these essential fats are sphingolipids, which are a component of the myelin sheath that enhances nerve transmission. Another example of these essential fats is the phospholipids that reside in cell membranes.

Deficiency

Naturally occurring pantothenic acid deficiency in humans is very rare and has been observed only in cases of severe malnutrition. World War II prisoners in the Philippines, Burma, and Japan experienced numbness and painful burning and tingling in their feet; these symptoms were relieved specifically by pantothenic acid.[4] Pantothenic acid deficiency in humans has been induced experimentally by coadministering a pantothenic acid antagonist and a pantothenic acid-deficient diet. Participants in this experiment complained of headache, fatigue, insomnia, intestinal disturbances, and numbness and tingling of their hands and feet.[6] In a more recent study, participants fed only a pantothenic acid-free diet did not develop clinical signs of deficiency, although some appeared listless and complained of fatigue.[7] Homopantothenate is a pantothenic acid antagonist with cholinergic effects (similar to those of the neurotransmitter acetylcholine). It was used in Japan to enhance mental function, especially in Alzheimer disease. A rare side effect was the development of hepatic encephalopathy, a condition of abnormal brain function resulting from failure of the liver to eliminate toxins. The encephalopathy was reversed by pantothenic acid supplementation, suggesting but not proving that it was due to pantothenic acid deficiency caused by the antagonist.[5]

As pantothenic acid deficiency is so rare in humans, most information about the effects of deficiency comes from experimental research in animals. Pantothenic acid-deficient rats developed damage to the adrenal glands, whereas monkeys developed anemia due to decreased synthesis of heme, a component of hemoglobin.

Dogs with pantothenic acid deficiency developed low blood glucose, rapid breathing and heart rates, and convulsions. Chickens developed skin irritation, feather abnormalities, and spinal nerve damage associated with the degeneration of the myelin sheath. Pantothenic acid-deficient mice showed decreased exercise tolerance and diminished storage of glucose (in the form of glycogen) in muscle and liver. Mice also developed skin irritation and graying of the fur, which was reversed by giving pantothenic acid. This finding led to the idea of adding pantothenic acid to shampoo, although it has not been successful in restoring hair color in humans.[4] The diversity of symptoms emphasizes the numerous functions of pantothenic acid in its coenzyme forms.

Adequate Intake

The Food and Nutrition Board (FNB) of the Institute of Medicine felt that the existing scientific evidence was insufficient to calculate a recommended dietary allowance (RDA) for pantothenic acid, so they set an adequate intake (AI). The AI for pantothenic acid (**Table 4.1**) was based on estimated dietary intakes in healthy population groups.[8]

Disease Prevention

Currently, there is insufficient evidence to support the use of pantothenic acid to prevent diseases or health conditions other than frank pantothenic acid deficiency, which appears to be quite rare in humans (see "Deficiency," p. 26).

Disease Treatment

Wound Healing

Administration of oral pantothenic acid and application of pantothenol ointment to the skin have been shown to accelerate the closure of skin wounds and increase the strength of scar tissue in animals. Adding calcium D-pantothenate to cultured human skin cells given an artificial wound increased the number of migrating skin cells and their speed of migration, effects likely to accelerate wound healing.[9] However, there are few data to support accelerated wound healing in humans. A randomized, double-blind study in patients undergoing surgery for tattoo removal found that supplementation with 1000 mg vitamin C and 200 mg pantothenic acid did not significantly improve the wound-healing process.[10]

High Cholesterol

A pantothenic acid derivative called *pantethine* has been reported by a number of investigators to have a cholesterol-lowering effect. Pantethine is actually two molecules of pantetheine joined by a disulfide bond (chemical bond between two molecules of sulfur). In the synthetic pathway of CoA, pantethine is closer to CoA than pantothenic acid and is the functional component of CoA and acyl-carrier proteins. Several studies found doses of 900 mg pantethine daily (300 mg three times daily) to be significantly more effective than placebo in lowering total cholesterol and triglyceride levels in the blood of both diabetic and nondiabetic individuals.[11] Pantethine was also found to lower cholesterol and triglyceride levels in

Table 4.1 Adequate intake for pantothenic acid

Life stage	Age	Males (mg/day)	Females (mg/day)
Infants	0–6 months	1.7	1.7
Infants	7–12 months	1.8	1.8
Children	1–3 years	2	2
Children	4–8 years	3	3
Children	9–13 years	4	4
Adolescents	14–18 years	5	5
Adults	≥19 years	5	5
Pregnancy	All ages	–	6
Breast-feeding	All ages	–	7

diabetic patients on hemodialysis with no adverse side effects. The fact that pantethine has few side effects was particularly attractive for hemodialysis patients as a result of the increased risk of drug toxicity in patients with renal (kidney) failure.[12] Pantethine is not a vitamin; it is a derivative of pantothenic acid. The decision to use pantethine to treat elevated blood cholesterol or triglycerides should be made in collaboration with a qualified health-care provider who can give appropriate follow-up.

Sources

Food Sources

Pantothenic acid is available in a variety of foods. Rich sources include liver and kidney, yeast, egg yolk, and broccoli. Fish, shellfish, chicken, milk, yogurt, legumes, mushrooms, avocados, and sweet potatoes are also good sources. Whole grains are good sources of pantothenic acid, but the processing and refining of grains may result in a 35%–75% loss. Freezing and canning of foods result in similar losses.[8] Large national, nutritional surveys were unable to estimate pantothenic acid intake due to the scarcity of data on the pantothenic acid content of food. Smaller studies estimate average daily intakes of pantothenic acid to be from 5 mg/day to 6 mg/day in adults. **Table 4.2** lists some rich sources of pantothenic acid along with their content.

Intestinal Bacteria

The bacteria that normally colonize the colon (large intestine) are capable of making their own pantothenic acid. It is not yet known whether humans can absorb the pantothenic acid synthesized by their own intestinal bacteria in meaningful amounts. However, a specialized process for the uptake of biotin and pantothenic acid was identified in cultured cells derived from the lining of the colon, suggesting that humans may be able to absorb pantothenic acid and biotin produced by intestinal bacteria.[13]

Supplements

Pantothenic acid. Supplements commonly contain pantothenol, a more stable alcohol derivative, which is rapidly converted to pantothenic

Table 4.2 Food sources of pantothenic acid

Food	Serving	Pantothenic acid (mg)
Avocado, California	1 whole	1.99
Yogurt	8 ounces	1.35
Chicken, cooked	3 ounces[a]	0.98
Sweet potato, cooked	1 medium (½ cup)	0.88
Milk	1 cup (8 ounces)	0.83
Lentils, cooked	½ cup	0.63
Egg, cooked	1 large	0.61
Split peas, cooked	½ cup	0.58
Mushrooms, raw	½ cup, chopped	0.52
Broccoli, cooked	½ cup, chopped	0.48
Lobster, cooked	3 ounces[a]	0.24
Bread, whole wheat	1 slice	0.19
Tuna, light, canned in water	3 ounces[a]	0.18
Fish, cod, cooked	3 ounces[a]	0.15

[a]A 3-ounce serving of meat or seafood is about the size of a deck of cards.

acid by humans. Calcium and sodium D-pantothenate, the calcium and sodium salts of pantothenic acid, are also available as supplements.[4]

Pantethine. Pantethine is used as a cholesterol-lowering agent in Europe and Japan and is available in the United States as a dietary supplement.[14]

Safety

Toxicity

Pantothenic acid is not known to be toxic in humans. The only adverse effect noted was diarrhea resulting from very high intakes of 10–20 g/day of calcium D-pantothenate.[15] However, there is one case report of life-threatening eosinophilic pleuropericardial effusion in an elderly woman who took a combination of 10 mg/day of biotin and 300 mg/day of pantothenic acid for 2 months.[16] Due to the lack of reports of adverse effects when the dietary reference intakes (DRIs) for pantothenic acid were established in 1998, the FNB did not establish a tolerable upper intake level (UL) for pantothenic acid.[8] Pantethine is generally well tolerated in doses up to 1200 mg/ day. However, gastrointestinal side effects, such as nausea and heartburn, have been reported.[14]

Drug Interactions

Oral contraceptives (birth control pills) containing estrogen and progestin may increase the requirement for pantothenic acid.[15] Use of pantethine in combination with hydroxymethylglutaryl (HMG)-CoA reductase inhibitors (statins) or nicotinic acid may produce additive effects on blood lipids.[14]

LPI Recommendation

Little is known about the amount of dietary pantothenic acid required to promote optimal health or prevent chronic disease. The Linus Pauling Institute supports the recommendation by the FNB of 5 mg/day of pantothenic acid for adults. A varied diet should provide enough pantothenic acid for most people. Following the Linus Pauling Institute recommendation to take a daily multivitamin/mineral supplement, containing 100% of the daily value, will ensure an intake of at least 5 mg/day of pantothenic acid.

Older Adults

Currently there is little evidence that older adults differ in their intake or requirement for pantothenic acid. Most multivitamin/multimineral supplements provide at least 5 mg/day of pantothenic acid.

References

1. Trumbo PR. Pantothenic acid. In: Shils ME, Shike M, Ross AC, Caballero B, Cousins RJ, eds. Modern Nutrition in Health and Disease, 10th ed. Philadelphia, PA: Lippincott Williams & Wilkins; 2006:462–469
2. Tahiliani AG, Beinlich CJ. Pantothenic acid in health and disease. Vitam Horm 1991;46:165–228
3. Brody T. Nutritional Biochemistry, 2nd ed. San Diego, CA: Academic Press, 1999
4. Plesofsky-Vig N. Pantothenic acid. In: Shils ME, Olson JA, Shike M, Ross AC, eds. Modern Nutrition in Health and Disease, 9th ed. Philadelphia, PA: Lippincott Williams & Wilkins; 1999:423–432
5. Bender DA. Optimum nutrition: thiamin, biotin and pantothenate. Proc Nutr Soc 1999;58(2):427–433
6. Hodges RE, Ohlson MA, Bean WB. Pantothenic acid deficiency in man. J Clin Invest 1958;37(11):1642–1657
7. Fry PC, Fox HM, Tao HG. Metabolic response to a pantothenic acid deficient diet in humans. J Nutr Sci Vitaminol (Tokyo) 1976;22(4):339–346
8. Food and Nutrition Board, Institute of Medicine. Pantothenic acid. In: Dietary Reference Intakes for Thiamin, Riboflavin, Niacin, Vitamin B-6, Vitamin B-12, Pantothenic Acid, Biotin, and Choline. Washington, DC: National Academy Press; 1998:357–373
9. Weimann BI, Hermann D. Studies on wound healing: effects of calcium D-pantothenate on the migration, proliferation and protein synthesis of human dermal fibroblasts in culture. Int J Vitam Nutr Res 1999; 69(2):113–119
10. Vaxman F, Olender S, Lambert A, et al. Effect of pantothenic acid and ascorbic acid supplementation on human skin wound healing process. A double-blind, prospective and randomized trial. Eur Surg Res 1995;27(3):158–166
11. Gaddi A, Descovich GC, Noseda G, et al. Controlled evaluation of pantethine, a natural hypolipidemic compound, in patients with different forms of hyperlipoproteinemia. Atherosclerosis 1984;50(1):73–83
12. Coronel F, Tornero F, Torrente J, et al. Treatment of hyperlipemia in diabetic patients on dialysis with a physiological substance. Am J Nephrol 1991;11(1):32–36
13. Said HM, Ortiz A, McCloud E, Dyer D, Moyer MP, Rubin S. Biotin uptake by human colonic epithelial NCM460 cells: a carrier-mediated process shared with pantothenic acid. Am J Physiol 1998;275(5 Pt 1):C1365–C1371
14. Hendler SS, Rorvik DR, eds. PDR for Nutritional Supplements. Montvale: Medical Economics Co., Inc.; 2001
15. Flodin N. Pharmacology of Micronutrients. New York: Alan R. Liss, Inc.; 1988
16. Debourdeau PM, Djezzar S, Estival JL, Zammit CM, Richard RC, Castot AC. Life-threatening eosinophilic pleuropericardial effusion related to vitamins B5 and H. Ann Pharmacother 2001;35(4):424–426

5 Riboflavin

Riboflavin is a water-soluble B vitamin, also known as vitamin B_2. In the body, riboflavin is primarily found as an integral component of the coenzymes, flavin adenine dinucleotide (FAD) and flavin mononucleotide (FMN).[1] Coenzymes derived from riboflavin are termed "flavocoenzymes," and enzymes that use a flavocoenzyme are called "flavoproteins."[2]

Function

Oxidation–Reduction (Redox) Reactions

Living organisms derive most of their energy from oxidation–reduction (redox) reactions, which are processes that involve the transfer of electrons. Flavocoenzymes participate in redox reactions in numerous metabolic pathways.[3] They are critical for the metabolism of carbohydrates, fats, and proteins. FAD is part of the electron transport (respiratory) chain, which is central to energy production. Together with cytochrome P450, flavocoenzymes also participate in the metabolism of drugs and toxins.[4]

Antioxidant Functions

Glutathione reductase. This is an FAD-dependent enzyme that participates in the redox cycle of glutathione. The glutathione redox cycle plays a major role in protecting organisms from reactive oxygen species, such as hydroperoxides. Glutathione reductase requires FAD to regenerate two molecules of reduced glutathione from oxidized glutathione. Riboflavin deficiency has been associated with increased oxidative stress.[4] Measurement of glutathione reductase activity in red blood cells is commonly used to assess riboflavin nutritional status.[5]

Glutathione peroxidase. This a selenium-containing enzyme, requiring two molecules of reduced glutathione to break down hydroperoxides (**Fig. 5.1**).

Xanthine oxidase. This is another FAD-dependent enzyme, which catalyzes the oxidation of hypoxanthine and xanthine to uric acid. Uric acid is one of the most effective water-soluble antioxidants in the blood. Riboflavin deficiency can result in decreased xanthine oxidase activity, reducing blood uric acid levels.[6]

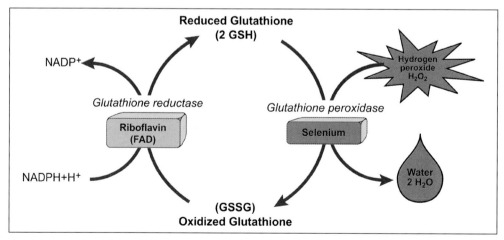

Fig. 5.1 The glutathione oxidation–reduction (redox) cycle. One molecule of hydrogen peroxide is reduced to two molecules of water, and two molecules of glutathione (GSH) are oxidized in a reaction catalyzed by the seleno-enzyme glutathione peroxidase. Oxidized glutathione (GSSG) may be reduced by the flavin adenine dinucleotide (FAD)-dependent enzyme glutathione reductase.

Nutrient Interactions

B-complex vitamins. As flavoproteins are involved in the metabolism of several other vitamins (vitamin B_6, niacin, and folic acid), severe
riboflavin deficiency may affect many enzyme
systems. Conversion of most naturally available
vitamin B_6 to its coenzyme form, pyridoxal
5'-phosphate (PLP), requires the FMN-dependent
enzyme, pyridoxine 5'-phosphate oxidase (PPO).[7]
At least two studies in elderly people have documented significant interactions between indicators of vitamin B_6 and riboflavin nutritional status.[8,9] The synthesis of the niacin-containing coenzymes, NAD and NADP, from the amino acid,
tryptophan, requires the FAD-dependent enzyme, kynurenine monooxygenase. Severe riboflavin deficiency can decrease the conversion of
tryptophan to NAD and NADP, increasing the risk
of niacin deficiency.[3] Methylene tetrahydrofolate
reductase (MTHFR) is an FAD-dependent enzyme
that plays an important role in maintaining the
specific folate coenzyme required to form methionine from homocysteine (**Fig. 5.2**). Along
with other B vitamins, increased riboflavin intake has been associated with decreased plasma
homocysteine levels.[10] Increased plasma riboflavin levels were associated with decreased plasma

homocysteine levels, mainly in individuals homozygous (T/T) for the C 677 T polymorphism of
the *MTHFR* gene and in individuals with low folate intake.[11] Such results illustrate that chronic
disease risk may be influenced by complex interactions between genetic and dietary factors.

Iron. Riboflavin deficiency alters iron metabolism. Although the mechanism is not clear, research in animals suggests that riboflavin deficiency may impair iron absorption, increase intestinal loss of iron, and/or impair iron utilization
for the synthesis of hemoglobin. In humans, improving riboflavin nutritional status has been
found to increase circulating hemoglobin levels.
Correction of riboflavin deficiency in individuals
who are both riboflavin and iron deficient improves the response of iron-deficiency anemia to
iron therapy.[12]

Deficiency

Ariboflavinosis is the medical name for clinical
riboflavin deficiency. Riboflavin deficiency is
rarely found in isolation; it occurs frequently in
combination with deficiencies of other water-
soluble vitamins. Symptoms of riboflavin defi-

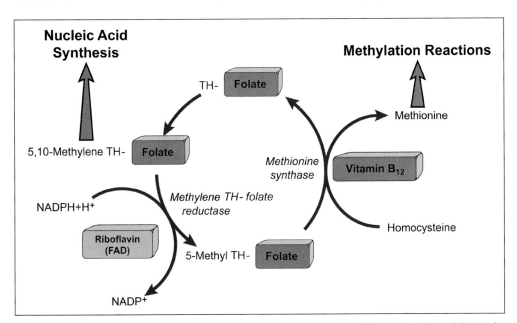

Fig. 5.2 Methylene tetrahydrofolate (THF) reductase.
Methylene TH-folate reductase is a flavin adenine dinucleotide (FAD)-dependent enzyme required to catalyze the
reduction of 5,10-methylene THF to 5-methyl THF, the
specific folate coenzyme required to form methionine
from homocysteine.

ciency include sore throat, redness and swelling of the lining of the mouth and throat, cracks or sores on the outsides of the lips (cheliosis) and at the corners of the mouth (angular stomatitis), inflammation and redness of the tongue (magenta tongue), and a moist, scaly skin inflammation (seborrheic dermatitis). Other symptoms may involve the formation of blood vessels in the clear covering of the eye (vascularization of the cornea) and a decreased red blood cell count, in which the existing red blood cells contain normal levels of hemoglobin and are of normal size (normochromic/normocytic anemia).[1,3] Severe riboflavin deficiency may result in decreased conversion of vitamin B_6 to its coenzyme form (PLP) and decreased conversion of tryptophan to niacin.

Pre-eclampsia is defined as the presence of elevated blood pressure, protein in the urine, and edema (significant swelling) during pregnancy. About 5% of women with pre-eclampsia may progress to eclampsia, a significant cause of maternal death. Eclampsia is characterized by seizures, in addition to high blood pressure and increased risk of hemorrhage (severe bleeding).[13] A study in 154 pregnant women at increased risk of pre-eclampsia found that those who were riboflavin deficient were 4.7 times more likely to develop pre-eclampsia than those who had adequate riboflavin nutritional status.[14] The cause of pre-eclampsia–eclampsia is not known. Decreased intracellular levels of flavocoenzymes could cause mitochondrial dysfunction, increase oxidative stress, and interfere with nitric oxide release and thus blood vessel dilation—all of these changes have been associated with pre-ec-

lampsia. However, a small randomized, placebo-controlled, double-blind trial in 450 pregnant women at high risk for pre-eclampsia found that supplementation with 15 mg riboflavin daily did not prevent the condition.[15]

Risk Factors for Riboflavin Deficiency

People with alcohol problems are at increased risk for riboflavin deficiency due to decreased intake, decreased absorption, and impaired utilization of riboflavin. In addition, anorexic individuals rarely consume adequate riboflavin, and lactose-intolerant individuals may not consume milk or other dairy products which are good sources of riboflavin. The conversion of riboflavin into FAD and FMN is impaired in hypothyroidism and adrenal insufficiency.[3,4] Further, people who are very active physically (athletes, laborers) may have a slightly increased riboflavin requirement. However, riboflavin supplementation has not generally been found to increase exercise tolerance or performance.[16]

Recommended Dietary Allowance

The recommended dietary allowance (RDA) for riboflavin, revised in 1998, was based on the prevention of deficiency (**Table 5.1**). Clinical signs of deficiency in humans appear at intakes of less than 0.5–0.6 mg/day, and urinary excretion of riboflavin is seen at intake levels of approximately 1 mg/day.[1]

Table 5.1 Recommended dietary allowance for riboflavin

Life stage	Age	Males (mg/day)	Females (mg/day)
Infants	0–6 months	0.3 (AI)	0.3 (AI)
Infants	7–12 months	0.4 (AI)	0.4 (AI)
Children	1–3 years	0.5	0.5
Children	4–8 years	0.6	0.6
Children	9–13 years	0.9	0.9
Adolescents	14–18 years	1.3	1.0
Adults	≥19 years	1.3	1.1
Pregnancy	All ages	–	1.4
Breast-feeding	All ages	–	1.6

AI, adequate intake.

Disease Prevention

Cataracts

Age-related cataracts are the leading cause of visual disability in the United States and other developed countries. Research has focused on the role of nutritional antioxidants because of evidence that light-induced oxidative damage of lens proteins may lead to the development of age-related cataracts. A case–control study found significantly decreased risk of age-related cataract (33%–51%) in men and women in the highest quintile of dietary riboflavin intake (median of 1.6–2.2 mg/day) compared with those in the lowest quintile (median of 0.08 mg/day in both men and women).[17] Another case–control study reported that individuals in the highest quintile of riboflavin nutritional status, as measured by red blood cell glutathione reductase activity, had approximately half the occurrence of age-related cataract as those in the lowest quintile of riboflavin status, although the results were not statistically significant.[18]

A cross-sectional study of 2900 Australian men and women, aged 49 years and older, found that those in the highest quintile of riboflavin intake were 50% less likely to have cataracts than those in the lowest quintile.[19] A prospective study of more than 50000 women did not observe a difference between rates of cataract extraction between women in the highest quintile of riboflavin intake (median of 1.5 mg/day) and women in the lowest quintile (median of 1.2 mg/day).[20] However, the range between the highest and lowest quintiles was small, and median intake levels for both quintiles were above the current RDA for riboflavin. Also, a study in 408 women found that higher dietary intakes of riboflavin were inversely associated with a 5-year change in lens opacification.[21] Although these observational studies provide support for the role of riboflavin in the prevention of cataracts, placebo-controlled intervention trials are needed to confirm the relationship.

Disease Treatment

Migraine Headaches

Some evidence indicates that impaired mitochondrial oxygen metabolism in the brain may play a role in the pathology of migraine headaches. As riboflavin is the precursor of the two flavocoenzymes (FAD and FMN) required by the flavoproteins of the mitochondrial electron transport chain, supplemental riboflavin has been investigated as a treatment for migraine. A randomized placebo-controlled trial examined the effect of 400 mg riboflavin/day for 3 months on migraine prevention in 54 men and women with a history of recurrent migraine headaches.[22] Riboflavin was significantly better than placebo in reducing attack frequency and the number of headache days, although the beneficial effect was most pronounced during the third month of treatment. A more recent study by the same investigators found that treatment with either a medication called a β-blocker or a high-dose riboflavin resulted in clinical improvement, but each therapy appeared to act on a distinct pathological mechanism: β-blockers on abnormal cortical information processing and riboflavin on decreased brain mitochondrial energy reserve.[23] A small study in 23 patients reported a reduction in median migraine attack frequency after supplementation with 400 mg riboflavin daily for 3 months.[24] In addition, a 3-month, randomized, double-blind, placebo-controlled study that administered a combination of riboflavin (400 mg/day), magnesium, and feverfew to migraine sufferers reported no therapeutic benefit of this supplement beyond that associated with taking a placebo containing 25 mg/day of riboflavin.[25] Compared with baseline measurements in this trial, both the placebo and treatment groups experienced some benefits with respect to the mean number of migraines, migraine days, or migraine index.[25] Although these findings are preliminary, data from most studies to date suggest that riboflavin supplementation might be a useful adjunct to pharmacological therapy in migraine prevention.

Sources

Food Sources

Most plant- and animal-derived foods contain at least small quantities of riboflavin. In the United States, wheat flour and bread have been enriched with riboflavin (as well as thiamin, niacin, and iron) since 1943. Data from large dietary surveys indicate that the average intake of riboflavin for men is about 2 mg/day and for women about 1.5 mg/day; both intakes are well above the RDA. Intake levels were similar for a population of elderly men and women.[1] Riboflavin is easily destroyed by exposure to light; for example, up to 50% of the riboflavin in milk contained in a clear glass bottle can be destroyed after 2 hours of exposure to bright sunlight.[6] Some foods with substantial amounts of riboflavin are listed in **Table 5.2** along with their riboflavin content.

Table 5.2 Food sources of riboflavin

Food	Serving	Riboflavin (mg)
Fortified cereal	1 cup	0.59–2.27
Milk, nonfat	1 cup (8 ounces)	0.34
Egg, cooked	1 large	0.27
Almonds	1 ounce	0.23
Spinach, boiled	½ cup	0.21
Chicken, dark meat, roasted	3 ounces[a]	0.16
Beef, cooked	3 ounces[a]	0.16
Asparagus, boiled	6 spears	0.13
Salmon, cooked	3 ounces[a]	0.12
Cheddar cheese	1 ounce	0.11
Broccoli, boiled	½ cup, chopped	0.10
Halibut, broiled	3 ounces[a]	0.08
Chicken, light meat, roasted	3 ounces[a]	0.08
Bread, white, enriched	1 slice	0.08
Bread, whole-wheat	1 slice	0.06

[a]A 3-ounce serving of meat or fish is about the size of a deck of cards.

Supplements

The most common forms of riboflavin available in supplements are riboflavin and riboflavin 5′-monophosphate. Riboflavin is most commonly found in multivitamin and vitamin B-complex preparations.[26]

Safety

Toxicity

No toxic or adverse effects of high riboflavin intake in humans are known. Studies in cell culture indicate that excess riboflavin may increase the risk of DNA strand breaks in the presence of chromium (IV), a known carcinogen.[27] This may be of concern to workers exposed to chrome, but no data in humans are available. High-dose riboflavin therapy has been found to intensify urine color to a bright yellow (flavinuria), but this is a harmless side effect. The FNB did not establish a tolerable upper intake level (UL) when the RDA was revised in 1998.[1]

Drug Interactions

Several early reports indicated that women taking high-dose oral contraceptives (OCs) had diminished riboflavin nutritional status. However, when investigators controlled for dietary riboflavin intake, no differences between OC users and nonusers were found.[1] Phenothiazine derivatives such as the antipsychotic medication chlorpromazine and tricyclic antidepressants inhibit the incorporation of riboflavin into FAD and FMN, as do the antimalarial medication, quinacrine, and the cancer chemotherapy agent, doxorubicin.[4] Long-term use of the anticonvulsant, phenobarbital may increase destruction of riboflavin, by liver enzymes, increasing the risk of deficiency.[3]

LPI Recommendation

The RDA for riboflavin (1.3 mg/day for men and 1.1 mg/day for women), which should prevent deficiency in most individuals, is easily met by eating a varied diet. Consuming a varied diet should supply 1.5–2.0 mg riboflavin a day. Following the Linus Pauling Institute recommendation to take a multivitamin/mineral supplement containing 100% of the daily values will ensure an intake of at least 1.7 mg riboflavin/day.

Older Adults

Some experts in nutrition and aging feel that the RDA (1.3 mg/day for men and 1.1 mg/day for women) leaves little margin for error in people aged over 50 years.[28,29] A study of independently living people aged between 65 and 90 years found that almost 25% consumed less than the recommended riboflavin intake, and 10% had biochemical evidence of deficiency.[30] In addition, epidemiological studies of cataract prevalence indicate that riboflavin intakes of 1.6–2.2 mg/day may reduce the risk of developing age-related cataracts. Individuals whose diets may not supply adequate riboflavin, especially those aged over 50, should consider taking a multivitamin/mineral supplement, which generally provides at least 1.7 mg riboflavin/day.

References

1. Food and Nutrition Board, Institute of Medicine. Riboflavin. In: Dietary Reference Intakes for Thiamin, Riboflavin, Niacin, Vitamin B$_6$, Vitamin B$_{12}$, Pantothenic Acid, Biotin, and Choline. Washington, DC: National Academy Press; 1998:87–122
2. Brody T. Nutritional Biochemistry, 2nd ed. San Diego, CA: Academic Press; 1999
3. McCormick DB. Riboflavin. In: Shils M, Olson JA, Shike M, Ross AC, eds. Modern Nutrition in Health and Disease, 9th ed. Baltimore, MD: Lippincott Williams & Wilkins; 1999:391–399
4. Powers HJ. Current knowledge concerning optimum nutritional status of riboflavin, niacin and pyridoxine. Proc Nutr Soc 1999;58(2):435–440
5. Rivlin RS. Riboflavin. In: Ziegler EE, Filer LJ, eds. Present Knowledge in Nutrition, 7th ed. Washington, DC: ILSI Press; 1996:167–173
6. Böhles H. Antioxidative vitamins in prematurely and maturely born infants. Int J Vitam Nutr Res 1997; 67(5):321–328
7. McCormick DB. Two interconnected B vitamins: riboflavin and pyridoxine. Physiol Rev 1989;69(4):1170–1198
8. Madigan SM, Tracey F, McNulty H, et al. Riboflavin and vitamin B-6 intakes and status and biochemical response to riboflavin supplementation in free-living elderly people. Am J Clin Nutr 1998;68(2):389–395
9. Löwik MR, van den Berg H, Kistemaker C, Brants HA, Brussaard JH. Interrelationships between riboflavin and vitamin B6 among elderly people (Dutch Nutrition Surveillance System). Int J Vitam Nutr Res 1994;64(3):198–203
10. Jacques PF, Bostom AG, Wilson PW, Rich S, Rosenberg IH, Selhub J. Determinants of plasma total homocysteine concentration in the Framingham Offspring cohort. Am J Clin Nutr 2001;73(3):613–621
11. Jacques PF, Kalmbach R, Bagley PJ, et al. The relationship between riboflavin and plasma total homocysteine in the Framingham Offspring cohort is influenced by folate status and the C677T transition in the methylenetetrahydrofolate reductase gene. J Nutr 2002;132(2):283–288
12. Powers HJ. Riboflavin-iron interactions with particular emphasis on the gastrointestinal tract. Proc Nutr Soc 1995;54(2):509–517
13. Crombleholme WR. Obstetrics. In: Tierney LM, McPhee SJ, Papadakis MA, eds. Current Medical Treatment and Diagnosis. 37th ed. Stamford, CA: Appleton & Lange; 1998: 731–734
14. Wacker J, Frühauf J, Schulz M, Chiwora FM, Volz J, Becker K. Riboflavin deficiency and preeclampsia. Obstet Gynecol 2000;96(1):38–44
15. Neugebauer J, Zanré Y, Wacker J. Riboflavin supplementation and preeclampsia. Int J Gynaecol Obstet 2006;93(2):136–137
16. Soares MJ, Satyanarayana K, Bamji MS, Jacob CM, Ramana YV, Rao SS. The effect of exercise on the riboflavin status of adult men. Br J Nutr 1993;69(2):541–551
17. Mares-Perlman JA, Brady WE, Klein BE, et al. Diet and nuclear lens opacities. Am J Epidemiol 1995; 141(4):322–334
18. Leske MC, Wu SY, Hyman L, et al; The Lens Opacities Case-Control Study Group. Biochemical factors in the lens opacities. Case-control study. Arch Ophthalmol 1995;113(9):1113–1119
19. Cumming RG, Mitchell P, Smith W. Diet and cataract: the Blue Mountains Eye Study. Ophthalmology 2000;107(3):450–456
20. Hankinson SE, Stampfer MJ, Seddon JM, et al. Nutrient intake and cataract extraction in women: a prospective study. BMJ 1992;305(6849):335–339
21. Jacques PF, Taylor A, Moeller S, et al. Long-term nutrient intake and 5-year change in nuclear lens opacities. Arch Ophthalmol 2005;123(4):517–526
22. Schoenen J, Jacquy J, Lenaerts M. Effectiveness of high-dose riboflavin in migraine prophylaxis. A randomized controlled trial. Neurology 1998;50(2):466–470
23. Sándor PS, Afra J, Ambrosini A, Schoenen J. Prophylactic treatment of migraine with beta-blockers and riboflavin: differential effects on the intensity dependence of auditory evoked cortical potentials. Headache 2000;40(1):30–35
24. Boehnke C, Reuter U, Flach U, Schuh-Hofer S, Einhäupl KM, Arnold G. High-dose riboflavin treatment is efficacious in migraine prophylaxis: an open study in a tertiary care centre. Eur J Neurol 2004;11(7):475–477
25. Maizels M, Blumenfeld A, Burchette R. A combination of riboflavin, magnesium, and feverfew for migraine prophylaxis: a randomized trial. Headache 2004; 44(9):885–890
26. Hendler SS, Rorvik DR, eds. PDR for Nutritional Supplements. Montvale: Medical Economics Co., Inc.; 2001
27. Sugiyama M. Role of physiological antioxidants in chromium(VI)-induced cellular injury. Free Radic Biol Med 1992;12(5):397–407
28. Russell RM, Suter PM. Vitamin requirements of elderly people: an update. Am J Clin Nutr 1993;58(1):4–14
29. Blumberg J. Nutritional needs of seniors. J Am Coll Nutr 1997;16(6):517–523
30. López-Sobaler AM, Ortega RM, Quintas ME, et al. The influence of vitamin B2 intake on the activation coefficient of erythrocyte glutation reductase in the elderly. J Nutr Health Aging 2002;6(1):60–62

6 Thiamin

Thiamin (also spelled *thiamine*) is a water-soluble B vitamin, previously known as vitamin B_1 or aneurine.[1] Isolated and characterized in the 1930s, thiamin was one of the first organic compounds to be recognized as a vitamin.[2] Thiamin occurs in the human body as free thiamin and as various phosphorylated forms: thiamin monophosphate (TMP), thiamin triphosphate (TTP), and thiamin pyrophosphate (TPP), which is also known as thiamin diphosphate.

Function

Coenzyme Function

TPP is a required coenzyme for a small number of very important enzymes. The synthesis of TPP from free thiamin requires magnesium, adenosine triphosphate (ATP), and the enzyme, thiamin pyrophosphokinase.

Pyruvate dehydrogenase, 2-oxoglutarate dehydrogenase, and branched-chain ketoacid (BCKA) dehydrogenase each comprise a different enzyme complex found within cellular organelles called *mitochondria*. They catalyze the decarboxylation of pyruvate, 2-oxoglutarate, and branched-chain amino acids to form acetyl-coenzyme A (CoA), succinyl-CoA, and derivatives of branched-chain amino acids, respectively; all products play critical roles in the production of energy from food.[2] In addition to the thiamin coenzyme (TPP), each dehydrogenase complex requires a niacin-containing coenzyme, a riboflavin-containing coenzyme, and lipoic acid.

Transketolase catalyzes critical reactions in another metabolic pathway known as the pentose phosphate pathway. One of the most important intermediates of this pathway is ribose 5-phosphate, a phosphorylated 5-carbon sugar required for the synthesis of the high-energy ribonucleotides, ATP and guanosine triphosphate (GTP). It is also required for the synthesis of the nucleic acids, DNA and RNA, and the niacin-containing coenzyme nicotinamide adenine dinucleotide phosphate (NADP), which is essential for a number of biosynthetic reactions.[1,3] As transketolase decreases early in thiamin deficiency, measurement of its activity in red blood cells has been used to assess thiamin nutritional status.[2]

Deficiency

Beriberi, the disease resulting from severe thiamin deficiency, was described in Chinese literature as early as 2600 BC. Thiamin deficiency affects the cardiovascular, nervous, muscular, and gastrointestinal systems.[2] Beriberi has been termed *dry*, *wet*, and *cerebral*, depending on the systems affected by severe thiamin deficiency.[1]

The main feature of dry (paralytic or nervous) beriberi is peripheral neuropathy. Early in the course of the neuropathy, "burning feet syndrome" may occur. Other symptoms include abnormal (exaggerated) reflexes as well as diminished sensation and weakness in the legs and arms. Muscle pain and tenderness and difficulty rising from a squatting position have also been observed. Severely thiamin-deficient individuals may experience seizures.

In addition to neurological symptoms, wet (cardiac) beriberi is characterized by cardiovascular manifestations of thiamin deficiency, which include rapid heart rate, enlargement of the heart, severe swelling (edema), difficulty breathing, and ultimately congestive heart failure.

Cerebral beriberi may lead to Wernicke encephalopathy and Korsakoff psychosis, especially in people who abuse alcohol. The diagnosis of Wernicke encephalopathy is based on a "triad" of signs, which include abnormal eye movements, stance and gait abnormalities, and abnormalities in mental function that may include a confused apathetic state or a profound memory disorder termed *Korsakoff amnesia* or *Korsakoff psychosis*. Thiamin deficiency affecting the central nervous system is referred to as Wernicke disease when the amnesic state is not present and Wernicke–Korsakoff syndrome (WKS) when the amnesic symptoms are present along with the eye movement and gait disorders. Most WKS sufferers are people who abuse alcohol, although it has been observed in other disorders of gross malnutrition, including stomach cancer and AIDS. Administration of intravenous thiamin to WKS patients generally results in prompt improvement of the eye symptoms, but improvements in motor coordination and memory may be less, depending on how long the symptoms have been present. Recent evidence of increased immune cell activation and increased free radical production in the areas of the brain that are selectively damaged suggests that oxidative stress plays an important role in the neurological pathology of thiamin deficiency.[4]

Causes of Thiamin Deficiency

Thiamin deficiency may result from inadequate thiamin intake, increased requirement for thiamin, excessive loss of thiamin from the body, consumption of anti-thiamin factors in food, or a combination of these factors.

Inadequate intake. Inadequate consumption of thiamin is the main cause of thiamin deficiency in less developed countries.[2] Thiamin deficiency is common in low-income populations whose diets are high in carbohydrate and low in thiamin (e.g., milled or polished rice). Breast-fed infants whose mothers are thiamin deficient are vulnerable to developing infantile beriberi. Alcoholism, which is associated with low intake of thiamin among other nutrients, is the primary cause of thiamin deficiency in industrialized countries.

Increased requirement. Conditions resulting in an increased requirement for thiamin include strenuous physical exertion, fever, pregnancy, breast-feeding, and adolescent growth. Such conditions place individuals with marginal thiamin intake at risk for developing symptomatic thiamin deficiency. Recently, malaria patients in Thailand were found to be severely thiamin deficient more frequently than noninfected individuals.[5] Malarial infection leads to a large increase in the metabolic demand for glucose. As thiamin is required for the enzymes involved in glucose metabolism, the stresses induced by malarial infection could exacerbate thiamin deficiency in predisposed individuals. HIV-infected individuals, whether or not they had developed AIDS, were also found to be at increased risk for thiamin deficiency.[6] The lack of association between thia-

min intake and evidence of deficiency in these HIV-infected individuals suggests that they had an increased requirement for thiamin. Further, chronic alcohol abuse impairs intestinal absorption and utilization of thiamin;[1] thus, people with alcohol problems have increased requirements for thiamin.

Excessive loss. Excessive loss of thiamin may precipitate thiamin deficiency. By increasing urinary flow, diuretics may prevent reabsorption of thiamin by the kidneys and increase its excretion in the urine,[7,8] although this remains quite controversial. Individuals with kidney failure requiring hemodialysis lose thiamin at an increased rate and are at risk for thiamin deficiency.[9] People with alcohol problems who maintain a high fluid intake and urine flow rate may also experience increased loss of thiamin, exacerbating the effects of low thiamin intake.[10]

Anti-thiamin factors. The presence of anti-thiamin factors (ATFs) in foods also contributes to the risk of thiamin deficiency. Certain plants contain ATFs, which react with thiamin to form an oxidized, inactive product. Consuming large amounts of tea and coffee (including decaffeinated), as well as chewing tea leaves and betel nuts, has been associated with thiamin depletion in humans due to the presence of ATFs. Thiaminases are enzymes that break down thiamin in food. Individuals who habitually eat certain raw freshwater fish, raw shellfish, and ferns are at higher risk of thiamin deficiency because these foods contain thiaminase that normally is inactivated by heat in cooking.[1] In Nigeria, an acute neurological syndrome (seasonal ataxia) has been associated with thiamin deficiency precipitated by a thiaminase in African silkworms, a traditional high-protein food for some Nigerians.[11]

Recommended Dietary Allowance

The recommended dietary allowance (RDA) for thiamin, revised in 1998, was based on the prevention of deficiency in generally healthy individuals (**Table 6.1**).[12]

Table 6.1 Recommended dietary allowance for thiamin

Life stage	Age	Males (mg/day)	Females (mg/day)
Infants	0–6 months	0.2 (AI)	0.2 (AI)
Infants	7–12 months	0.3 (AI)	0.3 (AI)
Children	1–3 years	0.5	0.5
Children	4–8 years	0.6	0.6
Children	9–13 years	0.9	0.9
Adolescents	14–18 years	1.2	1.0
Adults	≥19 years	1.2	1.1
Pregnancy	All ages	–	1.4
Breast-feeding	All ages	–	1.4

AI, adequate intake.

Disease Prevention

Cataracts

A cross-sectional study of 2900 Australian men and women, aged 49 years and older, found that those in the highest quintile of thiamin intake were 40% less likely to have nuclear cataracts than those in the lowest quintile.[13] In addition, a recent study in 408 US women found that higher dietary intakes of thiamin were inversely associated with five-year change in lens opacification.[14] However, these cross-sectional associations have yet to be elucidated by studies of causation.

Disease Treatment

Alzheimer Disease

As thiamin deficiency can result in a form of dementia (WKS), its relationship to Alzheimer disease and other forms of dementia has been investigated. A case–control study in 38 elderly women found that blood levels of thiamin, TPP, and TMP were lower in those with dementia of the Alzheimer type (DAT) compared with the those in the control group.[15] Interestingly, several investigators have found evidence of decreased activity of the thiamin pyrophosphate-dependent enzymes, 2-oxoglutarate dehydrogenase and transketolase, in the brains of patients who died of Alzheimer disease.[16] Such findings are consistent with evidence of reduced glucose metabolism found on positron emission tomography (PET) of the brains of Alzheimer disease patients.[17] The finding of decreased brain levels of TPP in the presence of normal levels of free thiamin and TMP suggests that the decreased enzyme activity is not likely a result of thiamin deficiency but rather of impaired TPP synthesis.[18,19] Currently, there is only slight and inconsistent evidence that thiamin supplements are of benefit in Alzheimer disease. A double-blind, placebo-controlled study of 15 patients (10 completed the study) reported no beneficial effect of 3 g thiamin/day on cognitive decline over a 12-month period. In 1993, a preliminary report from another study claimed a mild benefit of 3–8 g thiamin/day in DAT, but no additional data from that study are available.[20] A mild beneficial effect in patients with Alzheimer disease was reported after 12 weeks of treatment with 100 mg/day of a thiamin derivative (thiamin tetrahydrofurfuryl disulfide), but this study was not placebo controlled.[21] A recent systematic review of randomized, double-blind, placebo-controlled trials of thiamin in patients with DAT found no evidence that thiamin was a useful treatment for the symptoms of Alzheimer disease.[22]

Congestive Heart Failure

Severe thiamin deficiency (wet beriberi) can lead to impaired cardiac function and ultimately congestive heart failure (CHF). Although cardiac manifestations of beriberi are rarely encountered in industrialized countries, CHF due to other causes is common, especially in elderly people. Diuretics used in the treatment of CHF, notably furosemide, have been found to increase thiamin excretion, potentially leading to marginal thiamin deficiency. A number of studies have examined thiamin nutritional status in CHF patients and most found a fairly low incidence of thiamin deficiency, as measured by assays of transketolase activity. As in the general population, older CHF patients were found to be at higher risk of thiamin deficiency than younger ones.[23] An important measure of cardiac function in CHF is the left ventricular ejection fraction (LVEF), which can be assessed by echocardiography. One study in 25 patients found that furosemide use, at doses of 80 mg/day or more, was associated with a 98% prevalence of thiamin deficiency.[24]

In a randomized, double-blind study of 30 CHF patients, all of whom had been taking furosemide (80 mg/day) for at least 3 months, intravenous (IV) thiamin therapy (200 mg/day) for 7 days resulted in an improved LVEF compared with IV placebo.[25] When all 30 of the CHF patients in that study subsequently received 6 weeks of oral thiamin therapy (200 mg/day), the average LVEF improved by 22%. This finding may be relevant because improvements in LVEF have been associated with improved survival in CHF patients.[26] However, conclusions from studies published to date are limited due to small sample sizes of the studies, lack of randomization in some studies, and a need for more precise assays of thiamin nutritional status. Currently, the role of thiamin supplementation in maintaining cardiac function in CHF patients remains controversial.

Cancer

Thiamin deficiency has been observed in some cancer patients with rapidly growing tumors. However, research in cell culture and animal models indicates that rapidly dividing cancer cells have a high requirement for thiamin.[27] All rapidly dividing cells require nucleic acids at an increased rate, but some cancer cells appear to rely heavily on the TPP-dependent enzyme, transketolase, to provide the ribose 5-phosphate necessary for nucleic acid synthesis. Thiamin supplementation in cancer patients is common to prevent thiamin deficiency, but Boros et al. caution that too much thiamin may actually fuel the growth of some malignant tumors,[28] suggesting that thiamin supplementation be reserved for those cancer patients who are actually thiamin deficient. Currently, there is no evidence available from studies in humans to support or refute this theory. However, it would be prudent for individuals with cancer who are considering thiamin supplementation to discuss it with the clinicians managing their cancer therapy.

Sources

Food Sources

A varied diet should provide most individuals with adequate thiamin to prevent deficiency. In the United States the average dietary thiamin intake for young men is about 2 mg/day and 1.2 mg/day for young women. A survey of people aged below 60 found an average dietary thiamin intake of 1.4 mg/day for men and 1.1 mg/day for women.[12] However, institutionalization and poverty both increase the likelihood of inadequate thiamin intake in elderly people.[29] Whole-grain cereals, legumes (e.g., beans and lentils), nuts, lean pork, and yeast are rich sources of thiamin.[1] As most of the thiamin is lost during the production of white flour and polished (milled) rice, white rice and foods made from white flour (e.g., bread and pasta) are fortified with thiamin in many Western countries. A number of thiamin-rich foods are listed in **Table 6.2** along with their thiamin content.

Supplements

Thiamin is available in nutritional supplements and for fortification as thiamin hydrochloride and thiamin nitrate.[30]

Safety

Toxicity

The Food and Nutrition Board (FNB) of the Institute of Medicine did not set a tolerable upper intake level for thiamin because there are no well-established toxic effects from the consumption of excess thiamin in food or through long-term oral supplementation (up to 200 mg/day). A small number of life-threatening anaphylactic reactions have been observed with large intravenous doses of thiamin.[12]

Table 6.2 Food sources of thiamin

Food	Serving	Thiamin (mg)
Wheat germ breakfast cereal	1 cup	4.47
Fortified breakfast cereal	1 cup	0.5–2.0
Pork, lean, cooked	3 ounces[a]	0.72
Long grain white rice, enriched, cooked	1 cup	0.26
Peas, cooked	½ cup	0.21
Long grain brown rice, cooked	1 cup	0.19
Pecans	1 ounce	0.19
Brazil nuts	1 ounce	0.18
Lentils, cooked	½ cup	0.17
Cantaloupe	½ fruit	0.11
White bread, enriched	1 slice	0.11
Whole-wheat bread	1 slice	0.10
Orange	1 fruit	0.10
Milk	1 cup	0.10
Spinach, cooked	½ cup	0.09
Long grain white rice, unenriched, cooked	1 cup	0.04
Egg, cooked	1 large	0.03

[a] 3 ounces of meat (or fish) is a serving about the size of a deck of cards.

Drug Interactions

Reduced blood levels of thiamin have been reported in individuals with seizure disorders (epilepsy) taking the anticonvulsant medication, phenytoin, for long periods of time.[31] 5-Fluorouracil, a drug used in cancer therapy, inhibits the phosphorylation of thiamin to TPP.[32] Diuretics, especially furosemide, may increase the risk of thiamin deficiency in individuals with marginal thiamin intake due to increased urinary excretion of thiamin.[8] Moreover, chronic alcohol abuse is associated with thiamin deficiency due to low dietary intake, impaired absorption and utilization, and increased excretion of the vitamin.[1]

LPI Recommendation

The Linus Pauling Institute supports the recommendation by the FNB of 1.2 mg/day for men and 1.1 mg/day for women. A varied diet should provide enough thiamin for most people. Following the Linus Pauling Institute recommendation to take a daily multivitamin/mineral supplement, containing 100% of the daily values, will ensure an intake of at least 1.5 mg thiamin/day.

Older Adults

Currently, there is no evidence that the requirement for thiamin is increased in older adults, but some studies have found inadequate dietary intake and thiamin insufficiency to be more common in elderly populations.[29] Thus, it would be prudent for older adults to take a multivitamin/mineral supplement, which will generally provide at least 1.5 mg thiamin/day.

References

1. Tanphaichitr V. Thiamin. In: Shils M, Olson JA, Shike M, Ross AC, eds. Modern Nutrition in Health and Disease, 9th ed. Baltimore, MD: Lippincott Williams & Wilkins; 1999:381–389
2. Rindi G. Thiamin. In: Ziegler EE, Filer LJ, eds. Present Knowledge in Nutrition, 7th ed. Washington, DC: ILSI Press; 1996:160–166
3. Brody T. Nutritional Biochemistry, 2nd ed. San Diego, CA: Academic Press; 1999
4. Todd K, Butterworth RF. Mechanisms of selective neuronal cell death due to thiamine deficiency. Ann N Y Acad Sci 1999;893:404–411
5. Krishna S, Taylor AM, Supanaranond W, et al. Thiamine deficiency and malaria in adults from southeast Asia. Lancet 1999;353(9152):546–549
6. Müri RM, Von Overbeck J, Furrer J, Ballmer PE. Thiamin deficiency in HIV-positive patients: evaluation by erythrocyte transketolase activity and thiamin pyrophosphate effect. Clin Nutr 1999;18(6):375–378

7. Suter PM, Haller J, Hany A, Vetter W. Diuretic use: a risk for subclinical thiamine deficiency in elderly patients. J Nutr Health Aging 2000;4(2):69–71

8. Rieck J, Halkin H, Almog S, et al. Urinary loss of thiamine is increased by low doses of furosemide in healthy volunteers. J Lab Clin Med 1999;134(3): 238–243

9. Hung SC, Hung SH, Tarng DC, Yang WC, Chen TW, Huang TP. Thiamine deficiency and unexplained encephalopathy in hemodialysis and peritoneal dialysis patients. Am J Kidney Dis 2001;38(5):941–947

10. Wilcox CS. Do diuretics cause thiamine deficiency? J Lab Clin Med 1999;134(3):192–193

11. Nishimune T, Watanabe Y, Okazaki H, Akai H. Thiamin is decomposed due to *Anaphe* spp. entomophagy in seasonal ataxia patients in Nigeria. J Nutr 2000; 130(6):1625–1628

12. Food and Nutrition Board, Institute of Medicine. Thiamin. In: Dietary Reference Intakes for Thiamin, Riboflavin, Niacin, Vitamin B_6, Vitamin B_{12}, Pantothenic Acid, Biotin, and Choline. Washington, DC: National Academy Press; 1998:58–86

13. Cumming RG, Mitchell P, Smith W. Diet and cataract: the Blue Mountains Eye Study. Ophthalmology 2000;107(3):450–456

14. Jacques PF, Taylor A, Moeller S, et al. Long-term nutrient intake and 5-year change in nuclear lens opacities. Arch Ophthalmol 2005;123(4):517–526

15. Glasø M, Nordbø G, Diep L, Bøhmer T. Reduced concentrations of several vitamins in normal weight patients with late-onset dementia of the Alzheimer type without vascular disease. J Nutr Health Aging 2004;8(5):407–413

16. Bender DA. Optimum nutrition: thiamin, biotin and pantothenate. Proc Nutr Soc 1999;58(2):427–433

17. Kish SJ. Brain energy metabolizing enzymes in Alzheimer's disease: alpha-ketoglutarate dehydrogenase complex and cytochrome oxidase. Ann N Y Acad Sci 1997;826:218–228

18. Mastrogiacoma F, Bettendorff L, Grisar T, Kish SJ. Brain thiamine, its phosphate esters, and its metabolizing enzymes in Alzheimer's disease. Ann Neurol 1996;39(5):585–591

19. Héroux M, Raghavendra Rao VL, Lavoie J, Richardson JS, Butterworth RF. Alterations of thiamine phosphorylation and of thiamine-dependent enzymes in Alzheimer's disease. Metab Brain Dis 1996;11(1):81–88

20. Meador K, Loring D, Nichols M, et al. Preliminary findings of high-dose thiamine in dementia of Alzheimer's type. J Geriatr Psychiatry Neurol 1993;6(4): 222–229

21. Mimori Y, Katsuoka H, Nakamura S. Thiamine therapy in Alzheimer's disease. Metab Brain Dis 1996;11 (1): 89–94

22. Rodríguez-Martín JL, Qizilbash N, López-Arrieta JM. Thiamine for Alzheimer's disease. Cochrane Database Syst Rev 2001;2(2):CD 001498

23. Wilkinson TJ, Hanger HC, George PM, Sainsbury R. Is thiamine deficiency in elderly people related to age or co-morbidity? Age Ageing 2000;29(2):111–116

24. Zenuk C, Healey J, Donnelly J, Vaillancourt R, Almalki Y, Smith S. Thiamine deficiency in congestive heart failure patients receiving long term furosemide therapy. Can J Clin Pharmacol 2003;10(4):184–188

25. Shimon I, Almog S, Vered Z, et al. Improved left ventricular function after thiamine supplementation in patients with congestive heart failure receiving long-term furosemide therapy. Am J Med 1995;98(5): 485–490

26. Leslie D, Gheorghiade M. Is there a role for thiamine supplementation in the management of heart failure? Am Heart J 1996;131(6):1248–1250

27. Comín-Anduix B, Boren J, Martinez S, et al. The effect of thiamine supplementation on tumour proliferation. A metabolic control analysis study. Eur J Biochem 2001;268(15):4177–4182

28. Boros LG, Brandes JL, Lee WN, et al. Thiamine supplementation to cancer patients: a double edged sword. Anticancer Res 1998;18(1B):595–602

29. Russell RM, Suter PM. Vitamin requirements of elderly people: an update. Am J Clin Nutr 1993;58(1): 4–14

30. Hendler SS, Rorvik DR, eds. PDR for Nutritional Supplements. Montvale: Medical Economics Co., Inc.; 2001

31. Flodin N. Pharmacology of Micronutrients. New York: Alan R. Liss, Inc., 1988

32. Schümann K. Interactions between drugs and vitamins at advanced age. Int J Vitam Nutr Res 1999; 69(3):173–178

7 Vitamin A

Vitamin A is a generic term for a large number of related compounds. Retinol (an alcohol) and retinal (an aldehyde) are often referred to as *preformed vitamin A*. Retinal can be converted by the body to retinoic acid (RA), the form of vitamin A known to affect gene transcription. Retinol, retinal, RA, and related compounds are known as *retinoids*. β-Carotene and other carotenoids that can be converted by the body into retinol are referred to as *provitamin A* carotenoids. Hundreds of different carotenoids are synthesized by plants, but only about 10% of them are provitamin A carotenoids.[1] The following discussion focuses mainly on preformed vitamin A and RA.

Function

Vision

The retina is located at the back of the eye. When light passes through the lens, it is sensed by the retina and converted to a nerve impulse for interpretation by the brain. Retinol is transported to the retina via the circulation and accumulates in retinal pigment epithelial cells (**Fig. 7.1**). Here, retinol is esterified to form a retinyl ester, which can be stored. When needed, retinyl esters are broken apart (hydrolyzed) and isomerized to form 11-*cis*-retinol, which can be oxidized to form 11-*cis*-retinal. 11-*cis*-Retinal can be shuttled across the interphotoreceptor matrix to the rod cell where it binds to a protein called *opsin* to form the visual pigment rhodopsin (also known as visual purple). Rod cells with rhodopsin can detect very small amounts of light, making them important for night vision. Absorption of a photon of light catalyzes the isomerization of 11-*cis*-retinal to all-*trans*-retinal and results in its release. This isomerization triggers a cascade of events, leading to the generation of an electrical signal to the optic nerve. The nerve impulse generated by the optic nerve is conveyed to the brain where it can be interpreted as vision. Once released, all-*trans* retinal is converted to all-*trans*-

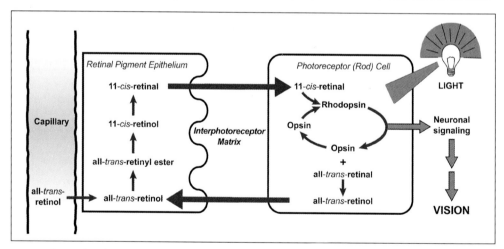

Fig. 7.1 The visual cycle: retinol is transported to the retina via the circulation, where it moves into retinal pigment epithelial cells. There, retinol is esterified to form a retinyl ester that can be stored. When needed, retinyl esters are broken apart (hydrolyzed) and isomerized to form 11-*cis*-retinol, which can be oxidized to form 11-*cis*-retinal. 11-*cis*-Retinal can be shuttled to the rod cell, where it binds to a protein called opsin to form the visual pigment rhodopsin (visual purple). Absorption of a photon of light catalyzes the isomerization of 11-*cis*-retinal to all-*trans*-retinal and results in its release. This isomerization triggers a cascade of events, leading to the generation of an electrical signal to the optic nerve. The nerve impulse generated by the optic nerve is conveyed to the brain where it can be interpreted as vision. Once released, all-*trans*-retinal is converted to all-*trans*-retinol, which can be transported across the interphotoreceptor matrix to the retinal epithelial cell to complete the visual cycle.

retinol, which can be transported across the interphotoreceptor matrix to the retinal epithelial cell, thereby completing the visual cycle.[2] Inadequate retinol available to the retina results in impaired dark adaptation, known as "night blindness."

Regulation of Gene Expression

Isomers of retinoic acid act as hormones to affect gene expression and thereby influence numerous physiological processes. All-*trans*-RA and 9-*cis*-RA are transported to the nucleus of the cell bound to cytoplasmic retinoic acid-binding proteins (CRABPs). Within the nucleus, RA binds to retinoic acid receptor proteins (**Fig. 7.2**). Specifically, all-*trans*-RA binds to retinoic acid receptors (RARs) and 9-*cis*-RA binds to retinoid X receptors (RXRs). RARs and RXRs form RAR/RXR heterodimers, which bind to regulatory regions of the chromosome called retinoic acid response elements (RAREs). A dimer is a complex of two protein molecules, heterodimers are complexes of two different proteins, and homodimers are complexes of two of the same protein. Binding of all-*trans*-RA and 9-*cis*-RA to an RAR and RXR, respectively, allows the complex to regulate the rate of gene transcription, thereby influencing the synthesis of certain proteins. RXRs may also form heterodimers with thyroid hormone receptors (THRs) or vitamin D receptors (VDRs). In this way, vitamin A, thyroid hormone, and vitamin D may interact to influence gene transcription.[3] Through the stimulation and inhibition of transcription of specific genes, RA plays a major role in cellular differentiation, the specialization of cells for highly specific physiological roles. Many of the physiological effects attributed to vitamin A appear to result from its role in cellular differentiation.

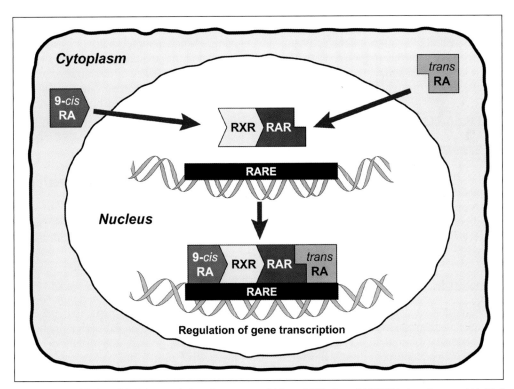

Fig. 7.2 A simplified model of the regulation of gene expression by retinoic acid (RA) isomers. All-*trans*-RA and 9-*cis*-RA are transported to the nucleus of the cell bound to cytoplasmic retinoic acid-binding proteins. Within the nucleus, all-*trans*-RA binds to retinoic acid receptors (RARs) and 9-*cis*-RA binds to retinoid receptors (RXRs). RARs and RXRs form RAR/RXR heterodimers, which bind to regulatory regions of the chromosome called retinoic acid response elements (RAREs). Binding of all-*trans*-RA and 9-*cis*-RA to RARs and RXRs, respectively, allows the complex to regulate the rate of gene transcription.

Immunity

Vitamin A is commonly known as the anti-infective vitamin, because it is required for normal functioning of the immune system.[4] The skin and mucosal cells (cells that line the airways, digestive tract, and urinary tract) function as a barrier and form the body's first line of defense against infection. Retinol and its metabolites are required to maintain the integrity and function of these cells.[5] Vitamin A and RA play a central role in the development and differentiation of white blood cells, such as lymphocytes, which play critical roles in the immune response. Activation of T lymphocytes, the major regulatory cells of the immune system, appears to require all-*trans*-RA binding of RARs.[3]

Growth and Development

Both vitamin A excess and deficiency are known to cause birth defects. Retinol and RA are essential for embryonic development.[4] During fetal development, RA functions in limb development and formation of the heart, eyes, and ears.[6] In addition, RA has been found to regulate expression of the gene for growth hormone.

Red Blood Cell Production

Red blood cells, similar to all blood cells, are derived from precursor cells called *stem cells*. Stem cells are dependent on retinoids for normal differentiation into red blood cells. In addition, vitamin A appears to facilitate the mobilization of iron from storage sites to the developing red blood cell for incorporation into hemoglobin, the oxygen carrier in red blood cells.[2,7]

Nutrient Interactions

Zinc. Zinc deficiency is thought to interfere with vitamin A metabolism in several ways:
- Zinc deficiency results in decreased synthesis of retinol-binding protein (RBP), which transports retinol through the circulation to tissues (e.g., the retina) and also protects the organism against the potential toxicity of retinol.
- Zinc deficiency results in decreased activity of the enzyme that releases retinol from its storage form, retinyl palmitate, in the liver.
- Zinc is required for the enzyme that converts retinol into retinal.[8,9]

At present, the health consequences of zinc deficiency on vitamin A nutritional status in humans are unclear.[10]

Iron. Vitamin A deficiency may exacerbate iron-deficiency anemia. Vitamin A supplementation has beneficial effects on iron-deficiency anemia and improves iron nutritional status among children and pregnant women. The combination of supplemental vitamin A and iron seems to reduce anemia more effectively than either supplemental iron or vitamin A alone.[11] Moreover, studies in rats have shown that iron deficiency alters plasma and liver levels of vitamin A.[12,13]

Deficiency

Vitamin A Deficiency and Vision

Vitamin A deficiency among children in less developed nations is the leading preventable cause of blindness.[14] The earliest evidence of vitamin A deficiency is impaired dark adaptation or night blindness. Mild vitamin A deficiency may result in changes in the conjunctiva (corner of the eye) called *Bitot spots*. Severe or prolonged vitamin A deficiency causes a condition called *xerophthalmia* (dry eye), characterized by changes in the cells of the cornea (clear covering of the eye) that ultimately result in corneal ulcers, scarring, and blindness.[4,9]

Vitamin A Deficiency and Infectious Disease

Vitamin A deficiency can be considered a nutritionally acquired immunodeficiency disease.[15] Even children who are only mildly deficient in vitamin A have a higher incidence of respiratory disease and diarrhea as well as a higher rate of mortality from infectious disease compared with children who consume sufficient vitamin A.[16] Vitamin A supplementation has been found to decrease both the severity and the incidence of deaths related to diarrhea and measles in less developed countries, where vitamin A deficiency is common.[17] The onset of infection reduces blood retinol levels very rapidly. This phenomenon is generally believed to be related to decreased synthesis of RBP by the liver. In this manner, infection stimulates a vicious cycle, because inadequate vitamin A nutritional status is related to increased severity and likelihood of death from infectious disease.[18] However, a review of four studies concluded that vitamin A supplementation is not beneficial in reducing the mother-to-child transmission of HIV.[19] One study found that HIV-infected women who were vitamin A deficient were three to four times more likely to transmit HIV to their infants.[20]

Recommended Dietary Allowance

The recommended dietary allowance (RDA) for vitamin A was revised by the Food and Nutrition Board (FNB) of the Institute of Medicine in 2001. The latest RDA is based on the amount needed to ensure adequate stores (4 months) of vitamin A in the body to support normal reproductive function, immune function, gene expression, and vision (**Table 7.1**).[21]

Disease Prevention

Cancer

Studies in cell culture and animal models have documented the capacity for natural and synthetic retinoids to reduce carcinogenesis significantly in skin, breast, liver, colon, prostate, and other sites.[2] However, the results of human studies examining the relationship between the consumption of preformed vitamin A and cancer are less clear.

Lung cancer. At least 10 prospective studies have compared blood retinol levels at baseline among people who subsequently developed lung cancer and those who did not. Only one of those studies found a statistically significant inverse association between serum retinol and lung cancer risk.[22] The results of the β-Carotene And Retinol Efficacy Trial (CARET) suggest that high-dose supplementation of vitamin A and β-carotene should be avoided in people at high risk of lung cancer.[23] About 9000 people (smokers and people with asbestos exposure) were assigned a daily regimen of 25 000 IU retinol and 30 mg β-carotene, while a similar number of people were assigned a placebo. After four years of follow-up, the incidence of lung cancer was 28% higher in the supplemented group compared with the placebo group. A possible explanation for such a finding is that the oxidative environment of the lung, created by smoke or asbestos exposure, gives rise to unusual carotenoid cleavage products, which are involved in carcinogenesis. Currently, it seems unlikely that increased retinol intake decreases the risk of lung cancer, although the effects of retinol may be different for nonsmokers than for smokers.[22]

Breast cancer. Retinol and its metabolites have been found to reduce the growth of breast cancer cells in vitro, but observational studies of dietary retinol intake in humans have not confirmed this.[24] Most epidemiological studies have failed to find significant associations between retinol intake and breast cancer risk in women,[25–28] although one large prospective study found that total vitamin A intake was inversely associated

Table 7.1 Recommended dietary allowance for vitamin A as preformed vitamin A (retinol)

Life stage	Age	Males µg/day (IU/day)	Females µg/day (IU/day)
Infants	0–6 months	400 (1333 IU) (AI)	400 (1333 IU) (AI)
Infants	7–12 months	500 (1667 IU) (AI)	500 (1667 IU) (AI)
Children	1–3 years	300 (1000 IU)	300 (1000 IU)
Children	4–8 years	400 (1333 IU)	400 (1333 IU)
Children	9–13 years	600 (2000 IU)	600 (2000 IU)
Adolescents	14–18 years	900 (3000 IU)	700 (2333 IU)
Adults	≥19 years	900 (3000 IU)	700 (2333 IU)
Pregnancy	≤18 years	–	750 (2500 IU)
Pregnancy	≥19 years	–	770 (2567 IU)
Breast-feeding	≤18 years	–	1200 (4000 IU)
Breast-feeding	≥19 years	–	1300 (4333 IU)

AI, adequate intake.

with the risk of breast cancer in premenopausal women with a family history of breast cancer.[29] Blood levels of retinol reflect the intake of both preformed vitamin A and provitamin A carotenoids such as β-carotene. Although a case–control study found serum retinol levels and serum antioxidant levels to be inversely related to the risk of breast cancer,[30] two prospective studies did not observe significant associations between blood retinol levels and subsequent risk of developing breast cancer.[31,32] Currently, there is little evidence in humans that increased intake of preformed vitamin A or retinol reduces breast cancer risk.

Disease Treatment

Pharmacological Doses of Retinoids

Retinoids are used at pharmacological doses to treat several conditions, including retinitis pigmentosa, acute promyelocytic leukemia, and various skin diseases. It is important to note that treatment with high doses of natural or synthetic retinoids overrides the body's own control mechanisms, so retinoid therapies are associated with potential side effects and toxicities. In addition, all of the retinoid compounds have been found to cause birth defects. Thus, women who have a chance of becoming pregnant should avoid treatment with these medications. Retinoids tend to be very long acting: side effects and birth defects have been reported to occur months after discontinuing retinoid therapy.[2] The retinoids discussed below are prescription drugs and should not be used without medical supervision.

Retinitis pigmentosa. Retinitis pigmentosa describes a broad spectrum of genetic disorders that result in the progressive loss of photoreceptor cells (rods and cones) in the eye's retina.[33] Early symptoms of retinitis pigmentosa include impaired dark adaptation and night blindness, followed by the progressive loss of peripheral and central vision over time. The results of a randomized controlled trial in more than 600 patients with common forms of retinitis pigmentosa indicated that supplementation with 4500 µg (15 000 IU)/day of preformed vitamin A (retinol) significantly slowed the loss of retinal function over a period of four to six years.[34] In contrast, supplementation with 400 IU/day of vi-

tamin E increased the loss of retinal function by a small but significant amount, suggesting that patients with common forms of retinitis pigmentosa may benefit from long-term vitamin A supplementation but should avoid vitamin E supplementation at levels higher than those found in a typical multivitamin. Up to 12 years of follow-up in these patients did not reveal any signs of liver toxicity as a result of excess vitamin A intake.[35] High-dose vitamin A supplementation to slow the course of retinitis pigmentosa requires medical supervision and must be discontinued if there is a possibility of pregnancy.

Acute promyelocytic leukemia. Normal differentiation of myeloid stem cells in the bone marrow gives rise to platelets, red blood cells, and white blood cells that are important for the immune response. Altered differentiation of those stem cells results in the proliferation of immature leukemic cells, giving rise to leukemia. A mutation of the RAR has been discovered in patients with a specific type of leukemia called acute promyelocytic leukemia (APL). Treatment with all-*trans*-RA or with high doses of all-*trans*-retinyl palmitate restores normal differentiation and leads to improvement in some APL patients.[2,18]

Diseases of the Skin

Both natural and synthetic retinoids have been used as pharmacological agents to treat disorders of the skin. Etretinate and acitretin are retinoids that have been useful in the treatment of psoriasis, whereas tretinoin and isotretinoin have been used successfully to treat severe acne. Retinoids most likely affect the transcription of skin growth factors and their receptors.[2] Use of pharmacological doses of retinoids by pregnant women causes birth defects.

Sources

Retinol Activity Equivalents

Different dietary sources of vitamin A have different potencies; for example, β-carotene is less easily absorbed than retinol and must be converted to retinal and retinol by the body. The most recent international standard of measure for vitamin A is retinol activity equivalents (RAE), which represent vitamin A activity as retinol:

Table 7.2 Retinol activity equivalent (RAE) ratios for β-carotene and other provitamin A carotenoids

Quantity consumed	Quantity bioconverted to retinol	RAE ratio
1 µg dietary or supplemental vitamin A	1 µg retinol	1:1
2 µg supplemental β-carotene	1 µg retinol	2:1
12 µg dietary β-carotene	1 µg retinol	12:1
24 µg dietary α-carotene	1 µg retinol	24:1
24 µg dietary β-cryptoxanthin	1 µg retinol	24:1

2 µg β-carotene in oil provided as a supplement can be converted by the body to 1 µg retinol, giving it an RAE ratio of 2:1. However, 12 µg β-carotene from foods are required to provide the body with 1 µg retinol, giving dietary β-carotene an RAE ratio of 12:1. Other provitamin A carotenoids in foods are less easily ab-

sorbed than β-carotene, resulting in RAE ratios of 24:1. The RAE ratios for β-carotene and other provitamin A carotenoids are shown in **Table 7.2**.[21] An older international standard, still commonly used, is the international unit (IU): 1 IU is equivalent to 0.3 µg retinol.

Food Sources

Free retinol is not generally found in foods. Retinyl palmitate, a precursor and storage form of retinol, is found in foods from animals. Plants contain carotenoids, some of which are precursors for vitamin A (e.g., α-carotene, β-carotene, and β-cryptoxanthin). Yellow and orange vegetables contain significant quantities of carotenoids. Green vegetables also contain carotenoids, although the pigment is masked by the green pigment of chlorophyll.[1] A number of good food sources of vitamin A are listed in **Table 7.3** along with their vitamin A content in RAEs. In those foods where retinol activity comes mainly from provitamin A carotenoids, the carotenoid content and the RAEs are presented.

Table 7.3 Food sources of vitamin A

Food	Serving	Vitamin A (µg RAE)	Vitamin A (IU)	Retinol (µg)	Retinol (IU)
Cod liver oil	1 teaspoon	1350	4500	1350	4500
Fortified breakfast cereals	1 serving	150–230	500–767	150–230	500–767
Egg	1 large	91	303	89	296
Butter	1 tablespoon	97	323	95	317
Whole milk	1 cup (8 fluid ounces)	68	227	68	227
2% fat milk (vitamin A added)	1 cup (8 fluid ounces)	134	447	134	447
Nonfat milk (vitamin A added)	1 cup (8 fluid ounces)	149	497	149	497
Sweet potato, canned	½ cup, mashed	555	1848	0	0
Sweet potato, baked	½ cup	961	3203	0	0
Pumpkin, canned	½ cup	953	3177	0	0
Carrot, raw	½ cup, chopped	538	1793	0	0
Cantaloupe	½ medium melon	467	1555	0	0
Mango	1 fruit	79	263	0	0
Spinach	½ cup, cooked	472	1572	0	0
Broccoli	½ cup, cooked	60	200	0	0
Kale	½ cup, cooked	443	1475	0	0
Collards	½ cup, cooked	386	1285	0	0
Squash, butternut	½ cup, cooked	572	1907	0	0

RAE, retinol activity equivalent.

Table 7.4 Tolerable upper intake level (UL) for preformed vitamin A (retinol)

Life stage	Age	UL (µg/day) (IU/day)
Infants	0–12 months	600 (2000)
Children	1–3 years	600 (2000)
Children	4–8 years	900 (3000)
Children	9–13 years	1700 (5667)
Adolescents	14–18 years	2800 (9333)
Adults	≥19 years	3000 (10 000)

Supplements

The principal forms of preformed vitamin A (retinol) in supplements are retinyl palmitate and retinyl acetate. β-Carotene is also a common source of vitamin A in supplements, and many supplements provide a combination of retinol and β-carotene.[36] If a percentage of the total vitamin A content of a supplement comes from β-carotene, this information is included in the Supplement Facts label under vitamin A. Most multivitamin supplements available in the United States provide 1500 µg (5000 IU) vitamin A, which is substantially more than the current RDA for vitamin A. This is due to the fact that the daily values used by the US Food and Drug Administration (FDA) for supplement labeling are based on the RDA established in 1968 rather than the most recent RDA, and multivitamin supplements typically provide 100% of the daily value for most nutrients. As retinol intakes of 5000 IU/day may be associated with an increased risk of osteoporosis in older adults, some companies have reduced the retinol content in their multivitamin supplements to 750 µg (2500 IU).

Safety

Toxicity

The condition caused by vitamin A toxicity is called *hypervitaminosis A*. It results from overconsumption of preformed vitamin A, not carotenoids. Preformed vitamin A is rapidly absorbed and slowly cleared from the body, so toxicity from it may result acutely from high-dose exposure over a short period of time or chronically from a much lower intake.[2] Acute vitamin A toxicity is relatively rare, and symptoms include nausea, headache, fatigue, loss of appetite, dizziness, dry skin, desquamation, and cerebral edema. Signs of chronic toxicity include dry itchy skin, desquamation, loss of appetite, headache, cerebral edema, and bone and joint pain. In addition, symptoms of vitamin A toxicity in infants include a bulging fontanel. Severe cases of hypervitaminosis A may result in liver damage, hemorrhage, and coma. Generally, signs of toxicity are associated with long-term consumption of vitamin A in excess of 10 times the RDA (8000–10 000 µg/day or 25 000–33 000 IU/day). However, more research is necessary to determine if subclinical vitamin A toxicity is a concern in certain populations.[37] There is evidence that some populations may be more susceptible to toxicity at lower doses, including elderly people, chronic alcohol users, and some people with a genetic predisposition to high cholesterol.[8] In January 2001, the FNB set the tolerable upper intake level (UL) of vitamin A intake for adults at 3000 µg (10 000 IU)/day of preformed vitamin A (**Table 7.4**).[21]

Safety in Pregnancy

Although normal fetal development requires sufficient vitamin A intake, consumption of excess preformed vitamin A (retinol) during pregnancy is known to cause birth defects. No increase in the risk of vitamin A-associated birth defects has been observed at doses of preformed vitamin A from supplements below 3000 µg/day (10 000 IU/day).[21] As a number of foods in the United States are fortified with preformed vitamin A, pregnant women should avoid multivitamin or prenatal supplements that contain more than 1500 µg (5000 IU) vitamin A. Vitamin A from β-carotene is not known to increase the risk of birth defects. Etretinate and isotretinoin, synthetic derivatives of retinol, are known to cause serious birth defects and should not be taken during pregnancy or if there is a possibility of becoming pregnant.[38] Tretinoin, another retinol derivative, is prescribed as a topical preparation that is applied to the skin. As a result of the potential for systemic absorption of topical tretinoin, its use during pregnancy is not recommended.

Effects on Bone

Results of some studies indicate that vitamin A intake is not associated with detrimental effects on bone mineral density (BMD) or fracture risk.[39-41] However, results of some prospective studies suggest that long-term intakes of preformed vitamin A in excess of 1500 µg/day (5000 IU/day) are associated with increased risk of osteoporotic fracture and decreased BMD in older men and women.[42-44] Although this level of intake is greater than the RDA of 700–900 µg/day (2300–3000 IU/day), it is substantially lower than the UL of 3000 µg/day (10 000 IU/day). Only excess intakes of preformed vitamin A (retinol), not β-carotene, were associated with adverse effects on bone health. Although these observational studies cannot provide the reason for the association between excess retinol intake and osteoporosis, limited experimental data suggest that excess retinol may stimulate bone resorption[45] or interfere with the ability of vitamin D to maintain calcium balance.[46]

In the United States, retinol intakes in excess of 5000 IU/day can be easily attained by those who regularly consume multivitamin supplements and/or fortified foods, including some breakfast cereals. At the other end of the spectrum, a significant number of elderly people have insufficient vitamin A intakes, which have also been associated with decreased BMD. One study of elderly men and women found that BMD was optimal at vitamin A intakes close to the RDA.[43] Until supplements and fortified foods are reformulated to reflect the current RDA for vitamin A, it makes sense to look for multivitamin supplements that contain 2500 IU or those that contain 5000 IU vitamin A, of which at least 50% comes from β-carotene.

Drug Interactions

Chronic alcohol consumption results in depletion of liver stores of vitamin A, and may contribute to alcohol-induced liver damage.[47] However, the liver toxicity of preformed vitamin A (retinol) is enhanced by chronic alcohol consumption, so narrowing the therapeutic window for vitamin A supplementation in those who abuse alcohol.[48] Oral contraceptives that contain estrogen and progestin increase RBP synthesis by the liver, increasing the export of the RBP–retinol complex in blood. Whether this increases the dietary requirement of vitamin A is not known. Retinoids or retinoid analogs, including acitretin, all-*trans*-RA, bexarotene, etretinate, and isotretinoin, should not be used in combination with vitamin A supplements, because they may increase the risk of vitamin A toxicity.[36]

LPI Recommendation

The RDA for vitamin A (2300 IU/day for women and 3000 IU/day for men) is sufficient to support normal gene expression, immune function, and vision. However, following the Linus Pauling Institute's recommendation to take a multivitamin/mineral supplement daily could supply as much as 5000 IU/day of vitamin A as retinol, the amount that has been associated with adverse effects on bone health in older adults. For this reason, we recommend taking a multivitamin/mineral supplement that provides no more than 2500 IU vitamin A or a supplement that provides 5000 IU vitamin A, of which at least 50% comes from β-carotene. High-potency vitamin A supplements should not be used without medical supervision due to the risk of toxicity.

Older Adults

Currently, there is little evidence that the requirement for vitamin A in older adults differs from that of younger adults. In addition, vitamin A toxicity may occur at lower doses in older adults than in younger adults. Following the Linus Pauling Institute's recommendation to take a multivitamin/mineral supplement daily could supply as much as 5000 IU/day of retinol, the amount that has been associated with adverse effects on bone health in older adults. For this reason, we recommend taking a multivitamin/mineral supplement that provides no more than 2500 IU vitamin A or a supplement that provides 5000 IU vitamin A, of which at least 50% comes from β-carotene. High-potency vitamin A supplements should not be used without medical supervision due to the risk of toxicity.

References

1. Groff JL. Advanced Nutrition and Human Metabolism, 2nd ed. St. Paul, MI: West Publishing; 1995
2. Ross AC. Vitamin A and retinoids. In: Shils M, ed. Modern Nutrition in Health and Disease. 9th ed. Baltimore, MD: Williams & Wilkins; 1999:305–327
3. Semba RD. The role of vitamin A and related retinoids in immune function. Nutr Rev 1998;56(1 Pt 2): S38–S48
4. Semba RD. Impact of vitamin A on immunity and infection in developing countries. In: Bendich A, Decklebaum RJ, eds. Preventive Nutrition: The Comprehensive Guide for Health Professionals, 2nd ed. Totowa, NJ: Humana Press Inc.; 2001:329–346
5. McCullough FS, Northrop-Clewes CA, Thurnham DI. The effect of vitamin A on epithelial integrity. Proc Nutr Soc 1999;58(2):289–293
6. Solomons NW. Vitamin A and carotenoids. In: Bowman BA, Russell RM, eds. Present Knowledge in Nutrition. 8th ed. Washington, DC: ILSI Press; 2001:127–145
7. Lynch SR. Interaction of iron with other nutrients. Nutr Rev 1997;55(4):102–110
8. Russell RM. The vitamin A spectrum: from deficiency to toxicity. Am J Clin Nutr 2000;71(4):878–884
9. Brody T. Nutritional Biochemistry, 2nd ed. San Diego, CA: Academic Press; 1999
10. Christian P, West KP Jr. Interactions between zinc and vitamin A: an update. Am J Clin Nutr 1998; 68(2, Suppl):435S–441S
11. Suharno D, West CE, Muhilal, Karyadi D, Hautvast JG. Supplementation with vitamin A and iron for nutritional anaemia in pregnant women in West Java, Indonesia. Lancet 1993;342(8883):1325–1328
12. Jang JT, Green JB, Beard JL, Green MH. Kinetic analysis shows that iron deficiency decreases liver vitamin A mobilization in rats. J Nutr 2000;130(5):1291–1296
13. Rosales FJ, Jang JT, Piñero DJ, Erikson KM, Beard JL, Ross AC. Iron deficiency in young rats alters the distribution of vitamin A between plasma and liver and between hepatic retinol and retinyl esters. J Nutr 1999;129(6):1223–1228
14. Underwood BA, Arthur P. The contribution of vitamin A to public health. FASEB J 1996;10(9):1040–1048
15. Semba RD. Vitamin A and human immunodeficiency virus infection. Proc Nutr Soc 1997;56(1B):459–469
16. Field CJ, Johnson IR, Schley PD. Nutrients and their role in host resistance to infection. J Leukoc Biol 2002;71(1):16–32
17. West CE. Vitamin A and measles. Nutr Rev 2000;58(2 Pt 2):S46–S54
18. Thurnham DI, Northrop-Clewes CA. Optimal nutrition: vitamin A and the carotenoids. Proc Nutr Soc 1999;58(2):449–457
19. Wiysonge CS, Shey MS, Sterne JA, Brocklehurst P. Vitamin A supplementation for reducing the risk of mother-to-child transmission of HIV infection. Cochrane Database Syst Rev 2005;(4):CD 003648
20. Ramasethu J. Semba RD, et al., Maternal vitamin A deficiency and mother-to-child transmission of HIV-1. Lancet 1994;343:1593-7. Pediatr AIDS HIV Infect 1995;6(5):303–304
21. Food and Nutrition Board, Institute of Medicine. Vitamin A. In: Dietary Reference Intakes for Vitamin A, Vitamin K, Arsenic, Boron, Chromium, Copper, Iodine, Iron, Manganese, Molybdenum, Nickel, Silicon, Vanadium, and Zinc. Washington, DC: National Academy Press; 2001:65–126
22. Comstock GW, Helzlsouer KJ. Preventive nutrition and lung cancer. In: Bendich A, Decklebaum RJ, eds. Preventive Nutrition: The Comprehensive Guide for Health Professionals, 2nd ed. Totowa, NJ: Humana Press Inc.; 2001:97–129
23. Omenn GS, Goodman GE, Thornquist MD, et al. Effects of a combination of beta carotene and vitamin A on lung cancer and cardiovascular disease. N Engl J Med 1996;334(18):1150–1155
24. Prakash P, Krinsky NI, Russell RM. Retinoids, carotenoids, and human breast cancer cell cultures: a review of differential effects. Nutr Rev 2000;58(6):170–176
25. Bohlke K, Spiegelman D, Trichopoulou A, Katsouyanni K, Trichopoulos D. Vitamins A, C and E and the risk of breast cancer: results from a case-control study in Greece. Br J Cancer 1999;79(1):23–29
26. Franceschi S. Micronutrients and breast cancer. Eur J Cancer Prev 1997;6(6):535–539
27. Longnecker MP, Newcomb PA, Mittendorf R, Greenberg ER, Willett WC. Intake of carrots, spinach, and supplements containing vitamin A in relation to risk of breast cancer. Cancer Epidemiol Biomarkers Prev 1997;6(11):887–892
28. Michels KB, Holmberg L, Bergkvist L, Ljung H, Bruce A, Wolk A. Dietary antioxidant vitamins, retinol, and breast cancer incidence in a cohort of Swedish women. Int J Cancer 2001;91(4):563–567
29. Zhang S, Hunter DJ, Forman MR, et al. Dietary carotenoids and vitamins A, C, and E and risk of breast cancer. J Natl Cancer Inst 1999;91(6):547–556
30. Ching S, Ingram D, Hahnel R, Beilby J, Rossi E. Serum levels of micronutrients, antioxidants and total antioxidant status predict risk of breast cancer in a case control study. J Nutr 2002;132(2):303–306
31. Hultén K, Van Kappel AL, Winkvist A, et al. Carotenoids, alpha-tocopherols, and retinol in plasma and breast cancer risk in northern Sweden. Cancer Causes Control 2001;12(6):529–537
32. Dorgan JF, Sowell A, Swanson CA, et al. Relationships of serum carotenoids, retinol, alpha-tocopherol, and selenium with breast cancer risk: results from a prospective study in Columbia, Missouri (United States). Cancer Causes Control 1998;9(1):89–97
33. van Soest S, Westerveld A, de Jong PT, Bleeker-Wagemakers EM, Bergen AA. Retinitis pigmentosa: defined from a molecular point of view. Surv Ophthalmol 1999;43(4):321–334
34. Berson EL, Rosner B, Sandberg MA, et al. A randomized trial of vitamin A and vitamin E supplementation for retinitis pigmentosa. Arch Ophthalmol 1993;111(6):761–772
35. Sibulesky L, Hayes KC, Pronczuk A, Weigel-DiFranco C, Rosner B, Berson EL. Safety of < 7500 RE (< 25000 IU) vitamin A daily in adults with retinitis pigmentosa. Am J Clin Nutr 1999;69(4):656–663
36. Hendler SS, Rorvik DR, eds. PDR for Nutritional Supplements. Montvale: Medical Economics Co., Inc.; 2001
37. Penniston KL, Tanumihardjo SA. The acute and chronic toxic effects of vitamin A. Am J Clin Nutr 2006;83(2):191–201
38. Chan A, Hanna M, Abbott M, Keane RJ. Oral retinoids and pregnancy. Med J Aust 1996;165(3):164–167
39. Rejnmark L, Vestergaard P, Charles P, et al. No effect of vitamin A intake on bone mineral density and frac-

ture risk in perimenopausal women. Osteoporos Int 2004;15(11):872–880

40. Sowers MF, Wallace RB. Retinol, supplemental vitamin A and bone status. J Clin Epidemiol 1990; 43(7):693–699

41. Ballew C, Galuska D, Gillespie C. High serum retinyl esters are not associated with reduced bone mineral density in the Third National Health And Nutrition Examination Survey, 1988–1994. J Bone Miner Res 2001;16(12):2306–2312

42. Michaëlsson K, Lithell H, Vessby B, Melhus H. Serum retinol levels and the risk of fracture. N Engl J Med 2003;348(4):287–294

43. Promislow JH, Goodman-Gruen D, Slymen DJ, Barrett-Connor E. Retinol intake and bone mineral density in the elderly: the Rancho Bernardo Study. J Bone Miner Res 2002;17(8):1349–1358

44. Feskanich D, Singh V, Willett WC, Colditz GA. Vitamin A intake and hip fractures among postmenopausal women. JAMA 2002;287(1):47–54

45. Rohde CM, DeLuca H. Bone resorption activity of all-trans retinoic acid is independent of vitamin D in rats. J Nutr 2003;133(3):777–783

46. Johansson S, Melhus H. Vitamin A antagonizes calcium response to vitamin D in man. J Bone Miner Res 2001;16(10):1899–1905

47. Wang XD. Chronic alcohol intake interferes with retinoid metabolism and signaling. Nutr Rev 1999;57(2):51–59

48. Leo MA, Lieber CS. Alcohol, vitamin A, and beta-carotene: adverse interactions, including hepatotoxicity and carcinogenicity. Am J Clin Nutr 1999;69(6):1071–1085

8 Vitamin B$_6$

Vitamin B$_6$ is a water-soluble vitamin that was first isolated in the 1930s. There are three traditionally considered forms of vitamin B$_6$: pyridoxal (PL), pyridoxine (PN), and pyridoxamine (PM). The phosphate ester derivative pyridoxal 5'-phosphate (PLP) is the principal coenzyme form and has the most importance in human metabolism.[1-3]

Function

Vitamin B$_6$ must be obtained from the diet because humans cannot synthesize it. PLP plays a vital role in the function of approximately 100 enzymes that catalyze essential chemical reactions in the human body,[1-5] for example, PLP functions as a coenzyme for glycogen phosphorylase, an enzyme that catalyzes the release of glucose from stored glycogen. Much of the PLP in the human body is found in muscle bound to glycogen phosphorylase. PLP is also a coenzyme for reactions used to generate glucose from amino acids, a process known as *gluconeogenesis*.[4,5]

Nervous System Function

In the brain, the synthesis of the neurotransmitter, serotonin, from the amino acid, tryptophan, is catalyzed by a PLP-dependent enzyme. Other neurotransmitters, such as dopamine, norepinephrine, and γ-aminobutyric acid (GABA), are also synthesized using PLP-dependent enzymes.[4]

Red Blood Cell Formation and Function

PLP functions as a coenzyme in the synthesis of heme, an iron-containing component of hemoglobin. Hemoglobin is found in red blood cells and is critical to their ability to transport oxygen throughout the body. Both PL and PLP are able to bind to the hemoglobin molecule and affect its ability to pick up and release oxygen. However, the impact of this on normal oxygen delivery to tissues is not known.[4]

Niacin Formation

The human requirement for another B vitamin, niacin, can be met in part by the conversion of the essential amino acid, tryptophan, to niacin, as well as through dietary intake. PLP is a coenzyme for a critical reaction in the synthesis of niacin from tryptophan, so adequate vitamin B$_6$ decreases the requirement for dietary niacin.[4]

Hormone Function

Steroid hormones, such as estrogen and testosterone, exert their effects in the body by binding to steroid hormone receptors in the nucleus of the cell and altering gene transcription. PLP binds to steroid receptors in a manner that inhibits the binding of steroid hormones, thus decreasing their effects. The binding of PLP to steroid receptors for estrogen, progesterone, testosterone, and other steroid hormones suggests that an individual's vitamin B$_6$ status may have implications for diseases affected by steroid hormones, including breast cancer and prostate cancers.[4]

Nucleic Acid Synthesis

PLP serves as a coenzyme for a key enzyme involved in the mobilization of single-carbon functional groups (one-carbon metabolism). Such reactions are involved in the synthesis of nucleic acids. The effect of vitamin B$_6$ deficiency on the function of the immune system may be partly related to the role of PLP in one-carbon metabolism.

Deficiency

Severe deficiency of vitamin B$_6$ is uncommon. People who abuse alcohol are thought to be most at risk of vitamin B$_6$ deficiency due to low dietary intakes and impaired metabolism of the vitamin. In the early 1950s, seizures were observed in infants as a result of severe vitamin B$_6$ deficiency caused by an error in the manufacture of infant formula. Abnormal electroencephalogram patterns have been noted in some studies of vitamin B_6 deficiency. Other neurological symptoms noted in severe vitamin B_6 deficiency include irritability, depression, and confusion; additional symptoms include inflammation of the tongue, sores or ulcers of the mouth, and ulcers of the skin at the corners of the mouth.[2]

Recommended Dietary Allowance

As vitamin B_6 is involved in many aspects of metabolism, several factors are likely to affect an individual's requirement for vitamin B_6. Of those factors, protein intake has been the most studied. Increased dietary protein results in an increased requirement for vitamin B_6, probably because PLP is a coenzyme for many enzymes involved in amino acid metabolism.[6] Unlike previous recommendations, the Food and Nutrition Board (FNB) of the Institute of Medicine did not express the most recent recommended dietary allowance (RDA) for vitamin B_6 in terms of protein intake, although the relationship was considered in setting the RDA.[7] The current RDA was revised by the FNB in 1998 (**Table 8.1**).

Disease Prevention

Cardiovascular Diseases

Even moderately elevated levels of homocysteine in the blood have been associated with increased risk for cardiovascular disease, including heart disease and stroke.[8] During protein digestion, amino acids, including methionine, are released. Homocysteine is an intermediate in the metabolism of methionine. Healthy individuals utilize two different pathways to metabolize homocysteine: one converts homocysteine back to methionine and is dependent on folic acid and vitamin B_{12}, and the other converts homocysteine to the amino acid cysteine and requires two vitamin B_6 (PLP)-dependent enzymes. Thus, the amount of homocysteine in the blood is regulated by at least three vitamins: folic acid, vitamin B_{12}, and vitamin B_6 (**Fig. 8.1**). Several large observational studies have demonstrated an association between low vitamin B_6 intake or status with increased blood homocysteine levels and increased risk of cardiovascular diseases.

A large prospective study found that the risk of heart disease in women who consumed, on average, 4.6 mg vitamin B_6 daily was only 67% of the risk in women who consumed an average of 1.1 mg daily.[9] Another large prospective study found that higher plasma levels of PLP were associated with a decreased risk of cardiovascular disease independent of homocysteine levels.[10] Further, several studies have reported that low plasma PLP status is a risk factor for coronary artery disease.[11-13] In contrast to folic acid supple-

Table 8.1 Recommended dietary allowance for vitamin B_6

Life stage	Age	Males (mg/day)	Females (mg/day)
Infants	0–6 months	0.1 (AI)	0.1 (AI)
Infants	7–12 months	0.3 (AI)	0.3 (AI)
Children	1–3 years	0.5	0.5
Children	4–8 years	0.6	0.6
Children	9–13 years	1.0	1.0
Adolescents	14–18 years	1.3	1.2
Adults	19–50 years	1.3	1.3
Adults	≥51 years	1.7	1.5
Pregnancy	All ages	–	1.9
Breast-feeding	All ages	–	2.0

AI, adequate intake.

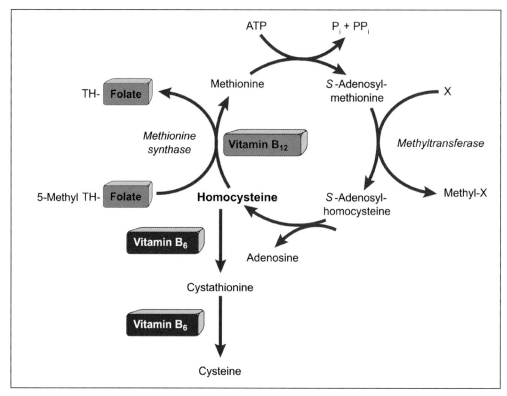

Fig. 8.1 Homocysteine metabolism. S-Adenosylhomocysteine is formed during S-adenosylmethionine-dependent methylation reactions, and the hydrolysis of S-adenosylhomocysteine results in homocysteine. Homocysteine may be remethylated to form methionine by a folate-dependent reaction that is catalyzed by methionine synthase, a vitamin B$_{12}$-dependent enzyme. Alternately, homocysteine may be metabolized to cysteine in reactions catalyzed by two vitamin B$_6$-dependent enzymes.

mentation, studies supplementing individuals with only vitamin B$_6$ have not resulted in significant decreases in basal (fasting) levels of homocysteine. However, one study found that vitamin B$_6$ supplementation was effective in lowering blood homocysteine levels after an oral dose of methionine (methionine load test) was given,[14] suggesting that vitamin B$_6$ may play a role in the metabolism of homocysteine after meals.

Immune Function

Low vitamin B$_6$ intake and nutritional status have been associated with impaired immune function, especially in elderly people. Decreased production of immune system cells known as lymphocytes, as well as decreased production of an important immune system protein called *interleukin-2* (IL-2), have been reported in vitamin B$_6$-deficient individuals.[15] Restoration of vitamin B$_6$ status has resulted in normalization of lymphocyte proliferation and IL-2 production, suggesting that adequate vitamin B$_6$ intake is important for optimal immune system function in older individuals.[15,16] However, one study found that the amount of vitamin B$_6$ required to reverse these immune system impairments in elderly people was 2.9 mg/day for men and 1.9 mg/day for women; these vitamin B$_6$ requirements are higher than the current RDA.[15]

Cognitive Function

A few studies have associated cognitive decline in elderly people or people with Alzheimer disease with inadequate nutritional status of folic acid, vitamin B$_{12}$, and vitamin B$_6$, and thus elevated levels of homocysteine.[17] One observational study found that higher plasma vitamin B$_6$ levels were associated with better performance on two measures of memory, but plasma vitamin B_6 levels were unrelated to performance on 18 other cognitive tests.[18] Similarly, a double-blind, placebo-controlled study in 38 healthy elderly men found that vitamin B_6 supplementation improved memory but had no effect on mood or mental performance.[19] Further, a placebo-controlled trial in 211 healthy younger, middle-aged, and older women found that vitamin B_6 supplementation (75 mg/day) for 5 weeks improved memory performance in some age groups but had no effect on mood.[20] Recently, a systematic review of randomized trials concluded that there is inadequate evidence that supplementation with vitamin B_6, vitamin B_{12}, or folic acid improves cognition in those with normal or impaired cognitive function.[21] As a result of mixed findings, it is currently unclear whether supplementation with B vitamins might blunt cognitive decline in elderly people. Further, it is not known if marginal B-vitamin deficiencies, which are relatively common in elderly people, even contribute to age-associated declines in cognitive function, or whether both result from processes associated with aging and/or disease.

Kidney Stones

A large prospective study examined the relationship between vitamin B_6 intake and the occurrence of symptomatic kidney stones in women. A group of more than 85 000 women without a prior history of kidney stones were followed over 14 years and those who consumed 40 mg or more of vitamin B_6 daily had only two-thirds the risk of developing kidney stones compared with those who consumed 3 mg or less.[22] However, in a group of more than 45 000 men followed over 6 years, no association was found between vitamin B_6 intake and the occurrence of kidney stones.[23] Limited data have shown that supplementation of vitamin B_6 at levels higher than the tolerable upper intake level (100 mg/day) decreases elevated urinary oxalate levels, an important determinant of calcium oxalate kidney stone formation in some individuals. However, it is less clear that supplementation actually resulted in decreased formation of calcium oxalate kidney stones. Currently, the relationship between vitamin B_6 intake and the risk of developing kidney stones requires further study before any recommendations can be made.

Disease Treatment

Vitamin B_6 supplements at pharmacological doses (i.e., doses much larger than those needed to prevent deficiency) have been used in an attempt to treat a wide variety of conditions, some of which are discussed below. In general, well-designed, placebo-controlled studies have shown little evidence that large supplemental doses of vitamin B_6 are beneficial.[24]

Side Effects of Oral Contraceptives

As vitamin B_6 is required for the metabolism of the amino acid tryptophan, the tryptophan load test (an assay of tryptophan metabolites after an oral dose of tryptophan) was used as a functional assessment of vitamin B_6 status. Abnormal tryptophan load tests in women taking high-dose oral contraceptives in the 1960s and 1970s suggested that these women were vitamin B_6 deficient. Abnormal results in the tryptophan load test led to a number of clinicians prescribing high doses (100–150 mg/day) of vitamin B_6 to women in order to relieve depression and other side effects sometimes experienced with oral contraceptives. However, most other indices of vitamin B_6 status were normal in women on high-dose oral contraceptives, and it is unlikely that the abnormality in tryptophan metabolism was due to vitamin B_6 deficiency.[24] A more recent placebo-controlled study in women on the lower-dose oral contraceptives, which are commonly prescribed today, found that doses up to 150 mg/day of vitamin B_6 (pyridoxine) had no benefit in preventing side effects, such as nausea, vomiting, dizziness, depression, and irritability.[25]

Premenstrual Syndrome

The use of vitamin B_6 to relieve the side effects of high-dose oral contraceptives led to its use in the treatment of the premenstrual syndrome (PMS). PMS refers to a cluster of symptoms, including but not limited to fatigue, irritability, moodiness/depression, fluid retention, and breast tenderness, that begin sometime after ovulation (midcycle) and subside with the onset of menstruation (the monthly period). A review of 12 placebo-controlled, double-blind trials on vitamin B_6 use for PMS treatment concluded that evidence for a beneficial effect was weak.[26] A more recent review of 25 studies suggested that supplemental vitamin B$_6$, up to 100 mg/day, may be of value to treat PMS; however, only limited conclusions could be drawn because most of the studies were of poor quality.[27]

Depression

Because a key enzyme in the synthesis of the neurotransmitters serotonin and norepinephrine is PLP dependent, it has been suggested that vitamin B$_6$ deficiency may lead to depression. However, clinical trials have not provided convincing evidence that vitamin B$_6$ supplementation is an effective treatment for depression,[24,28] although vitamin B$_6$ may have therapeutic efficacy in premenopausal women.[28]

Nausea and Vomiting in Pregnancy

Vitamin B$_6$ has been used since the 1940s to treat nausea during pregnancy. It was included in the medication Bendectin, which was prescribed for the treatment of morning sickness and later withdrawn from the market due to unproven concerns that it increased the risk of birth defects. Vitamin B$_6$ itself is considered safe during pregnancy and has been used in pregnant women without any evidence of fetal harm.[29] The results of two double-blind, placebo-controlled trials that used 25 mg pyridoxine every 8 hours for 3 days[30] or 10 mg pyridoxine every 8 hours for 5 days[29] suggest that vitamin B$_6$ may be beneficial in alleviating morning sickness. Each study found a slight but significant reduction in nausea or vomiting in pregnant women. A systematic review of placebo-controlled trials on nausea during early pregnancy found vitamin B$_6$ to be somewhat effective.[31] However, it should be noted that morning sickness also resolves without any treatment, making it difficult to perform well-controlled trials.

Carpal Tunnel Syndrome

Carpal tunnel syndrome causes numbness, pain, and weakness of the hand and fingers due to compression of the median nerve at the wrist. It may result from repetitive stress injury of the wrist or from soft-tissue swelling, which sometimes occurs with pregnancy or hypothyroidism.

Several early studies by the same investigator suggested that vitamin B$_6$ status was low in individuals with carpal tunnel syndrome and that supplementation with 100–200 mg/day over several months was beneficial.[32,33] A study in men not taking vitamin supplements found that decreased blood levels of PLP were associated with increased pain, tingling, and nocturnal wakening, all symptoms of carpal tunnel syndrome.[34] Studies using electrophysiological measurements of median nerve conduction have largely failed to find an association between vitamin B$_6$ deficiency and carpal tunnel syndrome. Although a few trials have noted some symptomatic relief with vitamin B$_6$ supplementation, double-blind, placebo-controlled trials have not generally found vitamin B$_6$ to be effective in treating carpal tunnel syndrome.[24,35]

Sources

Food Sources

Surveys in the United States have shown that dietary intake of vitamin B$_6$ averages about 2 mg/day for men and 1.5 mg/day for women. A survey of elderly individuals found that men and women aged over 60 years consumed about 1.2 mg/day and 1.0 mg/day, respectively; both intakes are lower than the current RDA. Certain plant foods contain a unique form of vitamin B$_6$ called *pyridoxine glucoside*; this form appears to be only about half as bioavailable as vitamin B$_6$ from other food sources or supplements. Vitamin B$_6$ in a mixed diet has been found to be approximately 75% bioavailable.[7] In most cases, including foods in the diet that are rich in vitamin B$_6$ should supply enough to prevent deficiency. However, those who follow a very restricted vegetarian diet might need to increase their vitamin B$_6$ intake by eating foods fortified with vitamin B$_6$ or by taking a supplement. Some foods that are relatively rich in vitamin B$_6$ and their vitamin B$_6$ content are listed in **Table 8.2**.

Supplements

Vitamin B$_6$ is available as pyridoxine hydrochloride in multivitamin, vitamin B-complex, and vitamin B$_6$ supplements.[36]

Table 8.2 Food sources of vitamin B_6

Food	Serving	Vitamin B_6 (mg)
Fortified cereal	1 cup	0.5–2.5
Potato, Russet, baked with skin	1 medium	0.70
Chicken, light meat without skin, cooked	3 ounces[a]	0.51
Salmon, wild, cooked	3 ounces[a]	0.48
Banana	1 medium	0.43
Turkey, without skin, cooked	3 ounces[a]	0.39
Spinach, cooked	1 cup	0.44
Vegetable juice cocktail	6 ounces	0.26
Hazelnuts, dry roasted	1 ounce	0.18

[a]A 3-ounce serving of meat or fish is about the size of a deck of cards.

Safety

Toxicity

As adverse effects have been documented only from vitamin B_6 supplements and never from food sources, only safety concerning the supplemental form of vitamin B_6 (pyridoxine) is discussed. Although vitamin B_6 is a water-soluble vitamin and is excreted in the urine, long-term supplementation with very high doses of pyridoxine may result in painful neurological symptoms known as sensory neuropathy. Symptoms include pain and numbness of the extremities and, in severe cases, difficulty walking. Sensory neuropathy typically develops at doses of pyridoxine in excess of 1000 mg/day. However, there have been a few case reports of individuals who developed sensory neuropathies at doses of more than 500 mg daily over a period of months. Yet, none of the studies in which an objective neurological examination was performed reported evidence of sensory nerve damage at intakes below 200 mg pyridoxine daily.[24] To prevent sensory neuropathy in virtually all individuals, the FNB set the tolerable upper intake level (UL) for pyridoxine at 100 mg/day for adults (**Table 8.3**).[7] As placebo-controlled studies have generally failed to show therapeutic benefits of high doses of pyridoxine, there is little reason to exceed the UL of 100 mg/day.

Table 8.3 Tolerable upper intake level (UL) for vitamin B_6

Life stage	Age	UL (mg/day)
Infants	0–12 months	Not possible to establish[a]
Children	1–3 years	30
Children	4–8 years	40
Children	9–13 years	60
Adolescents	14–18 years	80
Adults	≥19 years	100

[a]Source of intake should be from food and formula only.

Drug Interactions

Certain medications interfere with the metabolism of vitamin B_6, so some individuals may be vulnerable to a vitamin B_6 deficiency if supplemental vitamin B_6 is not taken. Anti-tuberculosis medications, including isoniazid and cycloserine, the metal chelator penicillamine, and anti-parkinsonian drugs including L-dopa, all form complexes with vitamin B_6 and thus create a functional deficiency. In addition, the efficacy of other medications may be altered by high doses of vitamin B_6, for example, high doses of vitamin B_6 have been found to decrease the efficacy of two anticonvulsants, phenobarbital and phenytoin, as well as levodopa.[4,24]

LPI Recommendation

Metabolic studies suggest that young women require 0.02 mg vitamin B_6/g protein consumed daily.[6,37,38] Using the upper boundary for acceptable levels of protein intake for women (100 g/day), the daily vitamin B_6 requirement for young women would be calculated at 2.0 mg/day. Older adults may also require at least 2.0 mg/day. For these reasons, the Linus Pauling Institute recommends that all adults consume at least 2.0 mg vitamin B_6 daily. Following the Linus Pauling Institute recommendation to take a daily multivitamin/mineral supplement containing 100% of the daily value for vitamin B_6 will ensure an intake of at least 2.0 mg/day of vitamin B_6. Although a vitamin B_6 intake of 2.0 mg/day is slightly higher than the most recent RDA, it is 50 times less than the UL set by the FNB (see **Table 8.3**).

Older Adults

Metabolic studies have indicated that the requirement for vitamin B$_6$ in older adults is approximately 2.0 mg/day;[39] this requirement could be even higher if the effect of marginally deficient vitamin B$_6$ intakes on immune function and homocysteine levels is clarified. Despite evidence that the requirement for vitamin B$_6$ may be slightly higher in older adults, several surveys have found that over half of individuals aged over 60 consume less than the current RDA (1.7 mg/day for men and 1.5 mg/day for women). For these reasons, the Linus Pauling Institute recommends that older adults take a multivitamin/mineral supplement, which generally provides at least 2.0 mg vitamin B$_6$ daily.

References

1. McCormick DB. Vitamin B$_6$. In: Bowman BA, Russell RM, eds. Present Knowledge in Nutrition, Vol. I. Washington, DC: International Life Sciences Institute; 2006:269–277

2. Leklem JE. Vitamin B$_6$. In: Machlin L, ed. Handbook of Vitamins. New York: Marcel Decker Inc.; 1991: 341–378

3. Dakshinamurti S, Dakshinamurti K. Vitamin B$_6$. In: Zempleni J, Rucker RB, McCormick DB, Suttie JW, eds. Handbook of Vitamins, 4th ed. New York: CRC Press (Taylor & Francis Group); 2007:315–359

4. Leklem JE. Vitamin B$_6$. In: Shils M, Olson JA, Shike M, Ross AC, eds. Modern Nutrition in Health and Disease, 9th ed. Baltimore, MD: Lippincott Williams & Wilkins; 1999:413–422

5. Mackey AD, Davis SR, Gregory JF III. Vitamin B$_6$. In: Shils ME, Shike M, Ross AC, Caballero B, Cousins RJ, eds. Modern Nutrition in Health and Disease, 10th ed. Philadelphia, PA: Lippincott Williams & Wilkins; 2006: 452–461

6. Hansen CM, Leklem JE, Miller LT. Vitamin B-6 status of women with a constant intake of vitamin B-6 changes with three levels of dietary protein. J Nutr 1996;126(7):1891–1901

7. Food and Nutrition Board, Institute of Medicine. Vitamin B$_6$. In: Dietary Reference Intakes for Thiamin, Riboflavin, Niacin, Vitamin B$_6$, Vitamin B$_{12}$, Pantothenic Acid, Biotin, and Choline. Washington, DC: National Academies Press; 1998:150–195

8. Boushey CJ, Beresford SA, Omenn GS, Motulsky AG. A quantitative assessment of plasma homocysteine as a risk factor for vascular disease. Probable benefits of increasing folic acid intakes. JAMA 1995; 274(13):1049–1057

9. Rimm EB, Willett WC, Hu FB, et al. Folate and vitamin B6 from diet and supplements in relation to risk of coronary heart disease among women. JAMA 1998; 279(5):359–364

10. Folsom AR, Nieto FJ, McGovern PG, et al. Prospective study of coronary heart disease incidence in relation to fasting total homocysteine, related genetic polymorphisms, and B vitamins: the Atherosclerosis Risk in Communities (ARIC) study. Circulation 1998; 98(3):204–210

11. Robinson K, Arheart K, Refsum H, et al; European COMAC Group. Low circulating folate and vitamin B6 concentrations: risk factors for stroke, peripheral vascular disease, and coronary artery disease. Circulation 1998;97(5):437–443

12. Robinson K, Mayer EL, Miller DP, et al. Hyperhomocysteinemia and low pyridoxal phosphate. Common and independent reversible risk factors for coronary artery disease. Circulation 1995;92(10):2825–2830

13. Lin PT, Cheng CH, Liaw YP, Lee BJ, Lee TW, Huang YC. Low pyridoxal 5'-phosphate is associated with increased risk of coronary artery disease. Nutrition 2006;22(11-12):1146–1151

14. Ubbink JB, Vermaak WJ, van der Merwe A, Becker PJ, Delport R, Potgieter HC. Vitamin requirements for the treatment of hyperhomocysteinemia in humans. J Nutr 1994;124(10):1927–1933

15. Meydani SN, Ribaya-Mercado JD, Russell RM, Sahyoun N, Morrow FD, Gershoff SN. Vitamin B-6 deficiency impairs interleukin 2 production and lymphocyte proliferation in elderly adults. Am J Clin Nutr 1991;53(5):1275–1280

16. Talbott MC, Miller LT, Kerkvliet NI. Pyridoxine supplementation: effect on lymphocyte responses in elderly persons. Am J Clin Nutr 1987;46(4):659–664

17. Selhub J, Bagley LC, Miller J, Rosenberg IH. B vitamins, homocysteine, and neurocognitive function in the elderly. Am J Clin Nutr 2000;71(2):614S–620S

18. Riggs KM, Spiro A III, Tucker K, Rush D. Relations of vitamin B-12, vitamin B-6, folate, and homocysteine to cognitive performance in the Normative Aging Study. Am J Clin Nutr 1996;63(3):306–314

19. Deijen JB, van der Beek EJ, Orlebeke JF, van den Berg H. Vitamin B-6 supplementation in elderly men: effects on mood, memory, performance and mental effort. Psychopharmacology (Berl) 1992;109(4):489–496

20. Bryan J, Calvaresi E, Hughes D. Short-term folate, vitamin B-12 or vitamin B-6 supplementation slightly affects memory performance but not mood in women of various ages. J Nutr 2002;132(6):1345–1356

21. Balk EM, Raman G, Tatsioni A, Chung M, Lau J, Rosenberg IH. Vitamin B6, B12, and folic acid supplementation and cognitive function: a systematic review of randomized trials. Arch Intern Med 2007;167(1): 21–30

22. Curhan GC, Willett WC, Speizer FE, Stampfer MJ. Intake of vitamins B6 and C and the risk of kidney stones in women. J Am Soc Nephrol 1999;10(4): 840–845

23. Curhan GC, Willett WC, Rimm EB, Stampfer MJ. A prospective study of the intake of vitamins C and B6, and the risk of kidney stones in men. J Urol 1996;155(6): 1847–1851

24. Bender DA. Non-nutritional uses of vitamin B6. Br J Nutr 1999;81(1):7–20

25. Villegas-Salas E, Ponce de León R, Juárez-Perez MA, Grubb GS. Effect of vitamin B6 on the side effects of a low-dose combined oral contraceptive. Contraception 1997;55(4):245–248

26. Kleijnen J, Ter Riet G, Knipschild P. Vitamin B6 in the treatment of the premenstrual syndrome—a review. Br J Obstet Gynaecol 1990;97(9):847–852

27. Wyatt KM, Dimmock PW, Jones PW, Shaughn O'Brien PM. Efficacy of vitamin B-6 in the treatment of premenstrual syndrome: systematic review. BMJ 1999;318(7195):1375–1381

28. Williams AL, Cotter A, Sabina A, Girard C, Goodman J, Katz DL. The role for vitamin B-6 as treatment for depression: a systematic review. Fam Pract 2005;22(5): 532–537

29. Vutyavanich T, Wongtrangan S, Ruangsri R. Pyridoxine for nausea and vomiting of pregnancy: a randomized, double-blind, placebo-controlled trial. Am J Obstet Gynecol 1995;173(3 Pt 1):881–884

30. Sahakian V, Rouse D, Sipes S, Rose N, Niebyl J. Vitamin B6 is effective therapy for nausea and vomiting of pregnancy: a randomized, double-blind placebo-controlled study. Obstet Gynecol 1991;78(1):33–36

31. Jewell D, Young G. Interventions for nausea and vomiting in early pregnancy. Cochrane Database Syst Rev 2002;(1):CD 000145

32. Ellis J, Folkers K, Watanabe T, et al. Clinical results of a cross-over treatment with pyridoxine and placebo of the carpal tunnel syndrome. Am J Clin Nutr 1979; 32(10):2040–2046

33. Ellis JM, Kishi T, Azuma J, Folkers K. Vitamin B6 deficiency in patients with a clinical syndrome including the carpal tunnel defect. Biochemical and clinical response to therapy with pyridoxine. Res Commun Chem Pathol Pharmacol 1976;13(4):743–757

34. Keniston RC, Nathan PA, Leklem JE, Lockwood RS. Vitamin B6, vitamin C, and carpal tunnel syndrome. A cross-sectional study of 441 adults. J Occup Environ Med 1997;39(10):949–959

35. Spooner GR, Desai HB, Angel JF, Reeder BA, Donat JR. Using pyridoxine to treat carpal tunnel syndrome. Randomized control trial. Can Fam Physician 1993;39:2122–2127

36. Hendler SS, Rorvik DR, eds. PDR for Nutritional Supplements. Montvale: Medical Economics Co., Inc.; 2001

37. Kretsch MJ, Sauberlich HE, Skala JH, Johnson HL. Vitamin B-6 requirement and status assessment: young women fed a depletion diet followed by a plant- or animal-protein diet with graded amounts of vitamin B-6. Am J Clin Nutr 1995;61(5):1091–1101

38. Hansen CM, Shultz TD, Kwak HK, Memon HS, Leklem JE. Assessment of vitamin B-6 status in young women consuming a controlled diet containing four levels of vitamin B-6 provides an estimated average requirement and recommended dietary allowance. J Nutr 2001;131(6):1777–1786

39. Ribaya-Mercado JD, Russell RM, Sahyoun N, Morrow FD, Gershoff SN. Vitamin B-6 requirements of elderly men and women. J Nutr 1991;121(7):1062–1074

9 Vitamin B$_{12}$

Vitamin B$_{12}$ has the largest and most complex chemical structure of all the vitamins. It is unique among vitamins in that it contains a metal ion, cobalt. For this reason *cobalamin* is the term used to refer to compounds with vitamin B$_{12}$ activity. Methylcobalamin and 5-deoxyadenosylcobalamin are the forms of vitamin B$_{12}$ used in the human body.[1] The form of cobalamin used in most supplements, cyanocobalamin, is readily converted to 5-deoxyadenosyl- and methylcobalamin in the body. In mammals, cobalamin is a cofactor for only two enzymes, methionine synthase and L-methylmalonyl-coenzyme A (CoA) mutase.[2]

Function

Cofactor for Methionine Synthase

Methylcobalamin is required for the function of the folate-dependent enzyme, methionine synthase. This enzyme is required for the synthesis of the amino acid, methionine, from homocysteine. Methionine in turn is required for the synthesis of S-adenosylmethionine, a methyl group donor used in many biological methylation reactions, including the methylation of a number of sites within DNA and RNA.[3] Methylation of DNA may be important in cancer prevention. Inadequate function of methionine synthase can lead to an accumulation of homocysteine, which may be associated with increased risk of cardiovascular diseases (**Fig. 9.1**).

Cofactor for Methylmalonyl-CoA Mutase

5-Deoxyadenosylcobalamin is required by methylmalonyl-CoA mutase, the enzyme that catalyzes the conversion of L-methylmalonyl-CoA to succinyl-CoA. This biochemical reaction plays an important role in the production of energy from fats and proteins. Succinyl-CoA is also required for the synthesis of hemoglobin, the oxygen-carrying pigment in red blood cells.[3]

Deficiency

Vitamin B$_{12}$ deficiency is estimated to affect 10%–15% of individuals aged over 60.[4] Absorption of vitamin B$_{12}$ from food requires normal function of the stomach, pancreas, and small intestine. Stomach acid and enzymes free vitamin B$_{12}$ from food, allowing it to bind to other proteins called *R proteins*.[3] In the alkaline environment of the small intestine, R proteins are degraded by pancreatic enzymes, freeing vitamin B$_{12}$ to bind to intrinsic factor (IF), a protein secreted by specialized cells in the stomach. Receptors on the surface of the small intestine take up the IF–B$_{12}$ complex only in the presence of calcium, which is supplied by the pancreas.[5] Vitamin B$_{12}$ can also be absorbed by passive diffusion, but this process is very inefficient—only about 1% absorption of the vitamin B$_{12}$ dose is passive.[2]

Causes of Vitamin B$_{12}$ Deficiency

The most common causes of vitamin B$_{12}$ deficiency are pernicious anemia and food-bound vitamin B$_{12}$ malabsorption. Although both causes become more common with increasing age, they are separate conditions.[4]

Pernicious anemia. Pernicious anemia has been estimated to be present in approximately 2% of individuals aged over 60.[6] Although anemia is often a symptom, the condition is actually the end-stage of an autoimmune inflammation of the stomach, resulting in destruction of stomach cells by one's own antibodies. Progressive destruction of the cells that line the stomach causes decreased secretion of acid and enzymes required to release food-bound vitamin B$_{12}$. Antibodies to IF bind to IF, preventing formation of the IF–B$_{12}$ complex, further inhibiting vitamin B$_{12}$ absorption. If the body's vitamin B$_{12}$ stores are adequate before the onset of pernicious anemia, it may take years for symptoms of deficiency to develop. About 20% of the relatives of pernicious anemia patients also have pernicious anemia, suggesting a genetic predisposition. Treat-

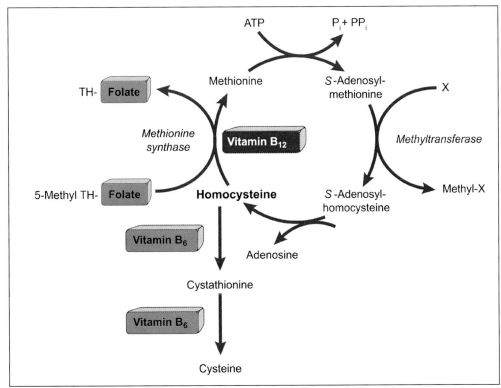

Fig. 9.1 Biological methylation reactions and homocysteine metabolism. Use of *S*-adenosylmethionine as the methyl donor for biological methylation reactions results in the formation of *S*-adenosylhomocysteine. Homocysteine is formed from the hydrolysis of *S*-adenosylhomocysteine. Homocysteine may be remethylated to form methionine by a folate-dependent reaction that is catalyzed by methionine synthase, a vitamin B_{12}-dependent enzyme. Alternately, homocysteine may be metabolized to cysteine in reactions catalyzed by two vitamin B_6-dependent enzymes.

ment of pernicious anemia generally requires injections of vitamin B_{12} to bypass intestinal absorption. High-dose oral supplementation is another treatment option, because consuming 1000 µg (1 mg)/day of vitamin B_{12} orally should result in the absorption of about 10 µg/day (about 1%) by passive diffusion.[4] In fact, high-dose oral therapy is considered to be as effective as intramuscular injection.[7–10]

Food-bound vitamin B_{12} malabsorption. Food-bound vitamin B_{12} malabsorption is defined as an impaired ability to absorb food or protein-bound vitamin B_{12}, although the free form is fully absorbable.[11] In elderly people, food-bound vitamin B_{12} malabsorption is thought to result mainly from atrophic gastritis, a chronic inflammation of the lining of the stomach that ultimately results in the loss of glands in the stomach (atrophy) and decreased stomach acid production. As stomach acid is required for the release of vitamin B_{12} from the proteins in food, vitamin B_{12} absorption is diminished. Decreased stomach acid production also provides an environment conducive to the overgrowth of anaerobic bacteria in the stomach, which further interferes with vitamin B_{12} absorption.[3] As vitamin B_{12} in supplements is not bound to protein, and as IF is still available, the absorption of supplemental vitamin B_{12} is not reduced as it is in pernicious anemia. Thus, individuals with food-bound vitamin B_{12} malabsorption do not have an increased requirement for vitamin B_{12}; they simply need it in the crystalline form found in fortified foods and dietary supplements.

Atrophic gastritis. Atrophic gastritis is thought to affect 10%–30% of people aged over 60 years, and the condition is frequently associated with infection by the bacterium, *Helicobacter pylori*. *H. pylori* infection induces chronic inflammation of the stomach, which may progress to peptic ulcer disease, atrophic gastritis, and/or gastric cancer in some individuals. The relationship of *H. pylori* infection to atrophic gastritis, gastric cancer, and vitamin B$_{12}$ deficiency is currently an area of active research.[4]

Other Causes of Vitamin B$_{12}$ Deficiency

Other causes of vitamin B$_{12}$ deficiency include surgical resection of the stomach or portions of the small intestine where receptors for the IF–B$_{12}$ complex are located. Conditions affecting the small intestine, such as malabsorption syndromes (celiac disease and tropical sprue), may also result in vitamin B$_{12}$ deficiency. As the pancreas provides critical enzymes as well as calcium needed for vitamin B$_{12}$ absorption, pancreatic insufficiency may contribute to vitamin B$_{12}$ deficiency. Because vitamin B$_{12}$ is found only in foods of animal origin, a strict vegetarian (vegan) diet has resulted in cases of vitamin B$_{12}$ deficiency. People who abuse alcohol may experience reduced intestinal absorption of vitamin B$_{12}$.[2] Individuals with acquired immune deficiency syndrome (AIDS) appear to be at increased risk of deficiency, possibly related to a failure of the IF–B$_{12}$ receptor to take up the IF–B$_{12}$ complex.[3] Long-term use of acid-reducing drugs has also been implicated in vitamin B$_{12}$ deficiency.

Symptoms of Vitamin B$_{12}$ Deficiency

Vitamin B$_{12}$ deficiency results in impairment of the activities of vitamin B$_{12}$-requiring enzymes. Impaired activity of methionine synthase may result in elevated homocysteine levels, whereas impaired activity of L-methylmalonyl-CoA mutase results in increased levels of a metabolite of methylmalonyl-CoA called *methylmalonic acid* (MMA). Individuals with mild vitamin B$_{12}$ deficiency may not experience symptoms, although blood levels of homocysteine and/or MMA may be elevated.[12]

Megaloblastic anemia. Diminished activity of methionine synthase in vitamin B$_{12}$ deficiency inhibits the regeneration of tetrahydrofolate (THF) and traps folate in a form that is not usable by the body (**Fig. 9.2**), resulting in symptoms of folate deficiency even in the presence of adequate folate levels. Thus, in both folate and vitamin B$_{12}$ deficiencies, folate is unavailable to participate in DNA synthesis. This impairment of DNA synthesis affects the rapidly dividing cells of the bone marrow earlier than other cells, resulting in the production of large, immature, hemoglobin-poor, red blood cells. The resulting anemia is known as *megaloblastic anemia* and is the symptom for which the disease, pernicious anemia, was named.[3] Supplementation with folic acid will provide enough usable folate to restore normal red blood cell formation. However, if vitamin B$_{12}$ deficiency is the cause, it will persist despite resolution of the anemia. Thus, megaloblastic anemia should not be treated with folic acid until the underlying cause has been determined.[5]

Neurological symptoms. The neurological symptoms of vitamin B$_{12}$ deficiency include numbness and tingling of the arms and, more commonly, the legs, difficulty walking, memory loss, disorientation, and dementia with or without mood changes. Although the progression of neurological complications is generally gradual, such symptoms are not always reversible with treatment of vitamin B$_{12}$ deficiency, especially if they have been present for a long time. Neurological complications are not always associated with megaloblastic anemia and are the only clinical symptom of vitamin B$_{12}$ deficiency in about 25% of cases.[6] Although vitamin B$_{12}$ deficiency is known to damage the myelin sheath covering cranial, spinal, and peripheral nerves, the biochemical processes leading to neurological damage in vitamin B$_{12}$ deficiency are not well understood.[3]

Gastrointestinal symptoms. Tongue soreness, appetite loss, and constipation have also been associated with vitamin B$_{12}$ deficiency. The origins of these symptoms are unclear, but they may be related to the stomach inflammation underlying some cases of vitamin B$_{12}$ deficiency, or to the increased vulnerability of rapidly dividing gastrointestinal cells to impaired DNA synthesis.[6]

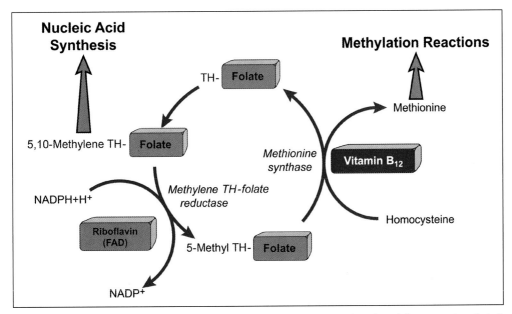

Fig. 9.2 Vitamin B_{12} and nucleic acid metabolism. 5,10-methylene tetrahydrofolate (THF) is required for the synthesis of nucleic acids, and 5-methyl THF is required for the formation of methionine from homocysteine by the vitamin B_{12}-dependent enzyme methionine synthase. Methionine, in the form of S-adenosylmethionine, is re-quired for many biological methylation reactions, includ-ing the methylation of DNA. Vitamin B_{12} deficiency traps folate in a form that is unusable by the body for DNA syn-thesis and results in a reduced capacity for DNA methyla-tion.

Recommended Dietary Allowance

The current recommended dietary allowance (RDA) was revised by the Food and Nutrition Board (FNB) of the Institute of Medicine in 1998 (**Table 9.1**). As a result of the increased risk of food-bound vitamin B_{12} malabsorption in older adults, the FNB recommended that adults over 50 years of age get most of the RDA from fortified food or vitamin B_{12}-containing supplements.[6]

Table 9.1 Recommended dietary allowance for vitamin B_{12}

Life stage	Age	Males (µg/day)	Females (µg/day)
Infants	0–6 months	0.4 (AI)	0.4 (AI)
Infants	7–12 months	0.5 (AI)	0.5 (AI)
Children	1–3 years	0.9	0.9
Children	4–8 years	1.2	1.2
Children	9–13 years	1.8	1.8
Adolescents	14–18 years	2.4	2.4
Adults	19–50 years	2.4	2.4
Adults	≥51 years	2.4[a]	2.4[a]
Pregnancy	All ages	–	2.6
Breast-feeding	All ages	–	2.8

AI, adequate intake.
[a]It is advisable for this amount to be obtained by consuming foods fortified with vitamin B_{12} or from a vitamin B_{12}-containing supplement.

Disease Prevention

Cardiovascular Diseases

The results of more than 80 studies indicate that even moderately elevated levels of homocysteine in the blood increase the risk of cardiovascular diseases,[13] although the mechanism by which homocysteine increases the disease risk remains the subject of a great deal of research. The amount of homocysteine in the blood is regulated by at least three vitamins: folate, vitamin B$_{12}$, and vitamin B$_6$ (see **Fig. 9.1**). Analysis of the results of 12 homocysteine-lowering trials showed that folic acid supplementation (0.5–5.0 mg/day) had the greatest lowering effect on blood homocysteine levels (25%); co-supplementation with folic acid and vitamin B$_{12}$ (mean 0.5 mg/day or 500 µg/day) provided an additional 7% reduction in blood homocysteine concentrations.[14] The results of a sequential supplementation trial in 53 men and women indicated that, after folic acid supplementation, vitamin B$_{12}$ became the major determinant of plasma homocysteine levels.[15]

Some evidence indicates that vitamin B$_{12}$ deficiency is a major cause of elevated homocysteine levels in people aged over 60. Two studies found blood MMA levels to be elevated in more than 60% of elderly individuals with elevated homocysteine levels. An elevated MMA level, together with elevated homocysteine, in the absence of impaired kidney function, suggests either a vitamin B$_{12}$ deficiency or a combined vitamin B$_{12}$ and folate deficiency.[16] Thus, it is important to evaluate vitamin B$_{12}$ status as well as kidney function in older individuals with elevated homocysteine levels before starting homocysteine-lowering therapy. For more information about homocysteine and cardiovascular diseases, see Chapter 2.

Although increased intake of folic acid and vitamin B$_{12}$ has been found to decrease homocysteine levels, it is not currently known whether increasing the intake of these vitamins will translate to reductions in risk for cardiovascular diseases. However, several randomized, placebo-controlled trials are presently being conducted to determine whether homocysteine lowering through folic acid and other B-vitamin supplementation reduces the incidence of cardiovascular diseases. A meta-analysis of data from four of the ongoing trials shows that B-vitamin supplementation had no significant effect on risk of coronary heart disease or stroke, but only about 14 000 participants were included in the analysis and thus any conclusions are limited.[17] Nevertheless, the completion of ongoing clinical trials should help to answer whether or not supplemental B vitamins lower risk for cardiovascular diseases.

Cancer

Folate is required for the synthesis of DNA, and there is evidence that decreased availability of folate results in strands of DNA that are more susceptible to damage. Deficiency of vitamin B$_{12}$ traps folate in a form that is unusable by the body for DNA synthesis. Both vitamin B$_{12}$ and folate deficiencies result in a diminished capacity for methylation reactions (see **Fig. 9.2**). Thus, vitamin B$_{12}$ deficiency may lead to an elevated rate of DNA damage and altered methylation of DNA, both of which are important risk factors for cancer. A series of studies in young adults and older men indicated that increased levels of homocysteine and decreased levels of vitamin B$_{12}$ in the blood were associated with a biomarker of chromosome breakage in white blood cells. In a double-blind, placebo-controlled study, the same biomarker of chromosome breakage was minimized in young adults who were supplemented with 700 µg folic acid and 7 µg vitamin B$_{12}$ daily in cereal for 2 months.[18]

Breast cancer. A case–control study compared prediagnostic levels of serum folate, vitamin B$_6$, and vitamin B$_{12}$ in 195 women later diagnosed with breast cancer and 195 age-matched women who were not diagnosed with breast cancer.[19] Among women who were postmenopausal at the time of blood donation, the association between blood levels of vitamin B$_{12}$ and breast cancer suggested a threshold effect. The risk of breast cancer was more than doubled in women with serum vitamin B$_{12}$ levels in the lowest quintile compared with women in the four highest quintiles. The investigators found no relationship between breast cancer and serum levels of vitamin B$_6$, folate, or homocysteine. A case–control study in Mexican women (475 cases and 1391 controls) reported that breast cancer risk for women in the highest quartile (a quarter) of vitamin B$_{12}$ intake was 68% lower than for those in the lowest quartile.[20] Stratification of the data revealed that the inverse association between dietary vitamin B_{12} intake and breast cancer risk was stronger in postmenopausal women compared with premenopausal women, although both associations were statistically significant. As these studies were observational, it cannot be determined whether decreased serum levels of vitamin B_{12} or low dietary vitamin B_{12} intakes were a cause or a result of breast cancer. Previously, there has been little evidence to suggest a relationship between vitamin B_{12} status and breast cancer risk. However, high dietary folate intakes have been associated with reduced risk for breast cancer in several studies, and some studies have reported that vitamin B_{12} intake may modify this association.[21,22]

Neural Tube Defects

Neural tube defects (NTDs) may result in anencephaly or spina bifida, devastating and sometimes fatal birth defects. The defects occur between days 21 and 27 after conception, a time when many women do not realize that they are pregnant.[23] Randomized controlled trials have demonstrated 60%–100% reductions in NTD cases when women consumed folic acid supplements, in addition to a varied diet, during the month before and the month after conception. Increasing evidence indicates that the homocysteine-lowering effect of folic acid plays a critical role in lowering the risk of NTDs.[24] Homocysteine may accumulate in the blood when there is inadequate folate and/or vitamin B_{12} for effective functioning of the methionine synthase enzyme. Decreased vitamin B_{12} levels in the blood and amniotic fluid of pregnant women have been associated with an increased risk of NTDs, suggesting that adequate vitamin B_{12} intake in addition to folic acid may be beneficial in the prevention of NTDs.

Alzheimer Disease and Dementia

Individuals with Alzheimer disease often have low blood levels of vitamin B_{12}. One study found lower vitamin B_{12} levels in the cerebrospinal fluid of patients with Alzheimer disease than in patients with other types of dementia, although blood levels of vitamin B_{12} did not differ.[25] The reason for the association of low vitamin B_{12} status with Alzheimer disease is not clear. Vitamin B_{12} deficiency, similar to folate deficiency, may lead to decreased synthesis of methionine and

S-adenosylmethionine, thereby adversely affecting methylation reactions. Methylation reactions are essential for the metabolism of components of the myelin sheath of nerve cells, as well as for neurotransmitters. Also, moderately increased homocysteine levels as well as decreased folate and vitamin B_{12} levels have been associated with Alzheimer disease and vascular dementia.

Some but not all studies have associated elevated homocysteine concentrations or decreased serum levels of vitamin B_{12} with an increased risk of Alzheimer disease. A case–control study of 164 patients with dementia of the Alzheimer type (DAT) included 76 patients in whom the diagnosis of Alzheimer disease was confirmed by examination of brain cells after death.[26] Compared with 108 control individuals with no evidence of dementia, the patients with DAT and confirmed Alzheimer disease had higher blood homocysteine levels and lower blood levels of folate and vitamin B_{12}. Measures of general nutritional status indicated that the association of increased homocysteine levels and diminished vitamin B_{12} status with Alzheimer disease was not due to dementia-related malnutrition.[26]

In another study, low serum vitamin B_{12} (≤ 150 pmol/L) or folate (≤ 10 nmol/L) levels were associated with a doubling of the risk of developing Alzheimer disease in 370 elderly men and women followed over 3 years.[27] In a sample of 1092 men and women without dementia followed for an average of 10 years, those with higher plasma homocysteine levels at baseline had a significantly higher risk of developing Alzheimer disease and other types of dementia.[28]

Specifically, those with plasma homocysteine levels of more than 14 μmol/L had nearly double the risk of developing Alzheimer disease. A study in 650 elderly men and women reported that the risk of elevated plasma homocysteine levels was significantly higher in those with lower cognitive function scores.[29] A prospective study in 816 elderly men and women reported that those with elevated homocysteine levels (> 15 μmol/L) had a significantly higher risk of developing Alzheimer disease or dementia, but vitamin B_{12} status was not related to risk of Alzheimer disease or dementia in this study.[30] Similarly, another prospective study in 965 older adults found that vitamin B_{12} status was not related to the risk of Alzheimer disease.[31] Further, a prospective study in 1041 older adults, followed for a median of 3.9 years, found that vitamin B_{12} dietary intake was not associated with risk of developing Alzheimer disease.[32]

B-vitamin supplementation is commonly used to treat hyperhomocysteinemia. A recent randomized, double-blind, placebo-controlled clinical trial in 253 older individuals with plasma homocysteine concentrations of 13 µmol/L or more found that daily B-vitamin supplementation (1 mg folic acid, 0.5 mg vitamin B$_{12}$, and 10 mg vitamin B$_6$) for 2 years did not affect measures of cognitive performance, despite an average 4.36 µmol/L reduction in plasma homocysteine concentrations.[33] Another randomized, double-blind, placebo-controlled study in 195 elderly adults reported that oral vitamin B$_{12}$ supplementation (1 mg daily) for 6 months had no effect on measures of cognitive function.[34] Several of the homocysteine-lowering trials primarily focused on assessing cardiovascular disease risk will also assess measures of cognitive function.[35] Thus, the findings of these ongoing trials may provide insight into whether long-term B-vitamin supplementation is protective against dementia.

Depression

Observational studies have found that as many as 30% of patients hospitalized for depression are deficient in vitamin B$_{12}$.[36] A cross-sectional study of 700 community-living, physically disabled women aged over 65 found that vitamin B$_{12}$-deficient women were twice as likely to be severely depressed as non-deficient women.[37] A population-based study in 3884 elderly men and women with depressive disorders found that those with vitamin B$_{12}$ deficiency were almost 70% more likely to experience depression than those with normal vitamin B$_{12}$ status.[38] The reasons for the relationship between vitamin B$_{12}$ deficiency and depression are not clear but may involve S-adenosylmethionine (SAM). Vitamin B$_{12}$ and folate are required for the synthesis of SAM, a methyl group donor essential for the metabolism of neurotransmitters, the bioavailability of which has been related to depression. This hypothesis is supported by several studies that have shown that supplementation with SAM improves depressive symptoms.[39–42] As few studies have examined the relationship of vitamin B$_{12}$ status and the development of depression over time, it cannot yet be determined if vitamin B$_{12}$ deficiency plays a causal role in depression. However, due to

the high prevalence of vitamin B$_{12}$ deficiency in older individuals, it may be beneficial to screen for vitamin B$_{12}$ deficiency as part of a medical evaluation for depression.

Sources

Food Sources

Only bacteria can synthesize vitamin B$_{12}$. Vitamin B$_{12}$ is present in animal products such as meat, poultry, fish (including shellfish), and to a lesser extent milk, but it is not generally present in plant products or yeast.[1] Fresh pasteurized milk contains 0.9 µg per cup and is an important source of vitamin B$_{12}$ for some vegetarians.[6] Those vegetarians who eat no animal products need supplemental vitamin B$_{12}$ to meet their requirements. Also, individuals aged over 50 should obtain their vitamin B$_{12}$ in supplements or fortified foods such as fortified cereal because of the increased likelihood of food-bound vitamin B$_{12}$ malabsorption.

Most people do not have a problem obtaining the RDA of 2.4 µg/day of vitamin B$_{12}$ from food. In the United States, the average intake of vitamin B$_{12}$ is about 4.5 µg/day for young men, and 3 µg/day for young women. In a sample of adults aged over 60, men were found to have an average dietary intake of 3.4 µg/day and women had an average dietary intake of 2.6 µg/day.[6] Some foods with substantial amounts of vitamin B$_{12}$ are

Table 9.2 Food sources of vitamin B$_{12}$

Food	Serving	Vitamin B$_{12}$ (µg)
Clams, steamed	3 ounces[a]	84.0
Mussels, steamed	3 ounces[a]	20.4
Crab, steamed	3 ounces[a]	8.8
Salmon, baked	3 ounces[a]	2.4
Beef, cooked	3 ounces[a]	2.1
Rockfish, baked	3 ounces[a]	1.0
Milk	8 ounces	0.9
Brie, cheese	1 ounce	0.5
Egg, poached	1 large	0.4
Chicken, roasted	3 ounces[a]	0.3
Turkey, roasted	3 ounces[a]	0.3

[a] A 3-ounce serving of meat, fish, or shellfish is about the size of a deck of cards.

listed in **Table 9.2**, along with their vitamin B_{12} content.

Supplements

Cyanocobalamin is the principal form of vitamin B_{12} used in supplements but methylcobalamin is also available as a supplement. Cyanocobalamin is available by prescription in an injectable form and as a nasal gel for the treatment of pernicious anemia. Over-the-counter preparations containing cyanocobalamin include multivitamin, vitamin B-complex, and vitamin B_{12} supplements.[43]

Safety

Toxicity

No toxic or adverse effects have been associated with large intakes of vitamin B_{12} from food or supplements in healthy people. Doses as high as 1 mg (1000 µg) daily by mouth or 1 mg monthly by intramuscular injection have been used to treat pernicious anemia without significant side effects. When high doses of vitamin B_{12} are given orally, only a small percentage can be absorbed, which may explain the low toxicity. As a result of the low toxicity of vitamin B_{12}, no tolerable upper intake level (UL) was set by the FNB in 1998 when the RDA was revised.[6]

Drug Interactions

A number of drugs reduce the absorption of vitamin B_{12}. Proton pump inhibitors (e.g., omeprazole and lansoprazole), used for therapy of Zollinger–Ellison syndrome and gastroesophageal reflux disease, markedly decrease stomach acid secretion required for the release of vitamin B_{12} from food but not from supplements. Long-term use of proton pump inhibitors has been found to decrease blood vitamin B_{12} levels. However, vitamin B_{12} deficiency does not generally develop until after at least 3 years of continuous therapy.[44] Another class of gastric acid inhibitors known as H_2-receptor antagonists (e.g., cimetidine, famotidine, ranitidine), often used to treat peptic ulcer disease, has also been found to decrease the absorption of vitamin B_{12} from food. As inhibition of gastric acid secretion is not as prolonged as with proton pump inhibitors, H_2-receptor antagonists have not been found to cause overt vitamin B_{12} deficiency even after long-term use.[45]

Individuals taking drugs that inhibit gastric acid secretion should consider taking vitamin B_{12} in the form of a supplement because gastric acid is not required for its absorption. Other drugs found to inhibit vitamin B_{12} absorption from food include cholestyramine (a bile acid-binding resin used in the treatment of high cholesterol), chloramphenicol and neomycin (antibiotics), and colchicine (anti-gout medicine). Metformin, a medication for individuals with type 2 diabetes, decreases vitamin B_{12} absorption by tying up free calcium required for absorption of the IF–B_{12} complex. This effect is correctable by drinking milk or taking calcium carbonate tablets along with food or supplements.[5] Previous reports that megadoses of vitamin C destroy vitamin B_{12} have not been supported[46] and may have been an artifact of the assay used to measure vitamin B_{12} levels.[6]

Nitrous oxide, a commonly used anesthetic, inhibits both the vitamin B_{12}-dependent enzymes and can produce many of the clinical features of vitamin B_{12} deficiency, such as megaloblastic anemia or neuropathy. As nitrous oxide is commonly used for surgery in elderly people, some experts feel that vitamin B_{12} deficiency should be ruled out before its use.[4,12]

Large doses of folic acid given to an individual with an undiagnosed vitamin B_{12} deficiency could correct megaloblastic anemia without correcting the underlying vitamin B_{12} deficiency, leaving the individual at risk of developing irreversible neurological damage.[6] For this reason the FNB advises that all adults limit their intake of folic acid (supplements and fortification) to 1000 µg (1 mg) daily.

LPI Recommendation
A varied diet should provide enough vitamin B_{12} to prevent deficiency in most individuals aged 50 years and younger. Individuals aged over 50, strict vegetarians, and women planning to become pregnant should take a multivitamin supplement daily or eat a fortified breakfast cereal, which would ensure a daily intake of 6–30 µg vitamin B_{12} in a form that is easily absorbed. Higher doses of vitamin B_{12} supplements are recommended for patients taking medications that interfere with its absorption.

Older Adults

As vitamin B$_{12}$ malabsorption and vitamin B$_{12}$ deficiency are more common in older adults, LPI recommends that adults aged over 50 years take 100–400 µg/day of supplemental vitamin B$_{12}$ daily.

References

1. Brody T. Nutritional Biochemistry, 2nd ed. San Diego, CA: Academic Press, 1999
2. Carmel R. Cobalamin (Vitamin B-12). In: Shils ME, Shike M, Ross AC, Caballero B, Cousins RJ, eds. Modern Nutrition in Health and Disease. Philadelphia, PA: Lippincott Williams & Wilkins; 2006:482–497
3. Shane B. Folic acid, vitamin B-12, and vitamin B-6. In: Stipanuk M, ed. Biochemical and Physiological Aspects of Human Nutrition. Philadelphia, PA: WB Saunders Co.; 2000:483–518
4. Baik HW, Russell RM. Vitamin B12 deficiency in the elderly. Annu Rev Nutr 1999;19:357–377
5. Herbert V. Vitamin B-12. In: Ziegler EE, Filer LJ, eds. Present Knowledge in Nutrition. 7th ed. Washington, DC: ILSI Press; 1996:191–205
6. Food and Nutrition Board, Institute of Medicine. Vitamin B$_{12}$. In: Dietary Reference Intakes for Thiamin, Riboflavin, Niacin, Vitamin B$_6$, Vitamin B$_{12}$, Pantothenic Acid, Biotin, and Choline. Washington, DC: National Academy Press; 1998:306–356
7. Kuzminski AM, Del Giacco EJ, Allen RH, Stabler SP, Lindenbaum J. Effective treatment of cobalamin deficiency with oral cobalamin. Blood 1998;92(4):1191–1198
8. Lederle FA. Oral cobalamin for pernicious anemia. Medicine's best kept secret? JAMA 1991;265(1):94–95
9. Hathcock JN, Troendle GJ. Oral cobalamin for treatment of pernicious anemia? JAMA 1991;265(1):96–97
10. Elia M. Oral or parenteral therapy for B12 deficiency. Lancet 1998;352(9142):1721–1722
11. Ho C, Kauwell GP, Bailey LB. Practitioners' guide to meeting the vitamin B-12 recommended dietary allowance for people aged 51 years and older. J Am Diet Assoc 1999;99(6):725–727
12. Weir DG, Scott JM. Vitamin B$_{12}$ "cobalamin". In: Shils M, Olson JA, Shike M, Ross AC, eds. Modern Nutrition in Health and Disease. 9th ed. Baltimore, MD: Lippincott Williams & Wilkins; 1999:447–458
13. Gerhard GT, Duell PB. Homocysteine and atherosclerosis. Curr Opin Lipidol 1999;10(5):417–428
14. Homocysteine Lowering Trialists' Collaboration. Lowering blood homocysteine with folic acid based supplements: meta-analysis of randomised trials. Homocysteine Lowering Trialists' Collaboration. BMJ 1998;316(7135):894–898
15. Quinlivan EP, McPartlin J, McNulty H, et al. Importance of both folic acid and vitamin B12 in reduction of risk of vascular disease. Lancet 2002;359(9302):227–228
16. Stabler SP, Lindenbaum J, Allen RH. Vitamin B-12 deficiency in the elderly: current dilemmas. Am J Clin Nutr 1997;66(4):741–749
17. Clarke R, Lewington S, Sherliker P, Armitage J. Effects of B-vitamins on plasma homocysteine concentrations and on risk of cardiovascular disease and dementia. Curr Opin Clin Nutr Metab Care 2007;10(1):32–39
18. Fenech M. Micronucleus frequency in human lymphocytes is related to plasma vitamin B12 and homocysteine. Mutat Res 1999;428(1-2):299–304
19. Wu K, Helzlsouer KJ, Comstock GW, Hoffman SC, Nadeau MR, Selhub J. A prospective study on folate, B12, and pyridoxal 5'-phosphate (B6) and breast cancer. Cancer Epidemiol Biomarkers Prev 1999;8(3):209–217
20. Lajous M, Lazcano-Ponce E, Hernandez-Avila M, Willett W, Romieu I. Folate, vitamin B(6), and vitamin B(12) intake and the risk of breast cancer among Mexican women. Cancer Epidemiol Biomarkers Prev 2006;15(3):443–448
21. Shrubsole MJ, Jin F, Dai Q, et al. Dietary folate intake and breast cancer risk: results from the Shanghai Breast Cancer Study. Cancer Res 2001;61(19):7136–7141
22. Lajous M, Romieu I, Sabia S, Boutron-Ruault MC, Clavel-Chapelon F. Folate, vitamin B12 and postmenopausal breast cancer in a prospective study of French women. Cancer Causes Control 2006;17(9):1209–1213
23. Eskes TK. Open or closed? A world of difference: a history of homocysteine research. Nutr Rev 1998;56(8):236–244
24. Mills JL, Scott JM, Kirke PN, et al. Homocysteine and neural tube defects. J Nutr 1996;126(3):756S–760S
25. Nourhashemi F, Gillette-Guyonnet S, Andrieu S, et al. Alzheimer disease: protective factors. Am J Clin Nutr 2000;71(2):643S–649S
26. Clarke R, Smith AD, Jobst KA, Refsum H, Sutton L, Ueland PM. Folate, vitamin B12, and serum total homocysteine levels in confirmed Alzheimer disease. Arch Neurol 1998;55(11):1449–1455
27. Wang HX, Wahlin A, Basun H, Fastbom J, Winblad B, Fratiglioni L. Vitamin B(12) and folate in relation to the development of Alzheimer's disease. Neurology 2001;56(9):1188–1194
28. Seshadri S, Beiser A, Selhub J, et al. Plasma homocysteine as a risk factor for dementia and Alzheimer's disease. N Engl J Med 2002;346(7):476–483
29. Ravaglia G, Forti P, Maioli F, et al. Homocysteine and cognitive function in healthy elderly community dwellers in Italy. Am J Clin Nutr 2003;77(3):668–673
30. Ravaglia G, Forti P, Maioli F, et al. Homocysteine and folate as risk factors for dementia and Alzheimer disease. Am J Clin Nutr 2005;82(3):636–643
31. Luchsinger JA, Tang MX, Miller J, Green R, Mayeux R. Relation of higher folate intake to lower risk of Alzheimer disease in the elderly. Arch Neurol 2007;64(1):86–92
32. Morris MC, Evans DA, Schneider JA, Tangney CC, Bienias JL, Aggarwal NT. Dietary folate and vitamins B-12 and B-6 not associated with incident Alzheimer's disease. J Alzheimers Dis 2006;9(4):435–443
33. McMahon JA, Green TJ, Skeaff CM, Knight RG, Mann JI, Williams SM. A controlled trial of homocysteine lowering and cognitive performance. N Engl J Med 2006;354(26):2764–2772
34. Eussen SJ, de Groot LC, Joosten LW, et al. Effect of oral vitamin B-12 with or without folic acid on cognitive function in older people with mild vitamin B-12 deficiency: a randomized, placebo-controlled trial. Am J Clin Nutr 2006;84(2):361–370
35. B-Vitamin Treatment Trialists' Collaboration. Homocysteine-lowering trials for prevention of cardiovascular events: a review of the design and power of the large randomized trials. Am Heart J 2006;151(2):282–287

36. Hutto BR. Folate and cobalamin in psychiatric illness. Compr Psychiatry 1997;38(6):305–314
37. Penninx BW, Guralnik JM, Ferrucci L, Fried LP, Allen RH, Stabler SP. Vitamin B(12) deficiency and depression in physically disabled older women: epidemiologic evidence from the Women's Health and Aging Study. Am J Psychiatry 2000;157(5):715–721
38. Tiemeier H, van Tuijl HR, Hofman A, Meijer J, Kiliaan AJ, Breteler MM. Vitamin B12, folate, and homocysteine in depression: the Rotterdam Study. Am J Psychiatry 2002;159(12):2099–2101
39. Bressa GM. S-Adenosyl-l-methionine (SAMe) as antidepressant: meta-analysis of clinical studies. Acta Neurol Scand Suppl 1994;154:7–14
40. Bell KM, Plon L, Bunney WE Jr, Potkin SG. S-Adenosylmethionine treatment of depression: a controlled clinical trial. Am J Psychiatry 1988;145(9):1110–1114
41. Delle Chiaie R, Pancheri P, Scapicchio P. Efficacy and tolerability of oral and intramuscular S-adenosyl-L-methionine 1,4-butanedisulfonate (SAMe) in the treatment of major depression: comparison with imipramine in 2 multicenter studies. Am J Clin Nutr 2002;76(5):1172S–1176S
42. Williams AL, Girard C, Jui D, Sabina A, Katz DL. S-Adenosylmethionine (SAMe) as treatment for depression: a systematic review. Clin Invest Med 2005;28(3):132–139
43. Hendler SS, Rorvik DR, eds. PDR for Nutritional Supplements. Montvale: Medical Economics Co., Inc.; 2001
44. Kasper H. Vitamin absorption in the elderly. Int J Vitam Nutr Res 1999;69(3):169–172
45. Termanini B, Gibril F, Sutliff VE, Yu F, Venzon DJ, Jensen RT. Effect of long-term gastric acid suppressive therapy on serum vitamin B12 levels in patients with Zollinger-Ellison syndrome. Am J Med 1998;104(5):422–430
46. Simon JA, Hudes ES. Relation of serum ascorbic acid to serum vitamin B12, serum ferritin, and kidney stones in US adults. Arch Intern Med 1999;159(6):619–624

10 Vitamin C

Vitamin C, also known as ascorbic acid, is a water-soluble vitamin. Unlike most mammals and other animals, humans do not have the ability to make their own vitamin C, so we must obtain vitamin C through our diet.

Function

Vitamin C is required for the synthesis of collagen, an important structural component of blood vessels, tendons, ligaments, and bone. It also plays an important role in the synthesis of the neurotransmitter, norepinephrine. Neurotransmitters are critical to brain function and are known to affect mood. In addition, vitamin C is required for the synthesis of carnitine, a small molecule that is essential for the transport of fat into cellular organelles called *mitochondria*, where the fat is converted to energy.[1] Research also suggests that vitamin C is involved in the metabolism of cholesterol to bile acids, which may have implications for blood cholesterol levels and the incidence of gallstones.[2]

Vitamin C is also a highly effective antioxidant. Even in small amounts vitamin C can protect indispensable molecules in the body, such as proteins, lipids (fats), carbohydrates, and nucleic acids (DNA and RNA), from damage by free radicals and reactive oxygen species that can be generated during normal metabolism as well as through exposure to toxins and pollutants (e.g., cigarette smoke). Vitamin C may also be able to regenerate other antioxidants such as vitamin E.[1] One recent study of cigarette smokers found that vitamin C regenerated vitamin E from its oxidized form.[3]

Deficiency

Scurvy

Severe vitamin C deficiency has been known for many centuries as the potentially fatal disease, scurvy. By the late 1700s the British navy were aware that scurvy could be cured by eating oranges or lemons, even though vitamin C would not be isolated until the early 1930s. Symptoms of scurvy include bleeding and bruising easily, hair and tooth loss, and joint pain and swelling. Such symptoms appear to be related to the weakening of blood vessels, connective tissue, and bone, which all contain collagen. Early symptoms of scurvy, such as fatigue, may result from diminished levels of carnitine, which is needed to derive energy from fat, or from decreased synthesis of the neurotransmitter norepinephrine. Scurvy is rare in developed countries because it can be prevented by as little as 10 mg vitamin C daily.[4] However, cases have occurred in children and elderly people on very restricted diets.[5,6]

Recommended Dietary Allowance

The recommended dietary allowance (RDA) for vitamin C was revised in 2000 upward from 60 mg/day for men and women to 75 mg/day for women and 90 mg/day for men (**Table 10.1**). The RDA continues to be based primarily on the prevention of deficiency disease, rather than the prevention of chronic disease and the promotion of optimum health. The recommended intake for smokers is 35 mg/day higher than for nonsmokers, because smokers are under increased oxidative stress from the toxins in cigarette smoke and generally have lower blood levels of vitamin C.[7]

Disease Prevention

The amount of vitamin C required to prevent chronic disease appears to be more than that required for prevention of scurvy. Much of the information about vitamin C and the prevention of chronic disease is based on prospective studies, in which vitamin C intake is assessed in large numbers of people who are followed over time to determine whether they develop specific chronic diseases.

Table 10.1 Recommended dietary allowance for vitamin C

Life stage	Age	Males (mg/day)	Females (mg/day)
Infants	0–6 months	40 (AI)	40 (AI)
Infants	7–12 months	50 (AI)	50 (AI)
Children	1–3 years	15	15
Children	4–8 years	25	25
Children	9–13 years	45	45
Adolescents	14–18 years	75	65
Adults	≥19 years	90	75
Smokers	≥19 years	125	110
Pregnancy	≤18 years	–	80
Pregnancy	≥19 years	–	85
Breast-feeding	≤18 years	–	115
Breast-feeding	≥19 years	–	120

AI, adequate intake.

Cardiovascular Diseases

Coronary heart disease. Until recently, the results of most prospective studies indicated that low or deficient intakes of vitamin C were associated with an increased risk of cardiovascular diseases, and that modest dietary intakes of about 100 mg/day were sufficient for maximal reduction of cardiovascular disease risk among non-smoking men and women.[1] A recent meta-analysis of 14 cohort studies concluded that dietary vitamin C intake, but not supplemental vitamin C intake, was inversely related to coronary heart disease (CHD) risk.[8] Thus, some studies did not find significant reductions in CHD risk among vitamin C supplement users in well-nourished populations.[9–11] One notable exception was the First National Health and Nutrition Examination Survey (NHANES I) Epidemiologic Follow-up Study.[12] This study found that the risk of death from cardiovascular diseases was 42% lower in men and 25% lower in women who consumed more than 50 mg/day of dietary vitamin C *and* regularly took vitamin C supplements, corresponding to a total vitamin C intake of about 300 mg/day.[13] Results from the Nurses' Health Study (NHS), based on the follow-up of more than 85 000 women over 16 years, also suggested that higher vitamin C intakes may be cardioprotective.[14] In this study, vitamin C intake of more than 359 mg/day from diet plus supplements or supplement use itself was associated with a 27%–

28% reduction in CHD risk. However, in those women who did not take vitamin C supplements, dietary vitamin C intake was not significantly associated with CHD risk. Hence, both the NHANES I Epidemiologic Follow-up Study[12,13] and the NHS[14] do not support the conclusions of the above-mentioned meta-analysis.[8]

Another pooled analysis of nine prospective cohort studies, including more than 290 000 adults who were free of CHD at baseline and followed for an average of 10 years, found that those who took more than 700 mg/day of supplemental vitamin C had a 25% lower risk of CHD than those who did not take vitamin C supplements.[15] In addition, a randomized, double-blind, placebo-controlled trial in more than 14 000 older men participating in the Physicians' Health Study (PHS) II found that vitamin C supplementation (500 mg/day) for an average of 8 years had no significant effect on major cardiovascular events, total myocardial infarction, or cardiovascular mortality.[16] However, this study had several limitations.[17] Data from pharmacokinetic studies of vitamin C at the National Institutes of Health (NIH) indicate that plasma and circulating cells—and thus, presumably, total body pool—in healthy, young individuals reach near maximal concentrations of vitamin C at a dose of about 400 mg/day.[18] Therefore, the results of the pooled analysis of prospective cohort studies as well as individual, large prospective studies, such as the

NHANES I Epidemiologic Follow-up Study[12,13] and the NHS,[14] together with pharmacokinetic data of vitamin C in humans,[18] suggest that maximal reduction of CHD risk may require vitamin C intakes of 400 mg/day or more.[19]

Stroke. With respect to vitamin C and cerebrovascular disease, a prospective study that followed more than 2000 residents of a rural Japanese community for 20 years found that the risk of stroke in those with the highest serum levels of vitamin C was 29% lower than in those with the lowest serum levels of vitamin C.[20] In addition, the risk of stroke in those who consumed vegetables 6–7 days of the week was 54% lower than in those who consumed vegetables 0–2 days of the week. In this population, serum levels of vitamin C were highly correlated with fruit and vegetable intake. Therefore, as in many studies of vitamin C intake and chronic disease risk, it is difficult to separate the effects of vitamin C on stroke risk from the effects of other components of fruit and vegetables, emphasizing the benefits of a diet rich in fruit and vegetables in reducing stroke risk. Hence, plasma vitamin C levels may be a good biomarker for fruit and vegetable intake and other lifestyle factors that contribute to a reduced risk of stroke. A recent 10-year prospective study in 20 649 adults found that those in the top quartile (one-fourth) of plasma vitamin C concentrations had a 42% lower risk of stroke compared with those in the lowest quartile.[21] A randomized, double-blind, placebo-controlled trial in more than 14 000 older men participating in the PHS II found that vitamin C supplementation (500 mg/day) for an average of 8 years had no significant effect on stroke death, ischemic stroke, or hemorrhagic stroke.[16] However, this study had numerous limitations that make it difficult to draw conclusions for the general population.[17]

Cancer

A large number of studies have shown that increased consumption of fresh fruit and vegetables is associated with a reduced risk for most types of cancer.[22] Such studies were the basis for dietary guidelines endorsed by the US Department of Agriculture and the National Cancer Institute, which recommended at least five servings of fruit and vegetables per day. US govern-ment organizations currently recommend eating a variety of fruit and vegetables daily; the recommended number of servings depends on total caloric intake, which is governed by age, gender, body composition, and physical activity level.[23] A number of case–control studies have investigated the role of vitamin C in cancer prevention. Most have shown that higher intakes of vitamin C are associated with decreased incidence of cancers of the mouth, throat and vocal folds, esophagus, stomach, colon–rectum, and lung. As the possibility of bias is greater in case–control studies, prospective cohort studies are generally given more weight when evaluating the effect of nutrient intake on disease. In general, prospective studies in which the lowest intake group consumed more than 86 mg vitamin C daily have not found differences in cancer risk, whereas studies finding significant cancer risk reductions found them in people consuming at least 80–110 mg vitamin C daily.[1]

A prospective study that followed 870 men over a period of 25 years found that those who consumed more than 83 mg vitamin C daily had a striking 64% reduction in lung cancer compared with those who consumed less than 63 mg/day.[24] However, a pooled analysis of eight prospective studies concluded that dietary vitamin C was not related to lung cancer when the analysis was controlled for other dietary factors.[25] Although most large prospective studies observed no association between breast cancer and vitamin C intake, two studies found dietary vitamin C intake to be inversely associated with breast cancer risk in certain subgroups. In the NHS, premenopausal women with a family history of breast cancer who consumed an average of 205 mg/day of vitamin C from foods had a 63% lower risk of breast cancer than those who consumed an average of 70 mg/day.[26] In the Swedish Mammography Cohort, overweight women who consumed an average of 110 mg/day of vitamin C had a 39% lower risk of breast cancer compared with overweight women who consumed an average of 31 mg/day.[27]

A number of observational studies have found increased dietary vitamin C intake to be associated with decreased risk of stomach cancer, and laboratory experiments indicate that vitamin C inhibits the formation of carcinogenic compounds in the stomach.[28,29] Infection with the bacterium *Helicobacter pylori* is known to increase the risk of stomach cancer and also appears to lower the vitamin C content of stomach secretions. Although two intervention studies did not find a decrease in the occurrence of stomach cancer with vitamin C supplementation,[7] more recent research suggests that vitamin C supplementation may be a useful addition to standard *H. pylori* eradication therapy in reducing the risk of gastric cancer.[30,31] Another intervention trial, a randomized, double-blind, placebo-controlled trial in more than 14 000 older men participating in the PHS II, reported that vitamin C supplementation (500 mg/day) for an average of 8 years had no significant effect on total cancer or site-specific cancers, including colorectal, lung, and prostate cancer.[32]

Cataracts

Cataracts are a leading cause of visual impairment throughout the world. In the United States, cataract-related expenditures are estimated to exceed US $3 billion annually.[33] Cataracts occur more frequently and become more severe as people age. Decreased vitamin C levels in the lens of the eye have been associated with increased severity of cataracts in humans. Some, but not all, studies have observed increased dietary vitamin C intake[34,35] and increased blood levels of vitamin C[36,37] to be associated with decreased risk of cataracts. In general, those studies that have found a relationship suggest that vitamin C intake may have to be higher than 300 mg/day for a number of years before a protective effect can be detected.[1] A 7-year controlled intervention trial in 4629 men and women found that a daily anti-oxidant supplement containing 500 mg vitamin C, 400 IU vitamin E, and 15 mg β-carotene had no effect on the development and progression of age-related cataracts compared with a placebo.[38] Therefore, the relationship between vitamin C intake and the development of cataracts requires further clarification before specific recommendations can be made.

Gout

Gout, a condition that afflicts more than 1% of US adults, is characterized by abnormally high blood levels of uric acid (urate).[39] Urate crystals may form in joints, resulting in inflammation and pain, as well as in the kidneys and urinary tract, resulting in kidney stones. The tendency to develop elevated blood uric acid levels and gout is often inherited; however, dietary and lifestyle modification may be helpful in both the prevention and the treatment of gout.[40] In an observational study that included 1387 men, higher intakes of vitamin C were associated with lower serum levels of uric acid.[41] More recently, a prospective study that followed a cohort of 46 994 men for 20 years found that total daily vitamin C intake was inversely associated with risk of gout, with higher intakes being associated with greater risk reductions.[42] The results of this study also indicate that supplemental vitamin C may be helpful in the prevention of gout.[42] Interestingly, a randomized, double-blind, placebo-controlled trial in 184 adult nonsmokers reported that vitamin C supplementation (500 mg/day) for two months lowered serum concentrations of uric acid compared with placebo.[43]

Lead Toxicity

Although the use of lead paint and leaded gasoline has been discontinued in the United States, lead toxicity continues to be a significant health problem, especially in children living in urban areas. Abnormal growth and development have been observed in infants of women exposed to lead during pregnancy, while children who are chronically exposed to lead are more likely to develop learning disabilities, behavioral problems, and to have a low IQ. In adults, lead toxicity may result in kidney damage, high blood pressure, and anemia. In a study of 747 older men, blood lead levels were significantly higher in those who reported total dietary vitamin C intakes averaging < 109 mg/day compared with those who reported higher vitamin C intakes.[44] A much larger study of 19 578 people, including 4214 children aged from 6 years to 16 years, found higher serum vitamin C levels to be associated with significantly lower blood lead levels.[45] A US national survey of more than 10 000 adults found that blood lead levels were inversely related to serum vitamin C levels.[46]

An intervention trial that examined the effects of vitamin C supplementation on blood lead levels in 75 adult male smokers found that 1000 mg/day of vitamin C resulted in significantly lower blood lead levels over a 4-week treatment period compared with placebo.[47] A lower dose of 200 mg/day did not significantly affect blood lead levels, despite the finding that serum vitamin C levels were no different than those in the group who took 1000 mg/day. The mechanism for the relationship between vitamin C intake and blood lead levels is not known, although it has been postulated that vitamin C may inhibit intestinal absorption or enhance urinary excretion of lead.

Role in Immunity

Vitamin C affects several components of the human immune system, for example, vitamin C has been shown to stimulate both the production[48–52] and the function[53,54] of leukocytes (white blood cells), especially neutrophils, lymphocytes, and phagocytes. Specific measures of functions stimulated by vitamin C include cellular motility,[54] chemotaxis,[53,54] and phagocytosis.[53] Neutrophils, which attack foreign bacteria and viruses, seem to be the primary cell type stimulated by vitamin C, but lymphocytes and other phagocytes are also affected.[55] In addition, several studies have shown that supplemental vitamin C increases serum levels of antibodies[56,57] and C1q complement proteins[58–60] in guinea pigs, which—similar to humans—cannot synthesize vitamin C and hence depend on dietary vitamin C. However, some studies have reported no beneficial changes in leukocyte production or function with vitamin C treatment.[61–64] Vitamin C may also protect the integrity of immune cells. Neutrophils, mononuclear phagocytes, and lymphocytes accumulate vitamin C to high concentrations, which can protect these cell types from oxidative damage.[52,65,66] In response to invading microorganisms, phagocytic leukocytes release nonspecific toxins, such as superoxide radicals, hypochlorous acid ("bleach"), and peroxynitrite; these reactive oxygen species kill pathogens and, in the process, can damage the leukocytes themselves.[67] Vitamin C, through its antioxidant functions, has been shown to protect leukocytes from such effects of autooxidation.[68] Phagocytic leukocytes also produce and release cytokines, including interferons, which have antiviral activity.[69] Vitamin C has been shown to increase interferon levels in vitro.[70]

It is widely thought by the general public that vitamin C boosts the function of the immune system and, accordingly, may protect against viral infections and perhaps other diseases. Although some studies suggest the biological plausibility of vitamin C as an immune enhancer, human studies published to date are conflicting. Further, controlled clinical trials of appropriate statistical power would be necessary to determine if supplemental vitamin C boosts the immune system.

Disease Treatment

Cardiovascular Diseases

Vasodilation. The ability of blood vessels to relax or dilate (vasodilation) is compromised in individuals with atherosclerosis. Damage to the heart muscle caused by a heart attack and damage to the brain caused by a stroke are related, in part, to the inability of blood vessels to dilate enough to allow blood flow to the affected areas. The pain of angina pectoris is also related to insufficient dilation of the coronary arteries. Impaired vasodilation has been identified as an independent risk factor for cardiovascular disease.[71] Many randomized, double-blind, placebo-controlled studies have shown that treatment with vitamin C consistently results in improved vasodilation in individuals with CHD as well as in those with angina pectoris, congestive heart failure, diabetes, high cholesterol, and high blood pressure.[1,72–74] Improved vasodilation has been demonstrated at an oral dose of 500 mg vitamin C daily.[72]

Hypertension. Individuals with high blood pressure (hypertension) are at increased risk of developing cardiovascular diseases. Several, but not all, studies have demonstrated a blood pressure-lowering effect of vitamin C supplementation.[75] A small study in individuals with hypertension found that vitamin C supplementation with 500 mg/day for 6 weeks slightly decreased systolic blood pressure (1.8 mmHg reduction) compared with a placebo.[76] Another study in individuals with elevated blood pressure found that a daily supplement of 500 mg vitamin C resulted in an average drop in systolic blood pressure of 9% after 4 weeks.[77] It should be noted that those participants who were taking antihypertensive medications continued taking them throughout the 4-week study. As the findings with regard to vitamin C and high blood pressure have not yet been replicated in larger studies, it is important for individuals with significantly elevated blood pressure to continue current therapy (medication, lifestyle changes, etc.) in consultation with their health-care provider.

Cancer

Studies in the 1970s and 1980s conducted by Linus Pauling, Ewan Cameron, and colleagues suggested that very large doses of vitamin C (10 g/day intravenously for 10 days followed by at least 10 g/day orally indefinitely) were helpful in increasing the survival time and improving the quality of life of terminal cancer patients.[78] However, two randomized placebo-controlled studies conducted at the Mayo Clinic found no differences in outcome between terminal cancer patients receiving 10 g/day of vitamin C orally or placebo.[79,80] There were significant methodological differences between the Mayo Clinic and Pauling's studies, and recently, researchers from the NIH suggested that the route of administration (intravenous versus oral) may have been the key to the discrepant results. Intravenous administration can result in much higher blood levels of vitamin C than oral administration, and vitamin C levels that are toxic to cancer cells in culture can be achieved in humans only with intravenous but not oral administration of vitamin C.[81] Mark Levine and his colleagues at NIH have investigated the anticancer mechanism responsible for vitamin C and reported that it involves production of hydrogen peroxide, which is selectively toxic to cancer cells.[82–84] Thus, it appears reasonable to re-evaluate the use of high-dose vitamin C as adjunctive cancer therapy.

Currently, there are no results from controlled clinical trials indicating that vitamin C would adversely affect the survival of cancer patients. Recently, two phase I clinical trials in patients with advanced cancer found that intravenous administration of vitamin C at doses up to 1.5 g/kg body weight was well tolerated and safe in prescreened patients;[85,86] other phase I trials are ongoing.[87] In addition, phase II clinical trials evaluating the efficacy of vitamin C in cancer treatment are currently under way.[87] Some case reports have suggested that intravenous vitamin C may aid in cancer treatment.[88,89] However, vitamin C should not be used in place of therapy that has been demonstrated to be effective in the treatment of a particular type of cancer, for example, chemo-

therapy or radiotherapy. If an individual with cancer chooses to take vitamin supplements, it is important that the clinician coordinating his or her treatment is aware of the type and dose of each supplement. Although research is under way to determine whether combinations of antioxidant vitamins might be beneficial as an adjunct to conventional cancer therapy, definitive conclusions are not yet possible.[90]

Diabetes Mellitus

Cardiovascular diseases (heart disease and stroke) are the leading cause of death in individuals with diabetes. Evidence that diabetes is a condition of increased oxidative stress led to the hypothesis that higher intakes of antioxidant nutrients could help decrease cardiovascular disease risk in diabetic individuals. In support of this hypothesis, a 16-year study of 85 000 women, 2% of whom were diabetic, found that vitamin C supplement use (400 mg/day or more) was associated with significant reductions in the risk of fatal and nonfatal CHD in the entire cohort as well as in those with diabetes.[14] In contrast, a 15-year study of postmenopausal women found that diabetic women who reported taking at least 300 mg/day of vitamin C from supplements when the study began were at significantly higher risk of death from CHD and stroke than those who did not take vitamin C supplements.[91] Vitamin C supplement use was not associated with a significant increase in cardiovascular disease mortality in the cohort as a whole. Although a number of observational studies have found that higher dietary intakes of vitamin C are associated with lower cardiovascular disease risk, randomized controlled trials have not found antioxidant supplementation that included vitamin C to reduce the risk of cardiovascular disease in diabetic or other high-risk individuals.[92,93]

It is possible that genetic differences may influence the effect of vitamin C supplementation on cardiovascular disease. When the results of one randomized controlled trial were reanalyzed based on haptoglobin genotype, antioxidant therapy (1000 mg/day of vitamin C + 800 IU/day of vitamin E) was associated with improvement of coronary atherosclerosis in diabetic women with two copies of the haptoglobin 1 gene but worsening of coronary atherosclerosis in those with two copies of the haptoglobin 2 gene.[94] The significance of these findings is not entirely clear, but they suggest that there may be a subpopulation of people with diabetes who will benefit from antioxidant therapy, whereas others may not benefit or could actually be harmed.

Common Cold

The work of Linus Pauling stimulated public interest in the use of large doses (> 1 g/day, also sometimes called mega-doses) of vitamin C to prevent the common cold.[95] In the past 30 years, numerous placebo-controlled trials have examined the effect of vitamin C supplementation on the prevention and treatment of colds. A meta-analysis of 30 placebo-controlled prevention trials found that vitamin C supplementation in doses up to 2 g/day did not decrease the incidence of colds.[96] However, in a subgroup of marathon runners, skiers, and soldiers training in the Arctic, doses ranging from 250 mg/day to 1 g/day decreased the incidence of colds by 50%. Overall, the preventive use of vitamin C supplementation reduced the duration of colds by about 8% in adults and 14% in children. Most of the prevention trials used a dose of 1 g/day. When treatment was started at the onset of symptoms, vitamin C supplementation did not shorten the duration of colds in seven placebo-controlled trials at doses ranging from 1 g/day to 4 g/day. In addition, the same authors completed a meta-analysis of the 15 trials that assessed the effect of vitamin C on cold severity, in which no consistent evidence that vitamin C was beneficial in ameliorating cold symptoms was found. Thus, the overall conclusion of this meta-analysis was that vitamin C is ineffective as a prophylactic against the common cold, but individuals under stress, such as those exposed to strenuous physical exercise or cold weather, may experience some therapeutic benefit.[96] More recently, a randomized, double-blind (but not placebo-controlled) study reported that those who took 500 mg/day of supplemental vitamin C had a 66% lower risk for contracting three or more colds in a 5-year period compared with those who took 50 mg/day of supplemental vitamin C.[97] The authors of this study did not find any significant differences in the two groups when analyzing data about cold severity or duration. However, the doses used in this study were smaller than those used in most of the previous studies.

Some authors have asserted that the studies included in the above-mentioned meta-analysis[96] utilized daily doses of vitamin C that would be too low to observe a therapeutic benefit.[98,99] In addition, results of a recent pharmacokinetic study suggest that dividing the daily dose and administering it several times throughout the day, thereby increasing dose frequency, would better sustain plasma ascorbate levels.[81] Large-scale, controlled clinical trials using pharmacological doses of vitamin C are necessary to determine whether or not higher doses of vitamin C have any therapeutic value in preventing or treating the common cold.

Sources

Food Sources

As shown in **Table 10.2**, different fruits and vegetables vary in their vitamin C content,[100] but five servings (2½ cups) of fruit and vegetables should average out to about 200 mg vitamin C.

Supplements

Vitamin C (L-ascorbic acid) is available in many forms, but there is little scientific evidence that any one form is better absorbed or more effective than another. Most experimental and clinical research uses ascorbic acid or sodium ascorbate.

Table 10.2 Food sources of vitamin C

Food	Serving	Vitamin C (mg)
Sweet red pepper	½ cup, raw chopped	95
Orange juice	¾ cup (6 ounces)	62–93
Strawberries	1 cup, whole	85
Orange	1 medium	70
Grapefruit juice	¾ cup (6 ounces)	62–70
Broccoli	½ cup, cooked	51
Grapefruit	½ medium	38
Potato	1 medium, baked	17
Tomato	1 medium	16

Natural versus synthetic vitamin C. Natural and synthetic L-ascorbic acid are chemically identical and there are no known differences in their biological activities or bioavailabilities.[101]

Mineral ascorbates. Mineral salts of ascorbic acid are buffered and, therefore, less acidic than ascorbic acid. Some people find them less irritating to the gastrointestinal tract than ascorbic acid. Sodium ascorbate and calcium ascorbate are the most common forms, although a number of other mineral ascorbates are available. Sodium ascorbate provides 111 mg of sodium (889 mg of ascorbic acid) per 1000 mg of sodium ascorbate, and calcium ascorbate generally provides 90–110 mg of calcium (890–910 mg of ascorbic acid) per 1000 mg of calcium ascorbate.

Vitamin C with bioflavonoids. Bioflavonoids are a class of water-soluble plant pigments that are often found in vitamin C-rich fruit and vegetables, especially citrus fruits. There is little evidence that the bioflavonoids in most commercial preparations increase the bioavailability or efficacy of vitamin C.[102] Studies in cell culture indicate that a number of flavonoids inhibit the transport of vitamin C into cells,[103-105] and supplementation of rats with quercetin and vitamin C decreased the intestinal absorption of vitamin C.[103] More research is needed to determine the significance of these findings in humans.

Ascorbate and vitamin C metabolites. One supplement, Ester-C, contains mainly calcium ascorbate, but also contains small amounts of the vitamin C metabolites dehydroascorbate (oxidized ascorbic acid), calcium threonate, and trace levels of xylonate and lyxonate. Although the metabolites are supposed to increase the bioavailability of vitamin C, the only published study in humans addressing this issue found no difference between Ester-C and commercially available ascorbic acid tablets with respect to the absorption and urinary excretion of vitamin C.[102]

Ascorbyl palmitate. Ascorbyl palmitate is actually a vitamin C ester (i.e., vitamin C that has been esterified to a fatty acid). In this case, vitamin C is esterified to the saturated fatty acid palmitic acid, resulting in a fat-soluble form of vitamin C. Ascorbyl palmitate has been added to a number of skin creams due to interest in its antioxidant properties as well as its importance in collagen synthesis.[106] Although ascorbyl palmitate is also available as an oral supplement, it is likely that most of it is hydrolyzed (broken apart) to ascorbic acid and palmitic acid in the digestive tract before it is absorbed.[107]

Safety

Toxicity

A number of possible problems with very large doses of vitamin C have been suggested, mainly based on in vitro experiments or isolated case reports, including genetic mutations, birth defects, cancer, atherosclerosis, kidney stones, "rebound scurvy," increased oxidative stress, excess iron absorption, vitamin B_{12} deficiency, and erosion of dental enamel. However, none of these alleged adverse health effects has been confirmed, and there is no reliable scientific evidence that large amounts of vitamin C (up to 10 g/day in adults) are toxic or detrimental to health. With the latest RDA published in 2000, a tolerable upper intake level (UL) for vitamin C was set for the first time (**Table 10.3**). A UL of 2 g (2000 mg) daily was recommended in order to prevent most adults from experiencing diarrhea and gastrointestinal disturbances.[7] Such symptoms are not generally serious, especially if they resolve with temporary discontinuation or reduction of high-dose vitamin C supplementation.

Table 10.3 Tolerable upper intake level (UL) for vitamin C

Life stage	Age	UL (mg/day)
Infants	0–12 months	Not possible to establish[a]
Children	1–3 years	400
Children	4–8 years	650
Children	9–13 years	1200
Adolescents	14–18 years	1800
Adults	≥19 years	2000

[a]Source of intake should be from food and formula only.

Does Vitamin C Promote Oxidative Damage under Physiological Conditions?

Vitamin C is known to function as a highly effective antioxidant in living organisms. However, in test tube experiments, vitamin C can interact with some free metal ions to produce potentially damaging free radicals. Although free metal ions are not generally found under physiological conditions, the idea that high doses of vitamin C might be able to promote oxidative damage in vivo has received a great deal of attention. Widespread publicity has been given to a few studies suggesting a prooxidant effect of vitamin C,[108,109] but these studies turned out to be either flawed or of no physiological relevance. A comprehensive review of the literature found no credible scientific evidence that supplemental vitamin C promotes oxidative damage under physiological conditions or in humans.[110] Studies that report a prooxidant effect for vitamin C should be evaluated carefully to determine whether the study system was physiologically relevant and to rule out the possibility of methodological and design flaws.

Kidney Stones

As oxalate is a metabolite of vitamin C, there is some concern that high vitamin C intake could increase the risk of oxalate kidney stones. Some,[111-113] but not all,[114-116] studies have reported that supplemental vitamin C increases urinary oxalate levels. Whether any increase in oxalate levels would translate to an elevation in risk for kidney stones has been examined in epidemiological studies. Two large prospective studies, one following 45 251 men for 6 years and the other following 85 557 women for 14 years, reported that consumption of 1500 mg or more vitamin C daily did not increase the risk of kidney stone formation compared with those consuming less than 250 mg daily. However, a more recent prospective study that followed 45 619 men for 14 years found that those who consumed 1000 mg/day or more of vitamin C had a 41% higher risk of kidney stones compared with men consuming less than 90 mg vitamin C daily—the current RDA.[117] In this study, low intakes (90–249 mg/day) of vitamin C (primarily from the diet) were also associated with a significantly elevated risk. Supplemental vitamin C intake was only weakly associated with increased risk of kidney stones.[117] Despite conflicting results, it may be prudent for individuals predisposed to oxalate kidney stone formation to avoid high-dose vitamin C supplementation.

Drug Interactions

A number of drugs are known to lower vitamin C levels, requiring an increase in its intake. Estrogen-containing contraceptives (birth control pills) are known to lower vitamin C levels in plasma and white blood cells. Aspirin can lower vitamin C levels if taken frequently, e.g., taking two aspirin tablets every 6 hours for a week has been reported to lower vitamin C levels in white blood cells by 50%, primarily by increasing urinary excretion of vitamin C.[118]

There is some evidence, although controversial, that vitamin C interacts with anticoagulant medications (blood thinners) such as warfarin (Coumadin). Large doses of vitamin C may block the action of warfarin, requiring an increase in dose to maintain its effectiveness. Individuals on anticoagulants should limit their vitamin C intake to 1 g/day and have their prothrombin time monitored by the clinician after their anticoagulant therapy. As high doses of vitamin C have also been found to interfere with the interpretation of certain laboratory tests (e.g., serum bilirubin, serum creatinine, and the guaiac assay for occult blood), it is important to inform one's healthcare provider of any recent supplement use.[119]

Antioxidant supplements and HMG-CoA reductase inhibitors (statins). A 3-year randomized controlled trial in 160 patients with documented CHD and low high-density lipoprotein (HDL) levels found that a combination of simvastatin and niacin increased HDL2 levels, inhibited the progression of coronary artery stenosis (narrowing), and decreased the frequency of cardiovascular events, such as myocardial infarction (heart attack) and stroke.[120] Surprisingly, when an antioxidant combination (1000 mg vitamin C, 800 IU α-tocopherol, 100 μg selenium, and 25 mg β-carotene daily) was taken with the simvastatin–niacin combination, the protective effects were diminished. As the antioxidants were taken together in this trial, the individual contribution of vitamin C cannot be determined. In contrast, a much larger randomized controlled trial in more than 20 000 men and women with CHD or diabetes found that simvastatin and an antioxidant combination (600 mg vitamin E, 250 mg vitamin C, and 20 mg β-carotene daily) did not diminish the cardioprotective effects of simvastatin therapy over a 5-year period.[121] These contradictory findings indicate that further research is needed on potential interactions between antioxidant supplements and cholesterol-lowering drugs, such as hydroxymethylglutaryl (HMG)-CoA reductase inhibitors (statins).

LPI Recommendation

For healthy men and women, the Linus Pauling Institute recommends a vitamin C intake of at least 400 mg daily. Consuming at least five servings (2½ cups) of fruit and vegetables daily provides about 200 mg vitamin C. Most multivitamin supplements provide 60 mg vitamin C. To make sure that you meet the Institute's recommendation, supplemental vitamin C in two separate 250-mg doses taken in the morning and evening is recommended.

Older Adults

Although it is not yet known with certainty whether older adults have higher requirements for vitamin C than younger people, some older populations have been found to have vitamin C intakes considerably below the RDA of 75 and 90 mg/day for women and men, respectively. A vitamin C intake of at least 400 mg daily may be particularly important for older adults who are at higher risk for chronic diseases. In addition, a meta-analysis of 36 publications examining the relationship between vitamin C intake and plasma concentrations of vitamin C concluded that older adults (age 60–96 years) have considerably lower plasma levels of vitamin C after a certain intake of vitamin C compared with younger individuals (age 15–65 years),[122] suggesting that older adults may have higher vitamin C requirements. Studies conducted at the National Institutes of Health indicated that plasma and circulating cells in healthy, young people attain linear-maximal concentrations of vitamin C at a dose of about 400 mg/day—much higher than the current RDA. Pharmacokinetic studies in older adults have not yet been conducted, but evidence suggests that the efficiency of one of the molecular mechanisms for the cellular uptake of vitamin C declines with age.[123] As maximizing blood levels of vitamin C may be important in protection against oxidative damage to cells and biological molecules, a vitamin C intake of at least 400 mg daily is particularly important for older adults who are at higher risk for chronic diseases caused, in part, by oxidative damage, such as heart disease, stroke, certain cancers, and cataract.

References

1. Carr AC, Frei B. Toward a new recommended dietary allowance for vitamin C based on antioxidant and health effects in humans. Am J Clin Nutr 1999;69(6): 1086–1107
2. Simon JA, Hudes ES. Serum ascorbic acid and gallbladder disease prevalence among US adults: the Third National Health and Nutrition Examination Survey (NHANES III). Arch Intern Med 2000;160(7): 931–936
3. Bruno RS, Leonard SW, Atkinson J, et al. Faster plasma vitamin E disappearance in smokers is normalized by vitamin C supplementation. Free Radic Biol Med 2006;40(4):689–697
4. Sauberlich HE. A history of scurvy and vitamin C. In: Packer L, Fuchs J, eds. Vitamin C in Health and Disease. New York: Marcel Decker, Inc.; 1997:1–24
5. Stephen R, Utecht T. Scurvy identified in the emergency department: a case report. J Emerg Med 2001;21(3):235–237
6. Weinstein M, Babyn P, Zlotkin S. An orange a day keeps the doctor away: scurvy in the year 2000. Pediatrics 2001;108(3):E55
7. Food and Nutrition Board, Institute of Medicine. Vitamin C. In: Dietary Reference Intakes for Vitamin C, Vitamin E, Selenium, and Carotenoids. Washington, DC: National Academy Press; 2000:95–185
8. Ye Z, Song H. Antioxidant vitamins intake and the risk of coronary heart disease: meta-analysis of cohort studies. Eur J Cardiovasc Prev Rehabil 2008;15(1):26–34
9. Losonczy KG, Harris TB, Havlik RJ. Vitamin E and vitamin C supplement use and risk of all-cause and coronary heart disease mortality in older persons: the Established Populations for Epidemiologic Studies of the Elderly. Am J Clin Nutr 1996;64(2):190–196
10. Kushi LH, Folsom AR, Prineas RJ, Mink PJ, Wu Y, Bostick RM. Dietary antioxidant vitamins and death from coronary heart disease in postmenopausal women. N Engl J Med 1996;334(18):1156–1162
11. Muntwyler J, Hennekens CH, Manson JE, Buring JE, Gaziano JM. Vitamin supplement use in a low-risk population of US male physicians and subsequent cardiovascular mortality. Arch Intern Med 2002; 162(13):1472–1476
12. Enstrom JE, Kanim LE, Klein MA. Vitamin C intake and mortality among a sample of the United States population. Epidemiology 1992;3(3):194–202
13. Enstrom JE. Counterpoint–vitamin C and mortality. Nutr Today 1993;28:28–32
14. Osganian SK, Stampfer MJ, Rimm E, et al. Vitamin C and risk of coronary heart disease in women. J Am Coll Cardiol 2003;42(2):246–252
15. Sesso HD, Buring JE, Christen WG, et al. Vitamins E and C in the prevention of cardiovascular disease in men: the Physicians' Health Study II randomized controlled trial. JAMA 2008;300(18):2123–2133
17. Roberts LJ II, Traber MG, Frei B. Vitamins E and C in the prevention of cardiovascular disease and cancer in men. Free Radic Biol Med 2009;46(11):1558
18. Levine M, Wang Y, Padayatty SJ, Morrow J. A new recommended dietary allowance of vitamin C for healthy young women. Proc Natl Acad Sci USA 2001; 98(17):9842–9846
19. Frei B. To C or not to C, that is the question! J Am Coll Cardiol 2003;42(2):253–255

20. Yokoyama T, Date C, Kokubo Y, Yoshiike N, Matsumura Y, Tanaka H. Serum vitamin C concentration was inversely associated with subsequent 20-year incidence of stroke in a Japanese rural community. The Shibata study. Stroke 2000;31(10):2287–2294

21. Myint PK, Luben RN, Welch AA, Bingham SA, Wareham NJ, Khaw KT. Plasma vitamin C concentrations predict risk of incident stroke over 10y in 20 649 participants of the European Prospective Investigation into Cancer Norfolk prospective population study. Am J Clin Nutr 2008;87(1):64–69

22. Steinmetz KA, Potter JD. Vegetables, fruit, and cancer prevention: a review. J Am Diet Assoc 1996;96(10):1027–1039

23. Centers for Disease Control and Prevention. Eating a Variety of Fruits & Vegetables Every Day. [Web page]. Available at: http://www.fruitsandveggiesmatter.gov/. Accessed 4 Jan 2011

24. Kromhout D. Essential micronutrients in relation to carcinogenesis. Am J Clin Nutr 1987; 45(5, Suppl) 1361–1367

25. Cho E, Hunter DJ, Spiegelman D, et al. Intakes of vitamins A, C and E and folate and multivitamins and lung cancer: a pooled analysis of 8 prospective studies. Int J Cancer 2006;118(4):970–978

26. Zhang S, Hunter DJ, Forman MR, et al. Dietary carotenoids and vitamins A, C, and E and risk of breast cancer. J Natl Cancer Inst 1999;91(6):547–556

27. Michels KB, Holmberg L, Bergkvist L, Ljung H, Bruce A, Wolk A. Dietary antioxidant vitamins, retinol, and breast cancer incidence in a cohort of Swedish women. Int J Cancer 2001;91(4):563–567

28. Tsugane S, Sasazuki S. Diet and the risk of gastric cancer: review of epidemiological evidence. Gastric Cancer 2007;10(2):75–83

29. Liu C, Russell RM. Nutrition and gastric cancer risk: an update. Nutr Rev 2008;66(5):237–249

30. Feiz HR, Mobarhan S. Does vitamin C intake slow the progression of gastric cancer in Helicobacter pylori-infected populations? Nutr Rev 2002;60(1):34–36

31. Chuang CH, Sheu BS, Kao AW, et al. Adjuvant effect of vitamin C on omeprazole-amoxicillin-clarithromycin triple therapy for Helicobacter pylori eradication. Hepatogastroenterology 2007;54(73):320–324

32. Gaziano JM, Glynn RJ, Christen WG, et al. Vitamins E and C in the prevention of prostate and total cancer in men: the Physicians' Health Study II randomized controlled trial. JAMA 2009;301(1):52–62

33. Jacques PF. The potential preventive effects of vitamins for cataract and age-related macular degeneration. Int J Vitam Nutr Res 1999;69(3):198–205

34. Jacques PF, Chylack LT Jr, Hankinson SE, et al. Long-term nutrient intake and early age-related nuclear lens opacities. Arch Ophthalmol 2001;119(7):1009–1019

35. Yoshida M, Takashima Y, Inoue M, et al; JPHC Study Group. Prospective study showing that dietary vitamin C reduced the risk of age-related cataracts in a middle-aged Japanese population. Eur J Nutr 2007; 46(2):118–124

36. Simon JA, Hudes ES. Serum ascorbic acid and other correlates of self-reported cataract among older Americans. J Clin Epidemiol 1999;52(12):1207–1211

37. Dherani M, Murthy GV, Gupta SK, et al. Blood levels of vitamin C, carotenoids and retinol are inversely associated with cataract in a North Indian population. Invest Ophthalmol Vis Sci 2008;49(8):3328–3335

38. Age-Related Eye Disease Study Research Group. A randomized, placebo-controlled, clinical trial of high-dose supplementation with vitamins C and E and beta carotene for age-related cataract and vision loss: AREDS report no. 9. Arch Ophthalmol 2001;119 (10):1439–1452

39. Saag KG, Choi H. Epidemiology, risk factors, and lifestyle modifications for gout. Arthritis Res Ther 2006;8(Suppl 1):S2

40. Choi HK, Curhan G. Gout: epidemiology and lifestyle choices. Curr Opin Rheumatol 2005;17(3):341–345

41. Gao X, Curhan G, Forman JP, Ascherio A, Choi HK. Vitamin C intake and serum uric acid concentration in men. J Rheumatol 2008;35(9):1853–1858

42. Choi HK, Gao X, Curhan C. Vitamin C intake and risk of gout in men: a prospective study. Arch Intern Med 2009;169(5):502–507

43. Huang HY, Appel LJ, Choi MJ, et al. The effects of vitamin C supplementation on serum concentrations of uric acid: results of a randomized controlled trial. Arthritis Rheum 2005;52(6):1843–1847

44. Cheng Y, Willett WC, Schwartz J, Sparrow D, Weiss S, Hu H. Relation of nutrition to bone lead and blood lead levels in middle-aged to elderly men. The Normative Aging Study. Am J Epidemiol 1998;147(12):1162–1174

45. Simon JA, Hudes ES. Relationship of ascorbic acid to blood lead levels. JAMA 1999;281(24):2289–2293

46. Lee DH, Lim JS, Song K, Boo Y, Jacobs DR Jr. Graded associations of blood lead and urinary cadmium concentrations with oxidative-stress-related markers in the U.S. population: results from the third National Health and Nutrition Examination Survey. Environ Health Perspect 2006;114(3):350–354

47. Dawson EB, Evans DR, Harris WA, Teter MC, McGanity WJ. The effect of ascorbic acid supplementation on the blood lead levels of smokers. J Am Coll Nutr 1999;18(2):166–170

48. Prinz W, Bortz R, Bregin B, Hersch M. The effect of ascorbic acid supplementation on some parameters of the human immunological defence system. Int J Vitam Nutr Res 1977;47(3):248–257

49. Vallance S. Relationships between ascorbic acid and serum proteins of the immune system. BMJ 1977; 2(6084):437–438

50. Kennes B, Dumont I, Brohee D, Hubert C, Neve P. Effect of vitamin C supplements on cell-mediated immunity in old people. Gerontology 1983;29(5):305–310

51. Panush RS, Delafuente JC, Katz P, Johnson J. Modulation of certain immunologic responses by vitamin C. III. Potentiation of in vitro and in vivo lymphocyte responses. Int J Vitam Nutr Res Suppl 1982;23:35–47

52. Jariwalla RJ, Harakeh S. Antiviral and immunomodulatory activities of ascorbic acid. In: Harris JR, ed. Subcellular Biochemistry, Vol. 25. Ascorbic Acid: Biochemistry and Biomedical Cell Biology. New York: Plenum Press; 1996:215–231

53. Levy R, Shriker O, Porath A, Riesenberg K, Schlaeffer F. Vitamin C for the treatment of recurrent furunculosis in patients with impaired neutrophil functions. J Infect Dis 1996;173(6):1502–1505

54. Anderson R, Oosthuizen R, Maritz R, Theron A, Van Rensburg AJ. The effects of increasing weekly doses of ascorbate on certain cellular and humoral im-

mune functions in normal volunteers. Am J Clin Nutr 1980;33(1):71–76

55. Anderson R. The immunostimulatory, antiinflammatory and anti-allergic properties of ascorbate. Adv Nutr Res 1984;6:19–45

56. Prinz W, Bloch J, Gilich G, Mitchell G. A systematic study of the effect of vitamin C supplementation on the humoral immune response in ascorbate-dependent mammals. I. The antibody response to sheep red blood cells (a T-dependent antigen) in guinea pigs. Int J Vitam Nutr Res 1980;50(3):294–300

57. Feigen GA, Smith BH, Dix CE, et al. Enhancement of antibody production and protection against systemic anaphylaxis by large doses of vitamin C. Res Commun Chem Pathol Pharmacol 1982;38(2):313–333

58. Haskell BE, Johnston CS. Complement component C1q activity and ascorbic acid nutriture in guinea pigs. Am J Clin Nutr 1991; 54(6, Suppl)1:228S–1230S

59. Johnston CS, Cartee GD, Haskell BE. Effect of ascorbic acid nutriture on protein-bound hydroxyproline in guinea pig plasma. J Nutr 1985;115(8):1089–1093

60. Johnston CS, Kolb WP, Haskell BE. The effect of vitamin C nutriture on complement component C1q concentrations in guinea pig plasma. J Nutr 1987; 117(4):764–768

61. Shilotri PG, Bhat KS. Effect of mega doses of vitamin C on bactericidal activity of leukocytes. Am J Clin Nutr 1977;30(7):1077–1081

62. Vogel RI, Lamster IB, Wechsler SA, Macedo B, Hartley LJ, Macedo JA. The effects of megadoses of ascorbic acid on PMN chemotaxis and experimental gingivitis. J Periodontol 1986;57(8):472–479

63. Ludvigsson J, Hansson LO, Stendahl O. The effect of large doses of vitamin C on leukocyte function and some laboratory parameters. Int J Vitam Nutr Res 1979;49(2):160–165

64. Delafuente JC, Prendergast JM, Modigh A. Immunologic modulation by vitamin C in the elderly. Int J Immunopharmacol 1986;8(2):205–211

65. Bergsten P, Amitai G, Kehrl J, Dhariwal KR, Klein HG, Levine M. Millimolar concentrations of ascorbic acid in purified human mononuclear leukocytes. Depletion and reaccumulation. J Biol Chem 1990;265(5):2584–2587

66. Evans RM, Currie L, Campbell A. The distribution of ascorbic acid between various cellular components of blood, in normal individuals, and its relation to the plasma concentration. Br J Nutr 1982;47(3):473–482

67. Alberts B, Bray D, Lewis J, Raff M, Roberts K, Watson JD. Differentiated cells and the maintenance of tissues. In: Molecular Biology of the Cell, 3rd ed. New York: Garland Publishing, Inc.; 1994:1139–1193

68. Jariwalla RJ, Harakeh S. Mechanisms underlying the action of vitamin C in viral and immunodeficiency disease. In: Packer L, Fuchs J, eds. Vitamin C in Health and Disease. New York: Marcel Dekker, Inc.; 1997: 309–322

69. Pauling L. The immune system. In: How to Live Longer and Feel Better, 20th anniversary ed. Corvallis: Oregon State University Press; 2006:105–111

70. Dahl H, Degré M. The effect of ascorbic acid on production of human interferon and the antiviral activity in vitro. Acta Pathol Microbiol Scand [B] 1976; 84B(5):280–284

71. Vita JA, Keaney JF Jr. Endothelial function: a barometer for cardiovascular risk? Circulation 2002;106(6):640–642

72. Gokce N, Keaney JF Jr, Frei B, et al. Long-term ascorbic acid administration reverses endothelial vasomotor dysfunction in patients with coronary artery disease. Circulation 1999;99(25):3234–3240

73. Versari D, Daghini E, Virdis A, Ghiadoni L, Taddei S. Endothelium-dependent contractions and endothelial dysfunction in human hypertension. Br J Pharmacol 2009;157(4):527–536

74. Frikke-Schmidt H, Lykkesfeldt J. Role of marginal vitamin C deficiency in atherogenesis: in vivo models and clinical studies. Basic Clin Pharmacol Toxicol 2009;104(6):419–433

75. Ness AR, Chee D, Elliott P. Vitamin C and blood pressure—an overview. J Hum Hypertens 1997;11(6):343–350

76. Ward NC, Hodgson JM, Croft KD, Burke V, Beilin LJ, Puddey IB. The combination of vitamin C and grape-seed polyphenols increases blood pressure: a randomized, double-blind, placebo-controlled trial. J Hypertens 2005;23(2):427–434

77. Duffy SJ, Gokce N, Holbrook M, et al. Treatment of hypertension with ascorbic acid. Lancet 1999; 354(9195):2048–2049

78. Cameron E, Pauling L. Supplemental ascorbate in the supportive treatment of cancer: Prolongation of survival times in terminal human cancer. Proc Natl Acad Sci U S A 1976;73(10):3685–3689

79. Creagan ET, Moertel CG, O'Fallon JR, et al. Failure of high-dose vitamin C (ascorbic acid) therapy to benefit patients with advanced cancer. A controlled trial. N Engl J Med 1979;301(13):687–690

80. Moertel CG, Fleming TR, Creagan ET, Rubin J, O'Connell MJ, Ames MM. High-dose vitamin C versus placebo in the treatment of patients with advanced cancer who have had no prior chemotherapy. A randomized double-blind comparison. N Engl J Med 1985;312(3):137–141

81. Padayatty SJ, Sun H, Wang Y, et al. Vitamin C pharmacokinetics: implications for oral and intravenous use. Ann Intern Med 2004;140(7):533–537

82. Chen Q, Espey MG, Krishna MC, et al. Pharmacologic ascorbic acid concentrations selectively kill cancer cells: action as a pro-drug to deliver hydrogen peroxide to tissues. Proc Natl Acad Sci USA 2005; 102(38):13604–13609

83. Chen Q, Espey MG, Sun AY, et al. Ascorbate in pharmacologic concentrations selectively generates ascorbate radical and hydrogen peroxide in extracellular fluid in vivo. Proc Natl Acad Sci U S A 2007;104(21): 8749–8754

84. Chen Q, Espey MG, Sun AY, et al. Pharmacologic doses of ascorbate act as a prooxidant and decrease growth of aggressive tumor xenografts in mice. Proc Natl Acad Sci U S A 2008;105(32):11105–11109

85. Riordan HD, Casciari JJ, González MJ, et al. A pilot clinical study of continuous intravenous ascorbate in terminal cancer patients. P R Health Sci J 2005;24(4): 269–276

86. Hoffer LJ, Levine M, Assouline S, et al. Phase I clinical trial of i.v. ascorbic acid in advanced malignancy. Ann Oncol 2008;19(11):1969–1974

87. U.S. National Institutes of Health. ClinicalTrials.gov [Web page]. Available at: http://www.clinicaltrials.gov/. Accessed 4 Jan 2011

88. Padayatty SJ, Riordan HD, Hewitt SM, Katz A, Hoffer LJ, Levine M. Intravenously administered vitamin C as cancer therapy: three cases. CMAJ 2006; 174(7):937–942

89. Drisko JA, Chapman J, Hunter VJ. The use of antioxidants with first-line chemotherapy in two cases of ovarian cancer. J Am Coll Nutr 2003;22(2):118–123

90. Kaegi E, Task Force on Alternative Therapeutics of the Canadian Breast Cancer Research Initiative. Unconventional therapies for cancer: 5. Vitamins A, C, and E. CMAJ 1998;158(11):1483–1488

91. Lee DH, Folsom AR, Harnack L, Halliwell B, Jacobs DR Jr. Does supplemental vitamin C increase cardiovascular disease risk in women with diabetes? Am J Clin Nutr 2004;80(5):1194–1200

92. Waters DD, Alderman EL, Hsia J, et al. Effects of hormone replacement therapy and antioxidant vitamin supplements on coronary atherosclerosis in postmenopausal women: a randomized controlled trial. JAMA 2002;288(19):2432–2440

93. Heart Protection Study Collaborative Group. MRC/BHF Heart Protection Study of antioxidant vitamin supplementation in 20,536 high-risk individuals: a randomised placebo-controlled trial. Lancet 2002; 360(9326):23–33

94. Levy AP, Friedenberg P, Lotan R, et al. The effect of vitamin therapy on the progression of coronary artery atherosclerosis varies by haptoglobin type in postmenopausal women. Diabetes Care 2004;27(4): 925–930

95. Pauling LC. Vitamin C and the Common Cold. San Francisco, CA: WH Freeman, 1970

96. Douglas RM, Hemila H, D'Souza R, Chalker EB, Treacy B. Vitamin C for preventing and treating the common cold. Cochrane Database Syst Rev 2004; (4):CD000980

97. Sasazuki S, Sasaki S, Tsubono Y, Okubo S, Hayashi M, Tsugane S. Effect of vitamin C on common cold: randomized controlled trial. Eur J Clin Nutr 2006;60(1): 9–17

98. Sardi W. Narrow scope of vitamin C review. PLoS Med 2005;2(9):e308; author reply e309

99. Hickey S, Roberts H. Misleading information on the properties of vitamin C. PLoS Med 2005;2(9):e307; author reply e309

100. US Department of Agriculture, Agricultural Research Service. USDA National Nutrient Database for Standard Reference, Release 22. 2009. Available at: http://www.nal.usda.gov/fnic/foodcomp/search/. Accessed 4 Jan 2011

101. Gregory JF III. Ascorbic acid bioavailability in foods and supplements. Nutr Rev 1993;51(10):301–303

102. Johnston CS, Luo B. Comparison of the absorption and excretion of three commercially available sources of vitamin C. J Am Diet Assoc 1994;94(7):779–781

103. Song J, Kwon O, Chen S, et al. Flavonoid inhibition of sodium-dependent vitamin C transporter 1 (SVCT1) and glucose transporter isoform 2 (GLUT2), intestinal transporters for vitamin C and Glucose. J Biol Chem 2002;277(18):15252–15260

104. Park JB, Levine M. Intracellular accumulation of ascorbic acid is inhibited by flavonoids via blocking of dehydroascorbic acid and ascorbic acid uptakes in HL-60, U937 and Jurkat cells. J Nutr 2000;130(5): 1297–1302

105. Kwon O, Eck P, Chen S, et al. Inhibition of the intestinal glucose transporter GLUT2 by flavonoids. FASEB J 2007;21(2):366–377

106. Austria R, Semenzato A, Bettero A. Stability of vitamin C derivatives in solution and topical formulations. J Pharm Biomed Anal 1997;15(6):795–801

107. De Ritter E, Cohen N, Rubin SH. Physiological availability of dehydro-L-ascorbic acid and palmitoyl-L-ascorbic acid. Science 1951;113(2944):628–631

108. Lee SH, Oe T, Blair IA. Vitamin C-induced decomposition of lipid hydroperoxides to endogenous genotoxins. Science 2001;292(5524):2083–2086

109. Podmore ID, Griffiths HR, Herbert KE, Mistry N, Mistry P, Lunec J. Vitamin C exhibits pro-oxidant properties. Nature 1998;392(6676):559

110. Carr A, Frei B. Does vitamin C act as a pro-oxidant under physiological conditions? FASEB J 1999;13(9): 1007–1024

111. Traxer O, Huet B, Poindexter J, Pak CY, Pearle MS. Effect of ascorbic acid consumption on urinary stone risk factors. J Urol 2003;170(2 Pt 1):397–401

112. Levine M, Conry-Cantilena C, Wang Y, et al. Vitamin C pharmacokinetics in healthy volunteers: evidence for a recommended dietary allowance. Proc Natl Acad Sci U S A 1996;93(8):3704–3709

113. Massey LK, Liebman M, Kynast-Gales SA. Ascorbate increases human oxaluria and kidney stone risk. J Nutr 2005;135(7):1673–1677

114. Auer BL, Auer D, Rodgers AL. The effect of ascorbic acid ingestion on the biochemical and physicochemical risk factors associated with calcium oxalate kidney stone formation. Clin Chem Lab Med 1998;36(3):143–147

115. Liebman M, Chai W, Harvey E, Boenisch L. Effect of supplemental ascorbate and orange juice on urinary oxalate. Nutr Res 1997;17(3):415–425

116. Wandzilak TR, D'Andre SD, Davis PA, Williams HE. Effect of high dose vitamin C on urinary oxalate levels. J Urol 1994;151(4):834–837

117. Taylor EN, Stampfer MJ, Curhan GC. Dietary factors and the risk of incident kidney stones in men: new insights after 14 years of follow-up. J Am Soc Nephrol 2004;15(12):3225–3232

118. Basu TK. Vitamin C-aspirin interactions. Int J Vitam Nutr Res Suppl 1982;23:83–90

119. Hendler SS, Rorvik DR, eds. PDR for Nutritional Supplements. Montvale: Medical Economics Co., Inc.; 2001

120. Brown BG, Zhao XQ, Chait A, et al. Simvastatin and niacin, antioxidant vitamins, or the combination for the prevention of coronary disease. N Engl J Med 2001;345(22):1583–1592

121. Collins R, Peto R, Armitage J. The MRC/BHF Heart Protection Study: preliminary results. Int J Clin Pract 2002;56(1):53–56

122. Brubacher D, Moser U, Jordan P. Vitamin C concentrations in plasma as a function of intake: a meta-analysis. Int J Vitam Nutr Res 2000;70(5):226–237

123. Michels AJ, Joisher N, Hagen TM. Age-related decline of sodium-dependent ascorbic acid transport in isolated rat hepatocytes. Arch Biochem Biophys 2003;410(1):112–120

11 Vitamin D

Vitamin D is a fat-soluble vitamin that is essential for maintaining normal calcium metabolism.[1] Vitamin D_3 (cholecalciferol) can be synthesized by humans in the skin on exposure to ultraviolet B (UVB) radiation from sunlight, or it can be obtained from the diet. Plants synthesize ergosterol, which is converted to vitamin D_2 (ergocalciferol) by UV light.[2] When exposure to UVB radiation is insufficient for the synthesis of adequate amounts of vitamin D_3 in the skin, adequate intake of vitamin D from the diet is essential for health.

Function

Activation of Vitamin D

Vitamin D is itself biologically inactive, and it must be metabolized to its biologically active forms. After it is consumed in the diet or synthesized in the epidermis of skin, vitamin D enters the circulation and is transported to the liver. In the liver, vitamin D is hydroxylated to form 25-hydroxyvitamin D (calcidiol, the major circulating form of vitamin D). Increased exposure to sunlight or increased dietary intake of vitamin D increases serum levels of 25-hydroxyvitamin D, making the serum concentration a useful indicator of vitamin D nutritional status. In the kidney, the enzyme 25-hydroxyvitamin D_3-1-hydroxylase catalyzes a second hydroxylation of 25-hydroxyvitamin D, resulting in the formation of 1,25-dihydroxyvitamin D (calcitriol, $1\alpha,25$-dihydroxyvitamin D)—the most potent form of vitamin D. Most of the physiological effects of vitamin D in the body are related to the activity of 1,25-dihydroxyvitamin D.[2]

Mechanisms of Action

Most if not all actions of vitamin D are mediated through a nuclear transcription factor known as the *vitamin D receptor* (VDR).[3] Upon entering the nucleus of a cell, 1,25-dihydroxyvitamin D associates with the VDR and promotes its association with the retinoic acid X receptor (RXR). In the presence of 1,25-dihydroxyvitamin D the VDR/RXR complex binds small sequences of DNA known as *vitamin D response elements* (VDREs) and initiates a cascade of molecular interactions that modulate the transcription of specific genes. More than 50 genes in tissues throughout the body are known to be regulated by 1,25-dihydroxyvitamin D.[4]

Calcium Balance

Maintenance of serum calcium levels within a narrow range is vital for normal functioning of the nervous system, as well as for bone growth and maintenance of bone density. Vitamin D is essential for the efficient utilization of calcium by the body.[1] The parathyroid glands sense serum calcium levels and secrete parathyroid hormone (PTH) if calcium levels drop too low (**Fig. 11.1**). Elevations in PTH increase the activity of the 25-hydroxyvitamin D_3-1-hydroxylase enzyme in the kidney, resulting in increased production of 1,25-dihydroxyvitamin D. This increased production in turn results in changes in gene expression that normalize serum calcium by:

- increasing the intestinal absorption of dietary calcium
- increasing the reabsorption of calcium filtered by the kidneys
- mobilizing calcium from bone when there is insufficient dietary calcium to maintain normal serum calcium levels.

PTH and 1,25-dihydroxyvitamin D are required for these last two effects.[5]

Cell Differentiation

Cells that are dividing rapidly are said to be proliferating. Differentiation results in the specialization of cells for specific functions. In general, differentiation of cells leads to a decrease in proliferation. Although cellular proliferation is essential for growth and wound healing, uncontrolled proliferation of cells with certain mutations may lead to diseases such as cancer. The

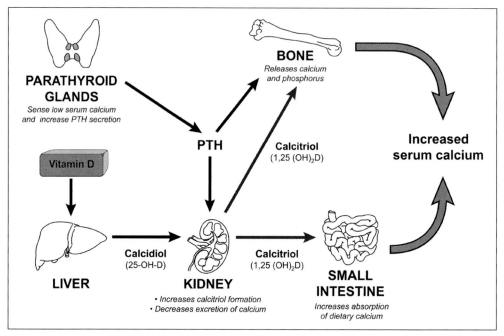

Fig. 11.1 The vitamin D endocrine system. Calcium-sensing proteins in the parathyroid glands sense serum calcium levels. In response to slight declines in serum calcium, the parathyroid glands secrete parathyroid hormone (PTH). PTH stimulates the activity of the 1-hydroxylase enzyme in the kidney, resulting in increased production of calcitriol, the biologically active form of vitamin D. Calcitriol acts to restore normal serum calcium levels in three ways: (1) by activating the vitamin D–dependent transport system in the small intestine, increasing the absorption of dietary calcium; (2) by increasing the mobilization of calcium from bone into the circulation; and (3) by increasing the reabsorption of calcium by the kidneys. PTH is also required to increase bone calcium mobilization and calcium reabsorption by the kidneys.

active form of vitamin D, 1,25-dihydroxyvitamin D, inhibits proliferation and stimulates the differentiation of cells.[1]

Immunity

Vitamin D in the form of 1,25-dihydroxyvitamin D is a potent immune system modulator. The VDR is expressed by most cells of the immune system, including T cells and antigen-presenting cells, such as dendritic cells and macrophages.[6] Under some circumstances, macrophages also produce 25-hydroxyvitamin D_3-1-hydroxylase which converts 25-hydroxyvitamin D to 1,25-dihydroxyvitamin D.[7] There is considerable scientific evidence that 1,25-dihydroxyvitamin D has a variety of effects on immune system function, which may enhance innate immunity and inhibit the development of autoimmunity.[8]

Insulin Secretion

The VDR is expressed by insulin-secreting cells of the pancreas, and the results of animal studies suggest that 1,25-dihydroxyvitamin D plays a role in insulin secretion under conditions of increased insulin demand.[9] Limited data in humans suggest that insufficient vitamin D levels may have an adverse effect on insulin secretion and glucose tolerance in type 2 diabetes.[10–12]

Blood Pressure Regulation

The renin–angiotensin system plays an important role in the regulation of blood pressure.[13] Renin is an enzyme that catalyzes the cleavage (splitting) of a small peptide (angiotensin I) from a larger protein (angiotensinogen) produced in the liver. Angiotensin-converting enzyme (ACE) catalyzes the cleavage of angiotensin I to angiotensin II, a peptide that can increase blood pressure by inducing the constriction of small arteries and increasing sodium and water retention. The rate of angiotensin II synthesis is dependent on renin.[14] Research in mice lacking the gene encoding the VDR indicates that 1,25-dihydroxyvitamin D decreases the expression of the gene encoding renin through its interaction with the VDR.[15] As inappropriate activation of the renin–angiotensin system is thought to play a role in some forms of human hypertension, adequate vitamin D levels may be important for decreasing the risk of high blood pressure.

Deficiency

In vitamin D deficiency, calcium absorption cannot be increased enough to satisfy the body's calcium needs.[2] Consequently, PTH production by the parathyroid glands is increased and calcium is mobilized from the skeleton to maintain normal serum calcium levels—a condition known as *secondary hyperparathyroidism*. Although it has long been known that severe vitamin D deficiency has serious consequences for bone health, recent research suggests that less obvious states of vitamin D deficiency are common and increase the risk of osteoporosis and other health problems.[16,17]

Severe Vitamin D Deficiency

Rickets. In infants and children, severe vitamin D deficiency results in the failure of bone to mineralize. Rapidly growing bones are most severely affected by rickets. The growth plates of bones continue to enlarge, but, in the absence of adequate mineralization, weight-bearing limbs (arms and legs) become bowed. In infants, rickets may result in delayed closure of the fontanel (soft spot) in the skull, and the ribcage may become deformed due to the pulling action of the diaphragm. In severe cases, low serum calcium levels (hypocalcemia) may cause seizures. Although fortification of foods has led to complacency about vitamin D deficiency, nutritional rickets is still being reported in cities throughout the world.[18,19]

Osteomalacia. Although adult bones are no longer growing, they are in a constant state of turnover, or "remodeling." In adults with severe vitamin D deficiency, the collagenous bone matrix is preserved but bone mineral is progressively lost, resulting in bone pain and osteomalacia (soft bones).

Muscle weakness and pain. Vitamin D deficiency causes muscle weakness and pain in children and adults. Muscle pain and weakness were prominent symptoms of vitamin D deficiency in a study of Arab and Danish Moslem women living in Denmark.[20] In a cross-sectional study of 150 consecutive patients referred to a clinic in Minnesota for the evaluation of persistent, nonspecific, musculoskeletal pain, 93% had serum 25-hydroxyvitamin D levels indicative of vitamin D deficiency.[21] A randomized controlled trial found that supplementation of elderly women with 800 IU/day of vitamin D and 1200 mg/day of calcium for 3 months increased muscle strength and decreased the risk of falling by almost 50% compared with supplementation with calcium alone.[22] More recently, a randomized controlled trial in 124 nursing home residents (average age 89 years) found that those taking 800 IU/day of supplemental vitamin D had a 72% lower fall rate than those taking a placebo.[23]

Risk Factors for Vitamin D Deficiency

Exclusively breast-fed infants. Infants who are exclusively breast-fed and do not receive vitamin D supplementation are at high risk of vitamin D deficiency, particularly if they have dark skin and/or receive little sun exposure.[19] Human milk generally provides 25 IU vitamin D per liter, which is not enough for an infant if it is the sole source of vitamin D. Older infants and toddlers exclusively fed milk substitutes and weaning foods that are not vitamin D fortified are also at risk of vitamin D deficiency.[18] The American Academy of Pediatrics recommends that all breast-fed and partially breast-fed infants be given a vitamin D supplement of 400 IU/day.[19]

Dark skin. People with dark-colored skin synthesize less vitamin D on exposure to sunlight than those with light-colored skin.[1] The risk of vitamin D deficiency is particularly high in dark-skinned people who live far from the equator. One US study reported that 42% of African–American women aged between 15 and 49 years were vitamin D deficient compared with 4% of white women.[24]

Elderly people. Elderly people have a reduced capacity to synthesize vitamin D in skin when exposed to UVB radiation, and they are more likely to stay indoors or use sunscreen, which blocks vitamin D synthesis. Institutionalized adults who are not supplemented with vitamin D are at extremely high risk of vitamin D deficiency.[25,26]

Covering all exposed skin or using sunscreen whenever outside. Osteomalacia has been documented in women who cover all their skin whenever they are outside for religious or cultural reasons.[27,28] The application of sunscreen with an SPF factor of 8 reduces production of vitamin D by 95%.[1]

Fat malabsorption syndromes. Cystic fibrosis and cholestatic liver disease impair the absorption of dietary vitamin D.[29]

Inflammatory bowel disease. People with an inflammatory bowel disease such as Crohn disease appear to be at increased risk of vitamin D deficiency, especially those who have had small bowel resections.[30]

Obesity. Obesity increases the risk of vitamin D deficiency.[31] Once vitamin D is synthesized in the skin or ingested, it is deposited in body fat stores, making it less bioavailable to people with large stores of body fat.

Assessing Vitamin D Nutritional Status

Growing awareness that vitamin D insufficiency has serious health consequences beyond rickets and osteomalacia highlights the need for accurate assessment of vitamin D nutritional status. Although there is general agreement that serum 25-hydroxyvitamin D level is the best indicator of vitamin D deficiency and sufficiency, the cutoff values have not been clearly defined.[18] While laboratory reference ranges for serum 25-hydroxyvitamin D levels are often based on average values from populations of healthy individuals, recent research suggests that health-based cutoff values aimed at preventing secondary hyperparathyroidism and bone loss should be consid-

erably higher. In general, serum 25-hydroxyvitamin D values less than 20–25 nmol/L (8–10 ng/mL) indicate severe deficiency associated with rickets and osteomalacia.[16,18] Although 50 nmol/L (20 ng/mL) has been suggested as the low end of the normal range,[32] more recent research suggests that PTH levels[33,34] and calcium absorption[35] are not optimized until serum 25-hydroxyvitamin D levels reach approximately 80 nmol/L (32 ng/mL). Thus, at least one vitamin D expert has argued that serum 25-hydroxyvitamin D values less than 80 nmol/L should be considered deficient,[17] whereas another suggests that a healthy serum 25-hydroxyvitamin D value is between 75 and 125 nmol/L (30 and 50 ng/mL).[36] With this latter cutoff value for insufficiency (i.e., 75 nmol/L or 30 ng/mL), it is estimated that one billion people in the world are currently vitamin D deficient.[37] Data from supplementation studies indicate that vitamin D intakes of at least 800–1000 IU/day are required by adults living in temperate latitudes to achieve serum 25-hydroxyvitamin D levels of at least 80 nmol/L.[38,39]

Recommended Dietary Allowance

In 2010, the Food and Nutrition Board (FNB) of the Institute of Medicine set a recommended dietary allowance (RDA) based on the amount of vitamin D needed for bone health. While the recommended intake was increased from the adequate intake set in 1997, some experts feel that this level is still too low to result in sufficient 25-hydroxyvitamin D levels[40–43]. The American Academy of Pediatrics currently recommends 400 IU/day for all infants, children, and adolescents.[19] The RDA for vitamin D is listed in **Table 11.1** by life stage and gender.

Table 11.1 Recommended dietary allowance (RDA) for vitamin D

Life stage	Age	Males (µg/day) (IU)	Females (µg/day) (IU)
Infants	0–6 months	10 (400) (AI)	10 (400) (AI)
Infants	6–12 months	10 (400) (AI)	10 (400) (AI))
Children	1–3 years	15 (600)	15 (600)
Children	4–8 years	15 (600)	15 (600)
Children	9–13 years	15 (600)	15 (600)
Adolescents	14–18 years	15 (600)	15 (600)
Adults	19–50 years	15 (600)	15 (600)
Adults	51–70 years	15 (600)	15 (600)
Adults	≥71 years	20 (800)	20 (800)
Pregnancy	All ages	–	15 (600)
Breast-feeding	All ages	–	15 (600)

AI, adequate intake.

Disease Prevention

Osteoporosis

Although osteoporosis is a multifactorial disease, vitamin D insufficiency can be an important contributing factor. A multinational (18 different countries with latitudes ranging from 64° north to 38° south) survey of more than 2600 postmenopausal women with osteoporosis revealed that 64% had 25-hydroxyvitamin D levels lower than 75 nmol/L (30 ng/mL).[44] Without sufficient vitamin D from sun exposure or dietary intake, intestinal calcium absorption cannot be maximized. This causes PTH secretion by the parathyroid glands; elevated PTH results in increased bone resorption, which may lead to osteoporotic fracture.[45] A prospective cohort study that followed more than 72000 postmenopausal women in the United States for 18 years found that those who consumed at least 600 IU/day of vitamin D from diet and supplements had a 37% lower risk of osteoporotic hip fracture than women who consumed less than 140 IU/day of vitamin D.[46]

The results of most clinical trials suggest that vitamin D supplementation can slow bone density losses or decrease the risk of osteoporotic fracture in men and women who are unlikely to be getting enough vitamin D. However, recent analyses indicate that there is a threshold of vitamin D intake that is necessary to observe reductions in fracture risk. For instance, a recent meta-analysis of randomized controlled trials in older adults found that supplementation with 700–800 IU vitamin D daily had a 26% and 23% lower risk of hip fracture and nonvertebral fracture, respectively. In contrast, supplementation with 400 IU vitamin D daily did not decrease risk of either hip or nonvertebral fracture.[47] In addition, recent results from the Women's Health Initiative trial in 36282 postmenopausal women showed that daily supplementation with 400 IU vitamin D_3, in combination with 1000 mg calcium, did not significantly reduce risk of hip fracture compared with a placebo.[48] Bischoff-Ferrari et al. suggest that daily intakes of more than 700 IU vitamin D may be necessary to optimize serum concentrations of 25-hydroxyvitamin D and thus reduce fracture risk.[40]

Support for such a threshold effect of vitamin D on bone health also comes from previous studies. One study in 247 postmenopausal US women reported that supplementation with 500 mg/day of calcium and either 100 IU/day or 700 IU/day of vitamin D_3 for 2 years slowed bone density losses at the hip only in the group taking 700 IU/day.[49] Another study found that daily supplementation of elderly men and women with 500 mg/day of calcium and 700 IU/day of vitamin D_3 for 3 years reduced bone density losses at the hip and spine and also reduced the frequency of nonvertebral fractures.[50] A subsequent analysis of this cohort revealed that, when the calcium and vitamin D_3 supplements were discontinued, the bone density benefits were lost within 2 years.[51] Another study found that oral supplementation with

800 IU/day of vitamin D_3 and 1200 mg/day of calcium for 3 years decreased the incidence of hip fracture in elderly French women.[52] Further, oral supplementation of elderly adults in the UK with 100 000 IU vitamin D_3 once every 4 months (equivalent to about 800 IU/day) for 5 years reduced the risk of osteoporotic fracture by 33% compared with placebo.[53] However, oral supplementation with 400 IU/day of vitamin D_3 for more than 3 years did not affect the incidence of fracture in a study of elderly Dutch men and women.[54] All of these studies indicate that at least 700 IU vitamin D_3 daily may be required to observe a beneficial effect on fracture incidence.

However, the Randomised Evaluation of Calcium Or vitamin D (RECORD) trial reported that oral supplemental vitamin D_3 (800 IU/day) alone, or in combination with calcium (1000 mg/day), did not prevent the occurrence of osteoporotic fractures in elderly adults who had already experienced a low-trauma, osteoporotic fracture.[55] The lack of an effect could possibly be due to low compliance in this study or the fact that vitamin D supplementation did not raise serum 25-hydroxyvitamin D levels to a level that would protect against fractures.[40]

To date, clinical trials have generally found that vitamin D_2 (ergocalciferol) is not effective at preventing fractures.[56] Overall, the current evidence suggests that vitamin D_3 supplements of at least 800 IU/day may be helpful in reducing bone loss and fracture rates in elderly people. For vitamin D supplementation to be effective in preserving bone health, adequate dietary calcium (1000–1200 mg/day) should also be consumed (see Chapter 14).

Cancer

Two characteristics of cancer cells are lack of differentiation (specialization) and rapid growth or proliferation. Many malignant tumors have been found to contain vitamin D receptors (VDRs), including breast, lung, skin (melanoma), colon, and bone. Biologically active forms of vitamin D, such as 1,25-dihydroxyvitamin D and its analogs, have been found to induce cell differentiation and/or inhibit proliferation of a number of cancerous and noncancerous cell types maintained in cell culture.[57] Results of some, but not all, human epidemiological studies suggest that vitamin D may protect against various cancers. However, it is important to note that epidemiological studies cannot prove such associations.

Colorectal cancer. The geographic distribution of colon cancer mortality resembles the historical geographic distribution of rickets,[58] providing circumstantial evidence that decreased sunlight exposure and diminished vitamin D nutritional status may be related to an increased risk of colon cancer. However, prospective cohort studies have not generally found total vitamin D intake to be associated with significant reductions in risk of colorectal cancer when other risk factors are taken into account.[59-62] However, some more recent studies have reported that higher vitamin D intakes and serum 25-hydroxyvitamin D levels are associated with reductions in colorectal cancer risk. One 5-year study of more than 120 000 people found that men with the highest vitamin D intakes had a risk of colorectal cancer that was 29% lower than men with the lowest vitamin D intakes.[63] Vitamin D intake in this study was not significantly associated with colorectal cancer risk in women. Moreover, serum 25-hydroxyvitamin D level, which reflects vitamin D intake and vitamin D synthesis, was inversely associated with the risk of potentially precancerous colorectal polyps [64] and indices of colonic epithelial cell proliferation,[65] two biomarkers for colon cancer risk.

More recently, a case–control analysis from the Nurses' Health Study cohort reported that plasma 25-hydroxyvitamin D levels were inversely associated with colorectal cancer.[66] A randomized, double-blind, placebo-controlled trial in 36 282 postmenopausal women participating in the Women's Health Initiative study found that a combination of supplemental vitamin D (400 IU/day) and calcium (1000 mg/day) did not lower the incidence of colorectal cancer.[67] However, it has been suggested that the daily vitamin D dose, 400 IU, was too low to detect any effect on cancer incidence.[68] In fact, a recent dose–response analysis estimated that 1000 IU oral vitamin D daily would lower one's risk of colorectal cancer by 50%.[69]

Breast cancer. Although breast cancer mortality follows a similar geographic distribution to that of colon cancer,[58,70] direct evidence of an association between vitamin D nutritional status and breast cancer risk is limited. A prospective study of women who participated in the first National Health and Nutrition Examination Survey (NHANES I) found that several measures of sunlight exposure and dietary vitamin D intake were associated with a reduced risk of breast cancer 20 years later.[71] More recently, a 16-year study of more than 88 000 women found that higher intakes of vitamin D were associated with significantly lower breast cancer risk in premenopausal women but not postmenopausal women.[72] Garland et al. conducted a pooled, dose–response analysis of two case–control studies in which women with breast cancer had significantly lower plasma 25-hydroxyvitamin D levels compared with controls.[73,74] These authors reported that women with a 25-hydroxyvitamin D level of 52 ng/mL (130 nmol/L) experienced a 50% lower risk of developing breast cancer compared with women with 25-hydroxyvitamin D levels lower than 13 ng/mL (32.5 nmol/L).[75] The authors state that, to obtain a 25-hydroxyvitamin D level of 52 ng/mL, around 4000 IU vitamin D_3 would need to be consumed daily, or 2000 IU vitamin D_3 daily plus very moderate sun exposure.[75] The current tolerable upper limit of intake (UL) for adults, set by the FNB of the Institute of Medicine, is 4000 IU/day (see "Safety," p. 91).

Prostate cancer. Epidemiological studies show correlations between risk factors for prostate cancer and conditions that can result in decreased vitamin D levels.[57] Increased age is associated with an increased risk of prostate cancer, as well as with decreased sun exposure and decreased capacity to synthesize vitamin D. The incidence of prostate cancer is higher in African-American men than in white American men, and the high melanin content of dark skin is known to reduce the efficiency of vitamin D synthesis. Geographically, mortality from prostate cancer is inversely associated with the availability of sunlight. Findings that prostate cells in culture can synthesize the 25-hydroxyvitamin D_3-1-hydroxylase enzyme and that, unlike the renal enzyme, its synthesis is not influenced by PTH or calcium levels also provide support for the idea that increasing 25-hydroxyvitamin D levels may be useful in preventing prostate cancer.[76] In contrast, prospective studies have not generally found significant relationships between serum 25-hydroxyvitamin D levels and subsequent risk of developing prostate cancer.[77–80] Although a pro-

spective study of Finnish men found that low serum 25-hydroxyvitamin D levels were associated with earlier and more aggressive prostate cancer development,[81] another prospective study of men from Finland, Norway, and Sweden found a U-shaped relationship between serum 25-hydroxyvitamin D levels and prostate cancer risk. In that study serum 25-hydroxyvitamin D concentrations of 19 nmol/L or lower and 80 nmol/L or higher were associated with higher prostate cancer risk.[82] Further research is needed to determine the nature of the relationship between vitamin D nutritional status and prostate cancer risk.

Autoimmune Diseases

Type 1 diabetes mellitus, multiple sclerosis (MS), and rheumatoid arthritis (RA) are examples of autoimmune diseases. Autoimmune diseases occur when the body mounts an immune response against its own tissue, rather than a foreign pathogen. In type 1 diabetes mellitus, insulin-producing β cells of the pancreas are the target of the inappropriate immune response. In MS, the target is the myelin-producing cells of the central nervous system and, in RA, the target is the collagen-producing cells of the joints.[83] Autoimmune responses are mediated by T lymphocytes (T cells). The biologically active form of vitamin D, 1,25-dihydroxyvitamin D, has been found to modulate T-cell responses, such that the autoimmune responses are diminished. Epidemiological studies have found that the prevalence of type 1 diabetes, MS, and RA increases as latitude increases, suggesting that lower exposure to UVB radiation and associated decreases in endogenous vitamin D synthesis may play a role in the pathology of these diseases. The results of several prospective cohort studies also suggest that adequate vitamin D intake could possibly decrease the risk of autoimmune diseases. A prospective cohort study of children born in Finland during the year 1966 and followed for 30 years found that those who received supplemental vitamin D during the first year of life had a significantly lower risk of developing type 1 diabetes, while children suspected of developing rickets (severe vitamin D deficiency) during the first year of life had a significantly higher risk of developing type 1 diabetes.[84] Vitamin D deficiency has also been implicated in MS.

A recent case–control study in US military personnel, including 257 cases of diagnosed MS, found that white individuals in the highest quintile (one-fifth) of serum 25-hydroxyvitamin D (> 99.1 nmol/L) had a 62% lower risk of developing MS.[85] A relationship between this indicator of vitamin D status and MS was not observed in black or Hispanic individuals, but the power to detect such an association was limited by small sample sizes and overall low serum 25-hydroxyvitamin D concentrations.[85] In two large cohorts of US women followed for at least 10 years, vitamin D supplement use was associated with a significant reduction in the risk of developing MS.[86] Similarly, postmenopausal women with the highest total vitamin D intakes were at significantly lower risk of developing RA after 11 years of follow-up than those with the lowest intakes.[87] Thus, evidence from both animal model studies and human epidemiological studies suggests that maintaining sufficient vitamin D levels could possibly help decrease the risk of several autoimmune diseases.

Hypertension

The results of epidemiological and clinical studies suggest an inverse relationship between serum 1,25-dihydroxyvitamin D levels and blood pressure, which may be explained by recent findings that 1,25-dihydroxyvitamin D decreases the expression of the gene encoding renin. Data from epidemiological studies suggest that conditions that decrease vitamin D synthesis in the skin, such as having dark-colored skin or living in temperate latitudes, are associated with increased prevalence of hypertension.[88] A controlled clinical trial in 18 hypertensive men and women living in the Netherlands found that exposure to UVB radiation three times weekly for 6 weeks during the winter increased serum 25-hydroxyvitamin D levels and significantly decreased 24-hour ambulatory systolic and diastolic blood pressure measurements by an average of 6 mmHg.[89] In randomized controlled trials of vitamin D supplementation, a combination of 1600 IU/day of vitamin D and 800 mg/day of calcium for 8 weeks significantly decreased systolic blood pressure in elderly women by 9% compared with calcium alone,[90] but supplementation with 400 IU vitamin D daily or a single dose of 100 000 IU vitamin D did not significantly lower blood pressure in elderly men and women over a 2-month period.[91,92] At present, data from controlled clinical trials are too limited to determine whether vitamin D supplementation will be effective in lowering blood pressure or preventing hypertension.

Sources

Sunlight

Solar UVB radiation (wavelengths of 290–315 nm) stimulates the production of vitamin D_3 in the epidermis of the skin.[93] Sunlight exposure can provide most people with their entire vitamin D requirement. Children and young adults who spend a short time outside two or three times a week will generally synthesize all the vitamin D that they need to prevent deficiency. One study reported that serum vitamin D concentrations after exposure to one minimal erythemal dose of simulated sunlight (the amount required to cause a slight pinkness of the skin) was equivalent to ingesting approximately 20 000 IU vitamin D_2.[94] People with dark-colored skin synthesize markedly less vitamin D on exposure to sunlight than those with light-colored skin.[1] In addition, elderly people have a diminished capacity to synthesize vitamin D from sunlight exposure and frequently use sunscreen or protective clothing in order to prevent skin cancer and sun damage. The application of sunscreen with an SPF factor of 8 reduces production of vitamin D by 95%. In latitudes around 40° north or 40° south (Boston is 42° north), there is insufficient UVB radiation available for vitamin D synthesis from November to early March. Ten degrees farther north or south (Edmonton, Canada) the "vitamin D winter" extends from mid-October to mid-March. According to Michael Holick, as little as 5–10 min of sun exposure on the arms and legs or face and arms three times weekly between 11 a. m. and 2 p. m. during the spring, summer, and fall at 42° latitude should provide a light-skinned individual with adequate vitamin D and allow for storage of any excess for use during the winter with minimal risk of skin damage.[36]

Table 11.2 Food sources of vitamin D

Food	Serving	Vitamin D (IU)	Vitamin D (µg)
Pink salmon, canned	3 ounces[a]	530	13.3
Sardines, canned	3 ounces[a]	231	5.8
Mackerel, canned	3 ounces[a]	213	5.3
Soy milk, fortified with vitamin D	8 ounces	100	2.5
Orange juice, fortified with vitamin D	8 ounces	100	2.5
Cow's milk, fortified with vitamin D	8 ounces	98	2.5
Cereal, fortified	1 serving (usually 1 cup)	40–50	1.0–1.3
Egg yolk	1 large	21	0.53

[a]A 3-ounce serving of meat or fish is about the size of a deck of cards.

Food Sources

Vitamin D is found naturally in very few foods. Foods containing vitamin D include some fatty fish (mackerel, salmon, sardines), fish liver oils, and eggs from hens that have been fed vitamin D. In the United States, milk and infant formula are fortified with vitamin D so that they contain 400 IU (10 µg) per quart. However, other dairy products, such as cheese and yogurt, are not always fortified with vitamin D. Some cereals and breads are also fortified with vitamin D. Recently, orange juice fortified with vitamin D has been made available in the United States. Accurate estimates of average dietary intakes of vitamin D are difficult because of the high variability of the vitamin D content of fortified foods.[29] Vitamin D contents of some vitamin D-rich foods are listed in **Table 11.2**.

Supplements

Most vitamin D supplements available without a prescription contain cholecalciferol (vitamin D₃). Multivitamin supplements generally provide 400 IU (10 µg) vitamin D. Single ingredient vitamin D supplements may provide 400–2000 IU vitamin D, but 400 IU is the most commonly available dose. A number of calcium supplements may also provide vitamin D.

Table 11.3 Tolerable upper intake level (UL) for vitamin D

Life stage	Age	UL (µg/day) (IU/day)
Infants	0–6 months	25 (1000)
Infants	6–12 months	37.5 (1500)
Children	1–3 years	62.5 (2500)
Children	4–8 years	75 (3000)
Children	9–13 years	100 (4000)
Adolescents	14–18 years	100 (4000)
Adults	≥19 years	100 (4000)

Safety

Toxicity

Vitamin D toxicity (hypervitaminosis D) induces abnormally high serum calcium levels (hypercalcemia), which could result in bone loss, kidney stones, and calcification of organs like the heart and kidneys if untreated over a long period. Hypercalcemia has been observed after daily doses of more than 50 000 IU vitamin D.[37] Overall, research suggests that vitamin D toxicity is very unlikely in healthy people at intake levels lower than 10 000 IU/day.[38,95,96] However, the FNB conservatively set a tolerable upper intake level (UL) of 4000 IU/day (100 µg/day) for all adults (**Table 11.3**). Vitamin D toxicity has not been observed to result from sun exposure.[37] Certain medical conditions can increase the risk of hypercalcemia in response to vitamin D, including primary hyperparathyroidism, sarcoidosis, tuberculosis, and lymphoma.[38] People with these conditions may develop hypercalcemia in response to any increase in vitamin D nutrition and should thus consult a qualified health-care provider regarding any increase in vitamin D intake.

Drug Interactions

The following medications increase the metabolism of vitamin D and may decrease serum 25-hydroxyvitamin D levels: phenytoin, fosphenytoin, phenobarbital, carbamazepine, and rifampin. The following medications should not be taken at the same time as vitamin D because they can decrease the intestinal absorption of vitamin D: cholestyramine, colestipol, orlistat, mineral oil, and the fat substitute olestra. The oral antifungal medication ketoconazole inhibits the 25-hydroxyvitamin D_3-1-hydroxylase enzyme and has been found to reduce serum levels of 1,25-hydroxyvitamin D in healthy men. The induction of hypercalcemia by toxic levels of vitamin D may precipitate cardiac arrhythmia in patients on digitalis.[97,98]

LPI Recommendation

The Linus Pauling Institute recommends that generally healthy adults take 2000 IU (50 µg) supplemental vitamin D daily. Most multivitamins contain 400 IU vitamin D, and single-ingredient vitamin D supplements are available for additional supplementation. Sun exposure, diet, skin color, and obesity have variable, substantial impacts on body vitamin D levels. To adjust for individual differences and ensure adequate body vitamin D status, the Linus Pauling Institute recommends aiming for a serum 25-hydroxyvitamin D level of at least 80 nmol/L (32 ng/mL). Numerous observational studies have found that serum 25-hydroxyvitamin D levels of 80 nmol/L (32 ng/mL) and above are associated with reduced risk of bone fractures, several cancers, MS, and type 1 (insulin-dependent) diabetes. Infants should have a minimum daily intake of 400 IU (10 µg) and children and adolescents should have a minimum daily intake of 600 IU (15 µg) vitamin D. Given the average vitamin D content of breast milk, infant formula, and the diets of children and adolescents, supplementation may be necessary to meet these recommendations.

Older Adults

Daily supplementation with 2000 IU (50 µg) vitamin D is especially important for older adults because aging is associated with a reduced capacity to synthesize vitamin D in the skin on sun exposure.

References

1. Holick MF. Vitamin D: importance in the prevention of cancers, type 1 diabetes, heart disease, and osteoporosis. Am J Clin Nutr 2004;79(3):362–371
2. Holick MF. Vitamin D: A millennium perspective. J Cell Biochem 2003;88(2):296–307
3. Sutton AL, MacDonald PN. Vitamin D: more than a "bone-a-fide" hormone. Mol Endocrinol 2003;17 (5): 777–791
4. Guyton KZ, Kensler TW, Posner GH. Vitamin D and vitamin D analogs as cancer chemopreventive agents. Nutr Rev 2003;61(7):227–238
5. DeLuca HF. Overview of general physiologic features and functions of vitamin D. Am J Clin Nutr 2004; 80(6, Suppl):1689S–1696S
6. Lin R, White JH. The pleiotropic actions of vitamin D. Bioessays 2004;26(1):21–28
7. Hayes CE, Nashold FE, Spach KM, Pedersen LB. The immunological functions of the vitamin D endocrine system. Cell Mol Biol (Noisy-le-grand) 2003;49(2): 277–300
8. Griffin MD, Xing N, Kumar R. Vitamin D and its analogs as regulators of immune activation and antigen presentation. Annu Rev Nutr 2003;23:117–145
9. Zeitz U, Weber K, Soegiarto DW, Wolf E, Balling R, Erben RG. Impaired insulin secretory capacity in mice lacking a functional vitamin D receptor. FASEB J 2003; 17(3):509–511
10. Borissova AM, Tankova T, Kirilov G, Dakovska L, Kovacheva R. The effect of vitamin D 3 on insulin secretion and peripheral insulin sensitivity in type 2 diabetic patients. Int J Clin Pract 2003;57(4):258–261
11. Orwoll E, Riddle M, Prince M. Effects of vitamin D on insulin and glucagon secretion in non-insulin-dependent diabetes mellitus. Am J Clin Nutr 1994;59(5): 1083–1087
12. Inomata S, Kadowaki S, Yamatani T, Fukase M, Fujita T. Effect of 1 alpha (OH)-vitamin D 3 on insulin secretion in diabetes mellitus. Bone Miner 1986;1(3): 187–192
13. Sheng H-W. Sodium, chloride and potassium. In: Stipanuk M, ed. Biochemical and Physiological Aspects of Human Nutrition. Philadelphia, PA: WB Saunders Co.; 2000:686–710
14. Sigmund CD. Regulation of renin expression and blood pressure by vitamin D(3). J Clin Invest 2002; 110(2):155–156
15. Li YC, Kong J, Wei M, Chen ZF, Liu SQ, Cao LP. 1,25-Dihydroxyvitamin D(3) is a negative endocrine regulator of the renin-angiotensin system. J Clin Invest 2002;110(2):229–238
16. Heaney RP. Long-latency deficiency disease: insights from calcium and vitamin D. Am J Clin Nutr 2003; 78(5):912–919
17. Zittermann A. Vitamin D in preventive medicine: are we ignoring the evidence? Br J Nutr 2003;89(5):552–572
18. Wharton B, Bishop N. Rickets. Lancet 2003;362(9393): 1389–1400
19. Wagner CL, Greer FR; American Academy of Pediatrics Section on Breastfeeding; American Academy of Pediatrics Committee on Nutrition. Prevention of rickets and vitamin D deficiency in infants, children, and adolescents. Pediatrics 2008;122(5):1142–1152 http://www.aap.org/new/VitaminDreport.pdf

20. Bringhurst FR, Demay MB, Kronenberg HM. Mineral metabolism. In: Larson PR, Kronenberg HM, Melmed S, Polonsky KS, eds. Larsen: Williams Textbook of Endocrinology: Elsevier; 2003:1317–1320

21. Plotnikoff GA, Quigley JM. Prevalence of severe hypovitaminosis D in patients with persistent, nonspecific musculoskeletal pain. Mayo Clin Proc 2003;78(12):1463–1470

22. Bischoff HA, Stähelin HB, Dick W, et al. Effects of vitamin D and calcium supplementation on falls: a randomized controlled trial. J Bone Miner Res 2003;18(2):343–351

23. Broe KE, Chen TC, Weinberg J, Bischoff-Ferrari HA, Holick MF, Kiel DP. A higher dose of vitamin d reduces the risk of falls in nursing home residents: a randomized, multiple-dose study. J Am Geriatr Soc 2007;55(2):234–239

24. Nesby-O'Dell S, Scanlon KS, Cogswell ME, et al. Hypovitaminosis D prevalence and determinants among African American and white women of reproductive age: third National Health and Nutrition Examination Survey, 1988–1994. Am J Clin Nutr 2002;76(1):187–192

25. Harris SS, Soteriades E, Coolidge JA, Mudgal S, Dawson-Hughes B. Vitamin D insufficiency and hyperparathyroidism in a low income, multiracial, elderly population. J Clin Endocrinol Metab 2000;85(11):4125–4130

26. Allain TJ, Dhesi J. Hypovitaminosis D in older adults. Gerontology 2003;49(5):273–278

27. Dawodu A, Agarwal M, Hossain M, Kochiyil J, Zayed R. Hypovitaminosis D and vitamin D deficiency in exclusively breast-feeding infants and their mothers in summer: a justification for vitamin D supplementation of breast-feeding infants. J Pediatr 2003;142(2):169–173

28. Glerup H, Mikkelsen K, Poulsen L, et al. Commonly recommended daily intake of vitamin D is not sufficient if sunlight exposure is limited. J Intern Med 2000;247(2):260–268

29. Food and Nutrition Board, Institute of Medicine. Vitamin D. In: Dietary Reference Intakes for Calcium, Phosphorus, Magnesium, Vitamin D, and Fluoride. Washington, DC: National Academies Press; 1999:250–287

30. Jahnsen J, Falch JA, Mowinckel P, Aadland E. Vitamin D status, parathyroid hormone and bone mineral density in patients with inflammatory bowel disease. Scand J Gastroenterol 2002;37:192–199

31. Arunabh S, Pollack S, Yeh J, Aloia JF. Body fat content and 25-hydroxyvitamin D levels in healthy women. J Clin Endocrinol Metab 2003;88(1):157–161

32. Malabanan A, Veronikis IE, Holick MF. Redefining vitamin D insufficiency. Lancet 1998;351(9105):805–806

33. Chapuy MC, Preziosi P, Maamer M, et al. Prevalence of vitamin D insufficiency in an adult normal population. Osteoporos Int 1997;7(5):439–443

34. Thomas MK, Lloyd-Jones DM, Thadhani RI, et al. Hypovitaminosis D in medical inpatients. N Engl J Med 1998;338(12):777–783

35. Heaney RP, Dowell MS, Hale CA, Bendich A. Calcium absorption varies within the reference range for serum 25-hydroxyvitamin D. J Am Coll Nutr 2003;22(2):142–146

36. Holick MF. Vitamin D deficiency: what a pain it is. Mayo Clin Proc 2003;78(12):1457–1459

37. Holick MF. Vitamin D deficiency. N Engl J Med 2007;357(3):266–281

38. Vieth R. Vitamin D supplementation, 25-hydroxyvitamin D concentrations, and safety. Am J Clin Nutr 1999;69(5):842–856

39. Tangpricha V, Koutkia P, Rieke SM, Chen TC, Perez AA, Holick MF. Fortification of orange juice with vitamin D: a novel approach for enhancing vitamin D nutritional health. Am J Clin Nutr 2003;77(6):1478–1483

40. Bischoff-Ferrari HA, Giovannucci E, Willett WC, Dietrich T, Dawson-Hughes B. Estimation of optimal serum concentrations of 25-hydroxyvitamin D for multiple health outcomes. Am J Clin Nutr 2006;84(1):18–28

41. Heaney RP. Vitamin D: how much do we need, and how much is too much? Osteoporos Int 2000;11(7):553–555

42. Hollis BW. Circulating 25-hydroxyvitamin D levels indicative of vitamin D sufficiency: implications for establishing a new effective dietary intake recommendation for vitamin D. J Nutr 2005;135(2):317–322

43. Vieth R. Why the optimal requirement for Vitamin D 3 is probably much higher than what is officially recommended for adults. J Steroid Biochem Mol Biol 2004;89–90(1–5):575–579

44. Lips P, Hosking D, Lippuner K, et al. The prevalence of vitamin D inadequacy amongst women with osteoporosis: an international epidemiological investigation. J Intern Med 2006;260(3):245–254

45. Lips P. Vitamin D deficiency and secondary hyperparathyroidism in the elderly: consequences for bone loss and fractures and therapeutic implications. Endocr Rev 2001;22(4):477–501

46. Feskanich D, Willett WC, Colditz GA. Calcium, vitamin D, milk consumption, and hip fractures: a prospective study among postmenopausal women. Am J Clin Nutr 2003;77(2):504–511

47. Bischoff-Ferrari HA, Willett WC, Wong JB, Giovannucci E, Dietrich T, Dawson-Hughes B. Fracture prevention with vitamin D supplementation: a meta-analysis of randomized controlled trials. JAMA 2005;293(18):2257–2264

48. Jackson RD, LaCroix AZ, Gass M, et al; Women's Health Initiative Investigators. Calcium plus vitamin D supplementation and the risk of fractures. N Engl J Med 2006;354(7):669–683

49. Dawson-Hughes B, Harris SS, Krall EA, Dallal GE, Falconer G, Green CL. Rates of bone loss in postmenopausal women randomly assigned to one of two dosages of vitamin D. Am J Clin Nutr 1995;61(5):1140–1145

50. Dawson-Hughes B, Harris SS, Krall EA, Dallal GE. Effect of calcium and vitamin D supplementation on bone density in men and women 65 years of age or older. N Engl J Med 1997;337(10):670–676

51. Dawson-Hughes B, Harris SS, Krall EA, Dallal GE. Effect of withdrawal of calcium and vitamin D supplements on bone mass in elderly men and women. Am J Clin Nutr 2000;72(3):745–750

52. Chapuy MC, Arlot ME, Delmas PD, Meunier PJ. Effect of calcium and cholecalciferol treatment for three years on hip fractures in elderly women. BMJ 1994;308(6936):1081–1082

53. Trivedi DP, Doll R, Khaw KT. Effect of four monthly oral vitamin D 3 (cholecalciferol) supplementation on fractures and mortality in men and women living in the community: randomised double blind controlled trial. BMJ 2003;326(7387):469–474

54. Lips P, Graafmans WC, Ooms ME, Bezemer PD, Bouter LM. Vitamin D supplementation and fracture incidence in elderly persons. A randomized, placebo-controlled clinical trial. Ann Intern Med 1996;124(4): 400–406

55. Grant AM, Avenell A, Campbell MK, et al; RECORD Trial Group. Oral vitamin D 3 and calcium for secondary prevention of low-trauma fractures in elderly people (Randomised Evaluation of Calcium Or vitamin D, RECORD): a randomised placebo-controlled trial. Lancet 2005;365(9471):1621–1628

56. Houghton LA, Vieth R. The case against ergocalciferol (vitamin D 2) as a vitamin supplement. Am J Clin Nutr 2006;84(4):694–697

57. Blutt SE, Weigel NL. Vitamin D and prostate cancer. Proc Soc Exp Biol Med 1999;221(2):89–98

58. Garland CF, Garland FC, Gorham ED. Calcium and vitamin D. Their potential roles in colon and breast cancer prevention. Ann N Y Acad Sci 1999;889:107–119

59. Terry P, Baron JA, Bergkvist L, Holmberg L, Wolk A. Dietary calcium and vitamin D intake and risk of colorectal cancer: a prospective cohort study in women. Nutr Cancer 2002;43(1):39–46

60. Martínez ME, Giovannucci EL, Colditz GA, et al. Calcium, vitamin D, and the occurrence of colorectal cancer among women. J Natl Cancer Inst 1996;88(19):1375–1382

61. Kearney J, Giovannucci E, Rimm EB, et al. Calcium, vitamin D, and dairy foods and the occurrence of colon cancer in men. Am J Epidemiol 1996;143(9):907–917

62. Bostick RM, Potter JD, Sellers TA, McKenzie DR, Kushi LH, Folsom AR. Relation of calcium, vitamin D, and dairy food intake to incidence of colon cancer among older women. The Iowa Women's Health Study. Am J Epidemiol 1993;137(12):1302–1317

63. McCullough ML, Robertson AS, Rodriguez C, et al. Calcium, vitamin D, dairy products, and risk of colorectal cancer in the Cancer Prevention Study II Nutrition Cohort (United States). Cancer Causes Control 2003;14(1):1–12

64. Peters U, McGlynn KA, Chatterjee N, et al. Vitamin D, calcium, and vitamin D receptor polymorphism in colorectal adenomas. Cancer Epidemiol Biomarkers Prev 2001;10(12):1267–1274

65. Holt PR, Arber N, Halmos B, et al. Colonic epithelial cell proliferation decreases with increasing levels of serum 25-hydroxy vitamin D. Cancer Epidemiol Biomarkers Prev 2002;11(1):113–119

66. Feskanich D, Ma J, Fuchs CS, et al. Plasma vitamin D metabolites and risk of colorectal cancer in women. Cancer Epidemiol Biomarkers Prev 2004;13(9): 1502–1508

67. Wactawski-Wende J, Kotchen JM, Anderson GL, et al; Women's Health Initiative Investigators. Calcium plus vitamin D supplementation and the risk of colorectal cancer. N Engl J Med 2006;354(7):684–696

68. Holick MF. Calcium plus vitamin D and the risk of colorectal cancer. N Engl J Med 2006;354(21):2287–2288, author reply 2287–2288

69. Gorham ED, Garland CF, Garland FC, et al. Vitamin D and prevention of colorectal cancer. J Steroid Biochem Mol Biol 2005;97(1–2):179–194

70. Grant WB. An ecologic study of dietary and solar ultraviolet-B links to breast carcinoma mortality rates. Cancer 2002;94(1):272–281

71. John EM, Schwartz GG, Dreon DM, Koo J. Vitamin D and breast cancer risk: the NHANES I Epidemiologic follow-up study, 1971–1975 to 1992. National Health and Nutrition Examination Survey. Cancer Epidemiol Biomarkers Prev 1999;8(5):399–406

72. Shin MH, Holmes MD, Hankinson SE, Wu K, Colditz GA, Willett WC. Intake of dairy products, calcium, and vitamin d and risk of breast cancer. J Natl Cancer Inst 2002;94(17):1301–1311

73. Lowe LC, Guy M, Mansi JL, et al. Plasma 25-hydroxy vitamin D concentrations, vitamin D receptor genotype and breast cancer risk in a UK Caucasian population. Eur J Cancer 2005;41(8):1164–1169

74. Bertone-Johnson ER, Chen WY, Holick MF, et al. Plasma 25-hydroxyvitamin D and 1,25-dihydroxyvitamin D and risk of breast cancer. Cancer Epidemiol Biomarkers Prev 2005;14(8):1991–1997

75. Garland CF, Gorham ED, Mohr SB, et al. Vitamin D and prevention of breast cancer: pooled analysis. J Steroid Biochem Mol Biol 2007;103(3–5):708–711

76. Young MV, Schwartz GG, Wang L, et al. The prostate 25-hydroxyvitamin D-1 alpha-hydroxylase is not influenced by parathyroid hormone and calcium: implications for prostate cancer chemoprevention by vitamin D. Carcinogenesis 2004;25(6):967–971

77. Corder EH, Guess HA, Hulka BS, et al. Vitamin D and prostate cancer: a prediagnostic study with stored sera. Cancer Epidemiol Biomarkers Prev 1993;2(5): 467–472

78. Braun MM, Helzlsouer KJ, Hollis BW, Comstock GW. Prostate cancer and prediagnostic levels of serum vitamin D metabolites (Maryland, United States). Cancer Causes Control 1995;6(3):235–239

79. Nomura AM, Stemmermann GN, Lee J, et al. Serum vitamin D metabolite levels and the subsequent development of prostate cancer (Hawaii, United States). Cancer Causes Control 1998;9(4):425–432

80. Gann PH, Ma J, Hennekens CH, Hollis BW, Haddad JG, Stampfer MJ. Circulating vitamin D metabolites in relation to subsequent development of prostate cancer. Cancer Epidemiol Biomarkers Prev 1996;5(2): 121–126

81. Ahonen MH, Tenkanen L, Teppo L, Hakama M, Tuohimaa P. Prostate cancer risk and prediagnostic serum 25-hydroxyvitamin D levels (Finland). Cancer Causes Control 2000;11(9):847–852

82. Tuohimaa P, Tenkanen L, Ahonen M, et al. Both high and low levels of blood vitamin D are associated with a higher prostate cancer risk: a longitudinal, nested case-control study in the Nordic countries. Int J Cancer 2004;108(1):104–108

83. Deluca HF, Cantorna MT. Vitamin D: its role and uses in immunology. FASEB J 2001;15(14):2579–2585

84. Hyppönen E, Läärä E, Reunanen A, Järvelin MR, Virtanen SM. Intake of vitamin D and risk of type 1 diabetes: a birth-cohort study. Lancet 2001;358 (9292):1500–1503

85. Munger KL, Levin LI, Hollis BW, Howard NS, Ascherio A. Serum 25-hydroxyvitamin D levels and risk of multiple sclerosis. JAMA 2006;296(23):2832–2838

86. Munger KL, Zhang SM, O'Reilly E, et al. Vitamin D intake and incidence of multiple sclerosis. Neurology 2004;62(1):60–65

87. Merlino LA, Curtis J, Mikuls TR, Cerhan JR, Criswell LA, Saag KG; Iowa Women's Health Study. Vitamin D intake is inversely associated with rheumatoid arthritis: results from the Iowa Women's Health Study. Arthritis Rheum 2004;50(1):72–77

88. Rostand SG. Ultraviolet light may contribute to geographic and racial blood pressure differences. Hypertension 1997;30(2 Pt 1):150–156

89. Krause R, Bühring M, Hopfenmüller W, Holick MF, Sharma AM. Ultraviolet B and blood pressure. Lancet 1998;352(9129):709–710

90. Pfeifer M, Begerow B, Minne HW, Nachtigall D, Hansen C. Effects of a short-term vitamin D(3) and calcium supplementation on blood pressure and parathyroid hormone levels in elderly women. J Clin Endocrinol Metab 2001;86(4):1633–1637

91. Pan WH, Wang CY, Li LA, Kao LS, Yeh SH. No significant effect of calcium and vitamin D supplementation on blood pressure and calcium metabolism in elderly Chinese. Chin J Physiol 1993;36(2):85–94

92. Scragg R, Khaw KT, Murphy S. Effect of winter oral vitamin D3 supplementation on cardiovascular risk factors in elderly adults. Eur J Clin Nutr 1995;49(9):640–646

93. Norman AW. Vitamin D. In: Bowman BA, Russell RM, eds. Present Knowledge in Nutrition, 8th ed. Washington, DC: ILSI Press; 2001:146–155

94. Holick MF. Vitamin D: the underappreciated D-lightful hormone that is important for skeletal and cellular health. Curr Opin Endocrinol Diabetes 2002;9(1):87–98

95. Heaney RP, Davies KM, Chen TC, Holick MF, Barger-Lux MJ. Human serum 25-hydroxycholecalciferol response to extended oral dosing with cholecalciferol. Am J Clin Nutr 2003;77(1):204–210

96. Vieth R, Chan PC, MacFarlane GD. Efficacy and safety of vitamin D3 intake exceeding the lowest observed adverse effect level. Am J Clin Nutr 2001;73(2):288–294

97. Hendler SS, Rorvik DR, eds. PDR for Nutritional Supplements. Montvale: Medical Economics Co., Inc.; 2001

98. Vitamin D. Natural Medicines Comprehensive Database [Website]. December 3, 2007. Available at: www.naturaldatabase.com. Accessed 4 Jan 2011

12 Vitamin E

The term *vitamin E* describes a family of eight antioxidants: four tocopherols (α-, β-, γ-, and δ-) and four tocotrienols (α-, β-, γ-, and δ-). α-Tocopherol is the only form of vitamin E that is actively maintained in the human body, so it is the form of vitamin E found in the largest quantities in blood and tissues.[1] As α-tocopherol is the form of vitamin E that appears to have the greatest nutritional significance, it is the primary topic of this chapter. It is also the only form that meets the latest recommended dietary allowance (RDA) for vitamin E.

Function

α-Tocopherol

The main function of α-tocopherol in humans appears to be that of an antioxidant. Free radicals are formed primarily in the body during normal metabolism and also upon exposure to environmental factors, such as cigarette smoke or pollutants. Fats, which are an integral part of all cell membranes, are vulnerable to destruction through oxidation by free radicals. The fat-soluble vitamin, α-tocopherol, is uniquely suited to intercept free radicals and thus prevent a chain reaction of lipid destruction. Aside from maintaining the integrity of cell membranes throughout the body, α-tocopherol also protects the fats in low-density lipoproteins (LDLs) from oxidation. Lipoproteins are particles composed of lipids and proteins that transport fats through the bloodstream. LDLs specifically transport cholesterol from the liver to the tissues of the body. Oxidized LDLs have been implicated in the development of cardiovascular diseases. When a molecule of α-tocopherol neutralizes a free radical, it is altered in such a way that its antioxidant capacity is lost. However, other antioxidants, such as vitamin C, are capable of regenerating the antioxidant capacity of α-tocopherol.[2,3]

Several other functions of α-tocopherol have been identified that are not likely related to its antioxidant capacity. For instance, α-tocopherol is known to inhibit the activity of protein kinase C, an important cell-signaling molecule. α-tocopherol appears also to affect the expression and activities of molecules and enzymes in immune and inflammatory cells. In addition, α-tocopherol has been shown to inhibit platelet aggregation and to enhance vasodilation.[4,5]

The isomeric form of α-tocopherol found in foods is *RRR*-α-tocopherol (also referred to as "natural" or *d*-α-tocopherol). Synthetic α-tocopherol, which is labeled *all-rac-* or *dl*-α-tocopherol, has only half the biological activity of *RRR*-α-tocopherol. Often vitamin E-fortified foods contain synthetic α-tocopherol, and the amounts are given as a percentage of the daily value of 30 IU. Throughout this chapter, amounts of α-tocopherol are expressed in both international units and milligrams.

γ-Tocopherol

The function of γ-tocopherol in humans is currently unclear. Although the most common form of vitamin E in the American diet is γ-tocopherol, blood levels of γ-tocopherol are generally 10 times lower than those of α-tocopherol. This phenomenon is apparently due to two mechanisms:

1. α-tocopherol is retained in the body by the action of the α-tocopherol transfer protein (α-TTP) in the liver, which preferentially incorporates α-tocopherol into lipoproteins that are circulated in the blood[1] and ultimately delivers α-tocopherol to different tissues in the body.[6]
2. Forms of vitamin E other than α-tocopherol are actively metabolized.[6] As γ-tocopherol is initially absorbed in the same manner as α-tocopherol, small amounts of γ-tocopherol are detectable in blood and tissue. Breakdown products of tocopherols, known as *metabolites*, can be detected in urine. More γ-tocopherol metabolites are excreted in urine than α-tocopherol metabolites, suggesting that less γ-tocopherol is needed for use by the body.[7]

Limited research in the test tube and in animals indicates that γ-tocopherol or its metabolites may play a role in protecting the body from free radical-induced damage,[8,9] but these effects have not been convincingly demonstrated in humans. Recently, concern has been raised about the fact that taking α-tocopherol supplements lowers γ-tocopherol levels in the blood. However, no adverse effects of moderate α-tocopherol supplementation have been demonstrated, although many benefits have been documented. In one prospective study, increased levels of plasma γ-tocopherol were associated with a significantly reduced risk of developing prostate cancer. In this study, increased levels of plasma α-tocopherol and toenail selenium were protective against prostate cancer development only when γ-tocopherol levels were also high.[10] These limited findings, in addition to the fact that α-tocopherol supplementation lowers γ-tocopherol levels in blood, have led some scientists to call for additional research on the effects of dietary and supplemental γ-tocopherol on health.[11] Importantly, relatively high plasma γ-tocopherol concentrations may indicate a high level of vegetable and vegetable oil intake.

Deficiency

Vitamin E deficiency has been observed in individuals with severe malnutrition, genetic defects affecting the α-TTP, and fat malabsorption syndromes. For example, children with cystic fibrosis or cholestatic liver disease, who have an impaired capacity to absorb dietary fat and therefore fat-soluble vitamins, may develop symptomatic vitamin E deficiency. Severe vitamin E deficiency results mainly in neurological symptoms, including impaired balance and coordination (ataxia), injury to the sensory nerves (peripheral neuropathy), muscle weakness (myopathy), and damage to the retina of the eye (pigmented retinopathy). For this reason, people who develop peripheral neuropathy, ataxia, or retinitis pigmentosa should be screened for vitamin E deficiency.[2] The developing nervous system appears to be especially vulnerable to vitamin E deficiency. For instance, children who have severe vitamin E deficiency from birth and are not treated with vitamin E rapidly develop neurological symptoms. In contrast, individuals who

develop malabsorption of vitamin E in adulthood may not develop neurological symptoms for 10–20 years. It should be noted that symptomatic vitamin E deficiency in healthy individuals who consume diets low in vitamin E has never been reported.[2,12]

Although true vitamin E deficiency is rare, marginal intake of vitamin E is relatively common in the United States. The National Health and Nutrition Examination Survey III (NHANES III) examined the dietary intake and blood levels of α-tocopherol in 16 295 adults (over the age of 18); 27% of white participants, 41% of African–Americans, 28% of Mexican–Americans, and 32% of the other participants were found to have blood levels of α-tocopherol less than 20 μmol/L. This cutoff value was chosen because the literature suggests an increased risk for cardiovascular disease below this level.[13] More recently, data from the NHANES 1999–2000 study indicate that mean dietary intake of α-tocopherol is 6.3 mg/day and 7.8 mg/day for women and men, respectively.[14] These intakes are well below the current intake recommendations of 15 mg/day. In fact, it has been estimated that more than 90% of Americans do not meet daily dietary recommendations for vitamin E.[15]

Recommended Dietary Allowance

The RDA for vitamin E was previously 8 mg/day for women and 10 mg/day for men. The RDA was revised by the Food and Nutrition Board (FNB) of the Institute of Medicine in 2000 (**Table 12.1**).[4] This new recommendation was based largely on the results of studies done in the 1950s in men fed vitamin E-deficient diets. In a test-tube analysis, hydrogen peroxide was added to blood samples and the breakdown of red blood cells, known as *hemolysis*, was used to indicate vitamin E deficiency. As hemolysis has also been reported in children with severe vitamin E deficiency, this analysis was considered to be a clinically relevant test of vitamin E status. Importantly, this means that the latest RDA for vitamin E continues to be based on the prevention of deficiency symptoms rather than on health promotion and prevention of chronic disease.

Table 12.1 Recommended dietary allowance for vitamin E

Life stage	Age	Males (mg/day)[a]	Females (mg/day)[a]
Infants	0–6 months	4 (AI)	4 (AI)
Infants	7–12 months	5 (AI)	5 (AI)
Children	1–3 years	6	6
Children	4–8 years	7	7
Children	9–13 years	11	11
Adolescents	14–18 years	15	15
Adults	≥19 years	15	15
Pregnancy	All ages	–	15
Breast-feeding	All ages	–	19

[a]Milligrams α-tocopherol.
AI, adequate intake.

Disease Prevention

Cardiovascular Diseases

The results of at least five large observational studies suggest that increased vitamin E consumption is associated with decreased risk of myocardial infarction (heart attack) or death from heart disease in both men and women. Each study was a prospective study that measured vitamin E consumption in presumably healthy people and followed them for a number of years to determine how many were diagnosed with or died as a result of heart disease. In two of the studies, individuals who consumed more than 7 mg/day of α-tocopherol in food were only approximately 35% as likely to die from heart disease as those who consumed less than 3–5 mg/day of α-tocopherol.[16,17] Two other large studies found a significant reduction in risk of heart disease only in women and men who consumed at least 100 IU supplemental *RRR*-α-tocopherol (67 mg *RRR*-α-tocopherol) daily.[18,19] More recently, several studies have observed plasma or red blood cell levels of α-tocopherol to be inversely associated with the presence or severity of carotid atherosclerosis detected using ultrasonography.[20–23] A randomized, placebo-controlled, intervention trial in 39 876 women participating in the Women's Health Study found that supplementation with 600 IU (400 mg) *RRR*-α-tocopherol every other day for 10 years had no effect on the incidence of various cardiovascular events (myocardial infarction and stroke), but

the vitamin E intervention decreased cardiovascular-related deaths by 24%.[24]

Analysis of data from the Women's Health Study also showed that women receiving the vitamin E intervention experienced a 21% reduction in risk of venous thromboembolism.[25] The benefits of vitamin E supplementation in chronic disease prevention are discussed in a recent review.[26] Intervention studies in patients with heart or renal disease, however, have not shown vitamin E supplements to be effective in preventing heart attacks or death (see below).

Cataracts

Cataracts appear to be formed by protein oxidation in the lens of the eye; such oxidation may be prevented by antioxidants like α-tocopherol. Several observational studies have examined the association between vitamin E consumption and the incidence and severity of cataracts. Results of these studies are mixed: some report that increased vitamin E intake protects against cataract development, whereas others report no association.[27] A placebo-controlled intervention trial in 4629 men and women found that a daily antioxidant supplement containing 500 mg vitamin C, 400 IU synthetic vitamin E (*dl*-α-tocopherol acetate; equivalent to 180 mg *RRR*-α-tocopherol), and 15 mg β-carotene did not affect development and progression of age-related cataracts over a 7-year period.[28] Similarly, antioxidant supplementation (500 mg vitamin C, 400 IU [268 mg] *RRR*-α-tocopherol, and 15 mg β-carotene) did not affect progression of cataracts in a 5-year intervention trial.[29] A 4-year, randomized, placebo-controlled trial reported that supplements containing 500 IU/day of natural vitamin E (335 mg *RRR*-α-tocopherol) did not reduce the incidence or progression of cataracts in older adults.[30] Another intervention trial found that a daily supplement of 50 mg synthetic α-tocopherol daily (equivalent to 25 mg *RRR*-α-tocopherol) did not alter the incidence of cataract surgery in male smokers.[31] Although results from some observational studies suggest that vitamin E may protect against cataract development, results from clinical trials do not support a preventive effect.

Immune Function

α-Tocopherol has been shown to enhance specific aspects of the immune response that appear to decline as people age. For example, elderly adults given 200 mg/day of synthetic α-tocopherol (equivalent to 100 mg or 150 IU *RRR*-α-tocopherol) for several months displayed increased formation of antibodies in response to hepatitis B vaccine and tetanus vaccine.[32] However, it is not known if such α-tocopherol-associated enhancements in the immune response of older adults actually translate to increased resistance to infections such as the flu (influenza virus).[33] A randomized, placebo-controlled trial in elderly nursing home residents reported that daily supplementation with 200 IU synthetic α-tocopherol (equivalent to 90 mg *RRR*-α-tocopherol) for 1 year significantly lowered the risk of contracting upper respiratory tract infections, especially the common cold, but had no effect on lower respiratory tract (lung) infections.[34] More research is needed to determine whether supplemental vitamin E may protect elderly people against the common cold or other infections.

Cancer

Many types of cancer are thought to result from oxidative damage to DNA caused by free radicals. The ability of α-tocopherol to neutralize free radicals has made it the subject of a number of cancer prevention studies. However, several large prospective studies have failed to find significant associations between α-tocopherol intake and the incidence of lung or breast cancer.[4] One study in a cohort of 77 126 men and women reported that use of vitamin E supplements over a 10-year period increased risk of lung cancer in current smokers.[35]

To date, most clinical trials have found that vitamin E supplementation has no effect on the risk of various cancers, except a possible benefit against development of prostate cancer. A randomized, placebo-controlled trial in 39 876 women participating in the Women's Health Study found that supplementation with 600 IU (400 mg) *RRR*-α-tocopherol every other day for 10 years had no effect on overall cancer incidence or cancer-related deaths.[24] This vitamin E intervention also did not affect the incidence of tissue-specific cancers, including breast, lung, and colon cancers. Moreover, a recently published meta-analysis of 12 randomized controlled trials concluded that vitamin E supplementation was not associated with overall cancer incidence, cancer mortality, or total mortality.[36] However, vitamin E supplementation may possibly reduce the risk of prostate cancer. A placebo-controlled intervention study that was designed to look at the effect of α-tocopherol supplementation on lung cancer development noted a 34% reduction in the incidence of prostate cancer in smokers given daily supplements of 50 mg synthetic α-tocopherol (equivalent to 25 mg *RRR*-α-tocopherol) daily.[37] A meta-analysis that combined the results of this study with three other randomized controlled trials associated vitamin E supplement use with a 15% lower risk of prostate cancer.[36] However, a large randomized, placebo-controlled intervention study using α-tocopherol and selenium supplementation (the SELECT trial), alone or in combination, was recently halted because there was no evidence of benefit in preventing prostate cancer.[38,39] After an average of 5.5 years of follow-up in the SELECT trial, participants taking vitamin E (400 IU/day *all-rac*-α-tocopherol) alone had a higher risk of prostate cancer, but the increase was not statistically significant.[40]

Disease Treatment

Cardiovascular Diseases

Observational studies have suggested that supplemental α-tocopherol might have value in the treatment of cardiovascular disease. For example, a small observational study of men who had previously undergone coronary artery bypass surgery found that those who took at least 100 IU supplemental α-tocopherol (67 mg RRR-α-tocopherol) daily had a reduction in the progression of coronary artery atherosclerosis measured by angiography compared with those who took less than 100 IU/day of α-tocopherol.[40] A randomized, placebo-controlled intervention trial in the United Kingdom (the CHAOS study) found that supplementing heart disease patients with either 400 or 800 IU synthetic α-tocopherol (equivalent to 180 or 360 mg RRR-α-tocopherol) for an average of 18 months dramatically reduced the occurrence of nonfatal heart attacks by 77%. However, α-tocopherol supplementation did not significantly reduce total deaths from heart disease.[41]

Chronic renal dialysis patients are at much greater risk of dying from cardiovascular disease than the general population, and there is evidence that they are also under increased oxidative stress. Supplementation of renal dialysis patients with 800 IU natural α-tocopherol (536 mg RRR-α-tocopherol) daily for an average of 1.4 years resulted in a significantly reduced risk of heart attack compared with placebo.[42] In contrast, three other intervention trials failed to find significant risk reductions with α-tocopherol supplementation. One study, which was designed mainly to examine cancer prevention, found that 50 mg synthetic α-tocopherol (equivalent to 25 mg RRR-α-tocopherol) daily resulted in a nonsignificant decrease in nonfatal heart attacks in participants who had had previous heart attacks.[43] However, two other large trials in individuals with evidence of cardiovascular disease (previous heart attack, stroke, or evidence of vascular disease) found that daily supplements of 400 IU natural α-tocopherol (equivalent to 268 mg RRR-α-tocopherol) or 300 mg synthetic α-tocopherol (equivalent to 150 mg RRR-α-tocopherol) did not significantly change the risk of a subsequent heart attack or stroke.[44,45] A trial in patients with either vascular disease or diabetes mellitus found that daily supplementation with 400 IU natural α-tocopherol for an average of 7 years had no effect on major cardiovascular events (myocardial infarction or stroke) or deaths; however, this study noted a slightly increased risk of heart failure in individuals taking vitamin E supplements.[46] Thus, results of clinical trials using vitamin E for the treatment of heart disease have been inconsistent.

Diabetes Mellitus

α-Tocopherol supplementation in individuals with diabetes has been proposed because diabetes appears to increase oxidative stress and because cardiovascular complications (heart attack and stroke) are among the leading causes of death in people with diabetes. One study found a biochemical marker of oxidative stress (urinary excretion of F_2-isoprostanes) was elevated in individuals with type 2 diabetes, and supplementation with 600 mg synthetic α-tocopherol (equivalent to 300 mg RRR-α-tocopherol) daily for 14 days reduced levels of the biomarker.[47] Studies of the effect of α-tocopherol supplementation on blood glucose control have been contradictory. Some studies have shown that supplemental vitamin E improves insulin action and glucose disposal in type 2 diabetic[48] and non-diabetic[48,49] individuals, whereas other studies have reported minimal to no improvements in glucose metabolism of patients with type 2 diabetes.[50,51] Increased oxidative stress has also been documented in type 1 diabetes.[47] One study reported that supplementing patients with type 1 diabetes with only 100 IU/day of synthetic α-tocopherol (equivalent to 45 mg RRR-α-tocopherol) for 1 month significantly improved both glycated hemoglobin and triglyceride levels.[52] This study also noted nonsignificant improvements in blood glucose levels after α-tocopherol supplementation.[52] Although there is reason to suspect that α-tocopherol supplementation may be beneficial in treatment for type 1 or 2 diabetes, evidence from well-controlled clinical trials is lacking.

Dementia (Impaired Cognitive Function)

The brain is particularly vulnerable to oxidative stress, which is thought to play a role in the pathology of neurodegenerative diseases such as Alzheimer disease.[53] In addition, some studies have documented low levels of vitamin E in cerebrospinal fluid of patients with Alzheimer disease.[54] A large placebo-controlled intervention trial in individuals with moderate neurological impairment found that supplementation with 2000 IU synthetic α-tocopherol daily for 2 years (equivalent to 900 mg/day *RRR*-α-tocopherol) significantly slowed progression of Alzheimer dementia.[55] In contrast, a placebo-controlled trial in patients with mild cognitive impairment reported that the same dosage of vitamin E did not slow progression to Alzheimer disease over a 3-year period.[56] After Alzheimer disease, vascular dementia (dementia resulting from strokes) is the most common type of dementia in the United States. A case–control study examining risk factors for vascular dementia in elderly Japanese–American men found that supplemental vitamin E and vitamin C intake was associated with a significantly decreased risk of vascular and other types of dementia but not Alzheimer dementia.[57] Among those without dementia, vitamin E supplement use was associated with better scores on cognitive tests. Although these findings are promising, further studies are required to determine the role of α-tocopherol supplementation in the treatment of Alzheimer disease and other types of dementia.

Cancer

Cancer cells proliferate rapidly and are resistant to death by apoptosis (programmed cell death). Cell culture studies indicate that the vitamin E ester, α-tocopheryl succinate, can inhibit proliferation and induce apoptosis in a number of cancer cell lines.[58,59] The ester form, α-tocopheryl succinate, not α-tocopherol, is required to effectively inhibit proliferation or induce cancer cell death.[60] Although the mechanisms for the effects of α-tocopheryl succinate on cancer cells are not yet clear, the fact that the ester form has no antioxidant activity argues against an antioxidant mechanism.[61] Limited data from animal models of cancer indicate that α-tocopheryl succinate administered by injection may inhibit tumor growth,[62–65] but much more research is required to determine whether α-tocopheryl succinate will be a useful adjunct to cancer therapy in humans. Certainly, administration by injection would be necessary for any benefit, because α-tocopheryl succinate taken orally is cleaved to form α-tocopherol in the intestine.[66] There is currently no evidence in humans that taking oral α-tocopheryl succinate supplements delivers α-tocopheryl succinate to tissues.

Sources

Food Sources

Major sources of α-tocopherol in the American diet include vegetable oils (olive, sunflower, and safflower oils), nuts, whole grains, and green leafy vegetables. All eight forms of vitamin E (α-, β-, γ-, and δ-tocopherols and tocotrienols) occur naturally in foods but in varying amounts. **Table 12.2** lists α-tocopherol and γ-tocopherol in some common foods.

Table 12.2 Food sources of vitamin E

Food	Serving	α-Tocopherol (mg)	γ-Tocopherol (mg)
Olive oil	1 tablespoon	1.9	0.1
Soybean oil	1 tablespoon	1.1	8.7
Corn oil	1 tablespoon	1.9	8.2
Canola oil	1 tablespoon	2.4	3.8
Safflower oil	1 tablespoon	4.6	0.1
Sunflower oil	1 tablespoon	5.6	0.7
Almonds	1 ounce	7.4	0.2
Hazelnuts	1 ounce	4.3	0
Peanuts	1 ounce	2.4	2.4
Spinach	½ cup, raw	0.3	0
Carrots	½ cup, raw chopped	0.4	0
Avocado (California)	1 fruit	2.7	0.4

Supplements

α-Tocopherol. In the United States, the average intake of α-tocopherol from food is approximately 8 mg daily for men and 6 mg daily for women;[14] these levels are well below the RDA of 15 mg/day of *RRR*-α-tocopherol.[4] Many scientists believe that it is difficult for an individual to consume more than 15 mg/day of α-tocopherol from food alone without increasing fat intake above recommended levels. All α-tocopherol in food is in the form of the isomer *RRR*-α-tocopherol. The same is not always true for supplements. Vitamin E supplements generally contain 100–1000 IU α-tocopherol. Supplements made from entirely natural sources contain only *RRR*-α-tocopherol (also labeled *d*-α-tocopherol). *RRR*-α-Tocopherol is the isomer preferred for use by the body, making it the most bioavailable form of α-tocopherol. Synthetic α-tocopherol, which is often found in fortified foods and nutritional supplements, is usually labeled *all-rac*-α-tocopherol or *dl*-α-tocopherol, meaning that all eight isomers of α-tocopherol are present in the mixture. Because half of the isomers of α-tocopherol present in *all-rac*-α-tocopherol are not usable by the body, synthetic α-tocopherol is less bioavailable and only half as potent. To calculate the number of milligrams of bioavailable α-tocopherol present in a supplement, use the following formulae.

RRR-α-tocopherol (natural or d-α-tocopherol):
$$IU \times 0.67 = mg \; RRR\text{-}\alpha\text{-tocopherol}$$
Example:
$$100 \; IU = 67 \; mg;$$
all-rac-α-tocopherol (synthetic or dl-α-tocopherol):
$$IU \times 0.45 = mg \; RRR\text{-}\alpha\text{-tocopherol}$$
Example:
$$100 \; IU = 45 \; mg.$$

α-Tocopheryl succinate and α-tocopheryl acetate (α-tocopheryl esters). α-Tocopherol supplements are available in the ester forms: α-tocopheryl succinate and α-tocopheryl acetate. Tocopherol esters are more resistant to oxidation during storage than unesterified tocopherols. When taken orally, the succinate or acetate moiety is removed from α-tocopherol in the intestine. The bioavailability of α-tocopherol from α-tocopheryl succinate and α-tocopheryl acetate is equivalent to that of free α-tocopherol. Because international units for α-tocopherol esters are adjusted for molecular weight, the conversion factors for determining the amount of bioavailable α-tocopherol provided by α-tocopheryl succinate and α-tocopheryl acetate are not different from those used for α-tocopherol.[4] The ester α-tocopheryl succinate, not α-tocopherol, is required to effectively inhibit growth and induce death in cancer cells grown in culture. However, there is currently no evidence in humans that taking oral α-tocopheryl succinate supplements delivers α-tocopheryl succinate to tissues.

α-Tocopheryl phosphates (Ester-E). There is currently no published evidence that supplements containing α-tocopheryl phosphates are more efficiently absorbed or have greater bioavailability in humans than supplements containing α-tocopherol.

γ-Tocopherol. γ-Tocopherol supplements and mixed tocopherol supplements are also commercially available.[67] The amounts of α- and γ-tocopherol in mixed tocopherol supplements vary, so it is important to read the label to determine the amount of each tocopherol present in supplements.

Safety

Toxicity

Few side effects have been noted in adults taking supplements of less than 2000 mg α-tocopherol daily (*RRR*- or *all-rac*-α-tocopherol). However, most studies of toxicity or side effects of α-tocopherol supplementation have lasted only a few weeks to a few months, and side effects occurring as a result of long-term α-tocopherol supplementation have not been adequately studied. The most worrisome possibility is that of impaired blood clotting, which may increase the likelihood of hemorrhage in some individuals. The FNB established a tolerable upper intake level (UL) for α-tocopherol supplements based on the prevention of hemorrhage (**Table 12.3**). The FNB felt that 1000 mg/day of α-tocopherol in any form (equivalent to 1500 IU/day of *RRR*-α-tocopherol or 1100 IU/day of *all-rac*-α-toco-pherol) would be the highest dose unlikely to result in hemorrhage in almost all adults.[4] Although only certain isomers of α-tocopherol are retained in the circulation, all forms are absorbed and me-

Table 12.3 Tolerable upper intake level (UL) for any form of supplementary α-tocopherol

Life stage	Age	UL (mg/day) α-tocopherol)
Infants	0–12 months	Not possible to establish[a]
Children	1–3 years	200
Children	4–8 years	300
Children	9–13 years	600
Adolescents	14–18 years	800
Adults	≥19	1000

[a]Source of intake should be from food and formula only.

tabolized by the liver. The rationale that any form of α-tocopherol (natural or synthetic) can be absorbed and thus could be potentially harmful is the basis for a UL that refers to all forms of α-tocopherol.

Some physicians recommend discontinuing high-dose vitamin E supplementation 1 month before elective surgery to decrease the risk of hemorrhage. Premature infants appear to be especially vulnerable to adverse effects of α-tocopherol supplementation, which should be used only under controlled supervision by a pediatrician.[67] Supplementation with 400 IU/day of vitamin E has been found to accelerate the progression of retinitis pigmentosa which is not associated with vitamin E deficiency.[68]

Vitamin E Supplementation and All-cause Mortality

A meta-analysis that combined the results of 19 clinical trials of vitamin E supplementation for various diseases, including heart disease, end-stage renal failure, and Alzheimer disease, reported that adults who took supplements of 400 IU/day or more were 6% more likely to die from any cause than those who did not take vitamin E supplements.[69] However, further breakdown of the risk by vitamin E dose and adjustment for other vitamin and mineral supplements revealed that the increased risk of death was statistically significant only at a dose of 2000 IU/day, which is higher than the UL for adults. In addition, three other meta-analyses that combined the results of randomized controlled trials designed to evaluate the efficacy of vitamin E supplementation for the prevention or treatment of

cardiovascular disease found no evidence that vitamin E supplementation up to 800 IU/day significantly increased or decreased cardiovascular disease mortality or all-cause mortality.[70,71,77] Additionally, a more recent meta-analysis of 57 randomized controlled trials found that vitamin E supplementation, up to doses of 5500 IU/day, had no effect on all-cause mortality.[72] Furthermore, a meta-analysis of 68 randomized trials found that supplemental vitamin E, singly or in combination with other antioxidant supplements, did not significantly alter risk of all-cause mortality.[73] At present, there is no convincing evidence that vitamin E supplementation up to 800 IU/day increases the risk of death from cardiovascular disease or other causes.

Drug Interactions

Use of vitamin E supplements may increase the risk of bleeding in individuals taking anticoagulant drugs, such as warfarin (Coumadin); antiplatelet drugs, such as clopidogrel (Plavix) and dipyridamole (Persantine); and nonsteroidal anti-inflammatory drugs (NSAIDs), including aspirin, ibuprofen, and others. Also, individuals on anticoagulant therapy (blood thinners) or individuals who are vitamin K deficient should not take α-tocopherol supplements without close medical supervision because of the increased risk of hemorrhage.[4] A number of medications may decrease the absorption of vitamin E, including cholestyramine, colestipol, isoniazid, mineral oil, orlistat, sucralfate, and the fat substitute olestra. Anticonvulsant drugs, such as phenobarbital, phenytoin, and carbamazepine, may decrease plasma levels of vitamin E.[4,67]

Antioxidants and HMG-CoA reductase inhibitors (statins). A 3-year randomized controlled trial in 160 patients with documented coronary heart disease (CHD) and low high-density lipoprotein (HDL) levels found that a combination of simvastatin and niacin increased HDL2 levels, inhibited the progression of coronary artery stenosis (narrowing), and decreased the frequency of cardiovascular events, such as myocardial infarction and stroke.[74] Surprisingly, when an antioxidant combination (1000 mg vitamin C, 800 IU α-tocopherol, 100 μg selenium, and 25 mg β-carotene daily) was taken with the simvastatin–niacin combination, the protective effects were diminished. However, in a much larger randomized controlled trial of simvastatin and an antioxidant combination (600 mg vitamin E, 250 mg vitamin C, and 20 mg β-carotene daily) in more than 20 000 men and women with coronary artery disease or diabetes, the antioxidant combination did not adversely affect the cardioprotective effects of simvastatin therapy over a 5-year period.[75] These contradictory findings indicate that further research is needed on potential interactions between antioxidant supplementation and cholesterol-lowering agents such as hydroxymethylglutaryl coenzyme A (HMG-CoA) reductase inhibitors (statins).

LPI Recommendation

Scientists at the Linus Pauling Institute feel that there is credible evidence that taking a supplement of 200 IU (134 mg) natural source *d*-α-tocopherol (*RRR*-α-tocopherol) daily with a meal may help protect adults from chronic diseases, such as heart disease, stroke, neurodegenerative diseases, and some types of cancer. The amount of α-tocopherol required for such beneficial effects appears to be much greater than that which could be achieved through diet alone. As supplements containing 200 IU *d*-α-tocopherol are often as expensive as supplements containing 400 IU *d*-α-tocopherol, a less expensive alternative may be to take 400 IU (268 mg) *d*-α-tocopherol every other day. α-Tocopherol supplements are unlikely to be absorbed unless taken with food.

Older Adults

The Linus Pauling Institute's recommendation of a supplement providing 200 IU natural source *d*-α-tocopherol daily (or 400 IU *d*-α-tocopherol every other day) with a meal is also appropriate for generally healthy older adults.

References

1. Traber MG. Utilization of vitamin E. Biofactors 1999;10(2-3):115–120
2. Traber MG. Vitamin E. In: Shils ME, Shike M, Ross AC, Caballero B, Cousins RJ, eds. Modern Nutrition in Health and Disease. Philadelphia, PA: Lippincott Williams & Wilkins; 2006:396–411
3. Bruno RS, Leonard SW, Atkinson J, et al. Faster plasma vitamin E disappearance in smokers is normalized by vitamin C supplementation. Free Radic Biol Med 2006;40(4):689–697
4. Food and Nutrition Board, Institute of Medicine. Vitamin E. In: Dietary Reference Intakes for Vitamin C, Vitamin E, Selenium, and Carotenoids. Washington, DC: National Academy Press; 2000:186–283
5. Traber MG. Does vitamin E decrease heart attack risk? summary and implications with respect to dietary recommendations. J Nutr 2001;131(2):395S–397S
6. Traber MG. Vitamin E regulatory mechanisms. Annu Rev Nutr 2007;27:347–362
7. Traber MG, Elsner A, Brigelius-Flohé R. Synthetic as compared with natural vitamin E is preferentially excreted as alpha-CEHC in human urine: studies using deuterated alpha-tocopheryl acetates. FEBS Lett 1998;437(1-2):145–148
8. Christen S, Woodall AA, Shigenaga MK, Southwell-Keely PT, Duncan MW, Ames BN. gamma-tocopherol traps mutagenic electrophiles such as NO(X) and complements alpha-tocopherol: physiological implications. Proc Natl Acad Sci USA 1997;94(7):3217–3222
9. Li D, Saldeen T, Mehta JL. gamma-tocopherol decreases ox-LDL-mediated activation of nuclear factor-kappaB and apoptosis in human coronary artery endothelial cells. Biochem Biophys Res Commun 1999;259(1):157–161
10. Helzlsouer KJ, Huang HY, Alberg AJ, et al. Association between alpha-tocopherol, gamma-tocopherol, selenium, and subsequent prostate cancer. J Natl Cancer Inst 2000;92(24):2018–2023
11. Jiang Q, Christen S, Shigenaga MK, Ames BN. gamma-tocopherol, the major form of vitamin E in the US diet, deserves more attention. Am J Clin Nutr 2001;74(6):714–722
12. Traber MG. Vitamin E. In: Bowman BA, Russell RM, eds. Present Knowledge in Nutrition, 9th ed. Vol. 1. Washington, DC: ILSI Press; 2006:211–219
13. Ford ES, Sowell A. Serum alpha-tocopherol status in the United States population: findings from the Third National Health and Nutrition Examination Survey. Am J Epidemiol 1999;150(3):290–300
14. Ahuja JK, Goldman JD, Moshfegh AJ. Current status of vitamin E nutriture. Ann N Y Acad Sci 2004;1031:387–390
15. Maras JE, Bermudez OI, Qiao N, Bakun PJ, Boody-Alter EL, Tucker KL. Intake of alpha-tocopherol is limited among US adults. J Am Diet Assoc 2004;104(4):567–575
16. Knekt P, Reunanen A, Järvinen R, Seppänen R, Heliövaara M, Aromaa A. Antioxidant vitamin intake and coronary mortality in a longitudinal population study. Am J Epidemiol 1994;139(12):1180–1189
17. Kushi LH, Folsom AR, Prineas RJ, Mink PJ, Wu Y, Bostick RM. Dietary antioxidant vitamins and death from coronary heart disease in postmenopausal women. N Engl J Med 1996;334(18):1156–1162
18. Rimm EB, Stampfer MJ, Ascherio A, Giovannucci E, Colditz GA, Willett WC. Vitamin E consumption and the risk of coronary heart disease in men. N Engl J Med 1993;328(20):1450–1456
19. Stampfer MJ, Hennekens CH, Manson JE, Colditz GA, Rosner B, Willett WC. Vitamin E consumption and the risk of coronary disease in women. N Engl J Med 1993;328(20):1444–1449
20. Cherubini A, Zuliani G, Costantini F, et al; VASA Study Group. High vitamin E plasma levels and low low-density lipoprotein oxidation are associated with the absence of atherosclerosis in octogenarians. J Am Geriatr Soc 2001;49(5):651–654
21. Gale CR, Ashurst HE, Powers HJ, Martyn CN. Antioxidant vitamin status and carotid atherosclerosis in the elderly. Am J Clin Nutr 2001;74(3):402–408

22. McQuillan BM, Hung J, Beilby JP, Nidorf M, Thompson PL. Antioxidant vitamins and the risk of carotid atherosclerosis. The Perth Carotid Ultrasound Disease Assessment study (CUDAS). J Am Coll Cardiol 2001;38(7):1788–1794

23. Simon E, Gariepy J, Cogny A, Moatti N, Simon A, Paul JL. Erythrocyte, but not plasma, vitamin E concentration is associated with carotid intima-media thickening in asymptomatic men at risk for cardiovascular disease. Atherosclerosis 2001;159(1):193–200

24. Lee IM, Cook NR, Gaziano JM, et al. Vitamin E in the primary prevention of cardiovascular disease and cancer: the Women's Health Study: a randomized controlled trial. JAMA 2005;294(1):56–65

25. Glynn RJ, Ridker PM, Goldhaber SZ, Zee RY, Buring JE. Effects of random allocation to vitamin E supplementation on the occurrence of venous thromboembolism: report from the Women's Health Study. Circulation 2007;116(13):1497–1503

26. Traber MG, Frei B, Beckman JS. Vitamin E revisited: do new data validate benefits for chronic disease prevention? Curr Opin Lipidol 2008;19(1):30–38

27. West AL, Oren GA, Moroi SE. Evidence for the use of nutritional supplements and herbal medicines in common eye diseases. Am J Ophthalmol 2006;141(1):157–166

28. Age-Related Eye Disease Study Research Group. A randomized, placebo-controlled, clinical trial of high-dose supplementation with vitamins C and E and beta carotene for age-related cataract and vision loss: AREDS report no. 9. Arch Ophthalmol 2001;119(10):1439–1452

29. Gritz DC, Srinivasan M, Smith SD, et al. The Antioxidants in Prevention of Cataracts Study: effects of antioxidant supplements on cataract progression in South India. Br J Ophthalmol 2006;90(7):847–851

30. McNeil JJ, Robman L, Tikellis G, Sinclair MI, McCarty CA, Taylor HR. Vitamin E supplementation and cataract: randomized controlled trial. Ophthalmology 2004;111(1):75–84

31. Teikari JM, Rautalahti M, Haukka J, et al. Incidence of cataract operations in Finnish male smokers unaffected by alpha tocopherol or beta carotene supplements. J Epidemiol Community Health 1998;52(7):468–472

32. Meydani SN, Meydani M, Blumberg JB, et al. Vitamin E supplementation and in vivo immune response in healthy elderly subjects. A randomized controlled trial. JAMA 1997;277(17):1380–1386

33. Han SN, Meydani SN. Vitamin E and infectious diseases in the aged. Proc Nutr Soc 1999;58(3):697–705

34. Meydani SN, Leka LS, Fine BC, et al. Vitamin E and respiratory tract infections in elderly nursing home residents: a randomized controlled trial. JAMA 2004;292(7):828–836

35. Slatore CG, Littman AJ, Au DH, Satia JA, White E. Long-term use of supplemental multivitamins, vitamin C, vitamin E, and folate does not reduce the risk of lung cancer. Am J Respir Crit Care Med 2008;177(5):524–530

36. Alkhenizan A, Hafez K. The role of vitamin E in the prevention of cancer: a meta-analysis of randomized controlled trials. Ann Saudi Med 2007;27(6):409–414

37. Heinonen OP, Albanes D, Virtamo J, et al. Prostate cancer and supplementation with alpha-tocopherol and beta-carotene: incidence and mortality in a controlled trial. J Natl Cancer Inst 1998;90(6):440–446

38. Klein EA, Thompson IM, Lippman SM, et al. SELECT: the next prostate cancer prevention trial. Selenium and Vitamin E Cancer Prevention Trial. J Urol 2001;166(4):1311–1315

39. National Cancer Institute. Review of Prostate Cancer Prevention Study Shows No Benefit for Use of Selenium and Vitamin E Supplements. [Web page]. Available at: www.cancer.gov/newscenter/pressreleases/SELECTresults2008. Accessed 4 Jan 2011

40. Azen SP, Qian D, Mack WJ, et al. Effect of supplementary antioxidant vitamin intake on carotid arterial wall intima-media thickness in a controlled clinical trial of cholesterol lowering. Circulation 1996;94(10):2369–2372

41. Stephens NG, Parsons A, Schofield PM, Kelly F, Cheeseman K, Mitchinson MJ. Randomised controlled trial of vitamin E in patients with coronary disease: Cambridge Heart Antioxidant Study (CHAOS). Lancet 1996;347(9004):781–786

42. Boaz M, Smetana S, Weinstein T, et al. Secondary prevention with antioxidants of cardiovascular disease in endstage renal disease (SPACE): randomised placebo-controlled trial. Lancet 2000;356(9237):1213–1218

43. Rapola JM, Virtamo J, Ripatti S, et al. Randomised trial of alpha-tocopherol and beta-carotene supplements on incidence of major coronary events in men with previous myocardial infarction. Lancet 1997;349(9067):1715–1720

44. Yusuf S, Dagenais G, Pogue J, Bosch J, Sleight P; The Heart Outcomes Prevention Evaluation Study Investigators. Vitamin E supplementation and cardiovascular events in high-risk patients. N Engl J Med 2000;342(3):154–160

45. Dietary supplementation with n-3 polyunsaturated fatty acids and vitamin E after myocardial infarction: results of the GISSI-Prevenzione trial. Gruppo Italiano per lo Studio della Sopravvivenza nell'Infarto miocardico. Lancet 1999;354(9177):447–455

46. Lonn E, Bosch J, Yusuf S, et al; HOPE and HOPE-TOO Trial Investigators. Effects of long-term vitamin E supplementation on cardiovascular events and cancer: a randomized controlled trial. JAMA 2005;293(11):1338–1347

47. Davì G, Ciabattoni G, Consoli A, et al. In vivo formation of 8-iso-prostaglandin f2alpha and platelet activation in diabetes mellitus: effects of improved metabolic control and vitamin E supplementation. Circulation 1999;99(2):224–229

48. Paolisso G, D'Amore A, Giugliano D, Ceriello A, Varricchio M, D'Onofrio F. Pharmacologic doses of vitamin E improve insulin action in healthy subjects and non-insulin-dependent diabetic patients. Am J Clin Nutr 1993;57(5):650–656

49. Paolisso G, Di Maro G, Galzerano D, et al. Pharmacological doses of vitamin E and insulin action in elderly subjects. Am J Clin Nutr 1994;59(6):1291–1296

50. Paolisso G, D'Amore A, Galzerano D, et al. Daily vitamin E supplements improve metabolic control but not insulin secretion in elderly type II diabetic patients. Diabetes Care 1993;16(11):1433–1437

51. Reaven PD, Herold DA, Barnett J, Edelman S. Effects of Vitamin E on susceptibility of low-density lipoprotein and low-density lipoprotein subfractions to oxidation and on protein glycation in NIDDM. Diabetes Care 1995;18(6):807–816

52. Jain SK, McVie R, Jaramillo JJ, Palmer M, Smith T. Effect of modest vitamin E supplementation on blood

glycated hemoglobin and triglyceride levels and red cell indices in type I diabetic patients. J Am Coll Nutr 1996;15(5):458–461

53. Meydani M. Antioxidants and cognitive function. Nutr Rev 2001;59(8 Pt 2):S75–80; discussion S80–72

54. Kontush K, Schekatolina S. Vitamin E in neurodegenerative disorders: Alzheimer's disease. Ann N Y Acad Sci 2004;1031:249–262

55. Sano M, Ernesto C, Thomas RG, et al. A controlled trial of selegiline, alpha-tocopherol, or both as treatment for Alzheimer's disease. The Alzheimer's Disease Cooperative Study. N Engl J Med 1997;336(17):1216–1222

56. Petersen RC, Thomas RG, Grundman M, et al; Alzheimer's Disease Cooperative Study Group. Vitamin E and donepezil for the treatment of mild cognitive impairment. N Engl J Med 2005;352(23):2379–2388

57. Masaki KH, Losonczy KG, Izmirlian G, et al. Association of vitamin E and C supplement use with cognitive function and dementia in elderly men. Neurology 2000;54(6):1265–1272

58. Yu W, Sanders BG, Kline K. RRR-alpha-tocopheryl succinate-induced apoptosis of human breast cancer cells involves Bax translocation to mitochondria. Cancer Res 2003;63(10):2483–2491

59. You H, Yu W, Munoz-Medellin D, Brown PH, Sanders BG, Kline K. Role of extracellular signal-regulated kinase pathway in RRR-alpha-tocopheryl succinate-induced differentiation of human MDA-MB-435 breast cancer cells. Mol Carcinog 2002;33(4):228–236

60. Neuzil J, Weber T, Schröder A, et al. Induction of cancer cell apoptosis by alpha-tocopheryl succinate: molecular pathways and structural requirements. FASEB J 2001;15(2):403–415

61. Brigelius-Flohé R, Kelly FJ, Salonen JT, Neuzil J, Zingg JM, Azzi A. The European perspective on vitamin E: current knowledge and future research. Am J Clin Nutr 2002;76(4):703–716

62. Weber T, Lu M, Andera L, et al. Vitamin E succinate is a potent novel antineoplastic agent with high selectivity and cooperativity with tumor necrosis factor-related apoptosis-inducing ligand (Apo2 ligand) in vivo. Clin Cancer Res 2002;8(3):863–869

63. Malafa MP, Fokum FD, Mowlavi A, Abusief M, King M. Vitamin E inhibits melanoma growth in mice. Surgery 2002;131(1):85–91

64. Malafa MP, Neitzel LT. Vitamin E succinate promotes breast cancer tumor dormancy. J Surg Res 2000; 93(1):163–170

65. Quin J, Engle D, Litwiller A, et al. Vitamin E succinate decreases lung cancer tumor growth in mice. J Surg Res 2005;127(2):139–143

66. Cheeseman KH, Holley AE, Kelly FJ, Wasil M, Hughes L, Burton G. Biokinetics in humans of RRR-alpha-tocopherol: the free phenol, acetate ester, and succinate ester forms of vitamin E. Free Radic Biol Med 1995;19(5):591–598

67. Hendler SS, Rorvik DR, eds. PDR for Nutritional Supplements. Montvale, NJ: Medical Economics Co.; Inc., 2001

68. Berson EL, Rosner B, Sandberg MA, et al. A randomized trial of vitamin A and vitamin E supplementation for retinitis pigmentosa. Arch Ophthalmol 1993;111(6):761–772

69. Miller ER III, Pastor-Barriuso R, Dalal D, Riemersma RA, Appel LJ, Guallar E. Meta-analysis: high-dosage vitamin E supplementation may increase all-cause mortality. Ann Intern Med 2005;142(1):37–46

70. Shekelle PG, Morton SC, Jungvig LK, et al. Effect of supplemental vitamin E for the prevention and treatment of cardiovascular disease. J Gen Intern Med 2004;19(4):380–389

71. Eidelman RS, Hollar D, Hebert PR, Lamas GA, Hennekens CH. Randomized trials of vitamin E in the treatment and prevention of cardiovascular disease. Arch Intern Med 2004;164(14):1552–1556

72. Vivekananthan DP, Penn MS, Sapp SK, Hsu A, Topol EJ. Use of antioxidant vitamins for the prevention of cardiovascular disease: meta-analysis of randomised trials. Lancet 2003;361(9374):2017–2023

73. Bjelakovic G, Nikolova D, Gluud LL, Simonetti RG, Gluud C. Mortality in randomized trials of antioxidant supplements for primary and secondary prevention: systematic review and meta-analysis. JAMA 2007;297(8):842–857

74. Brown BG, Zhao XQ, Chait A, et al. Simvastatin and niacin, antioxidant vitamins, or the combination for the prevention of coronary disease. N Engl J Med 2001;345(22):1583–1592

75. Collins R, Peto R, Armitage J. The MRC/BHF Heart Protection Study: preliminary results. Int J Clin Pract 2002;56(1):53–56

76. Lippman SM, Klein EA, Goodman PJ, et al. Effect of selenium and vitamin E on risk of prostate cancer and other cancers: the Selenium and Vitamin E Cancer Prevention Trial (SELECT). JAMA 2009;301(1):39–51

77. Abner EL, Schmitt FA, Mendiondo MS, Marcum JL, Kryscio RJ. Vitamin E and all-cause mortality: a meta-analysis. Curr Aging Sci 2011 Jan 14 [e pub ahead of print]

13 Vitamin K

Vitamin K is a fat-soluble vitamin. The "K" is derived from the German word *koagulation*. Coagulation refers to the process of blood clot formation, and vitamin K is essential for the functioning of several proteins involved in blood clotting.[1] There are two naturally occurring forms of vitamin K. Plants synthesize phylloquinone, which is also known as vitamin K_1. Bacteria synthesize a range of vitamin K forms using repeating 5-carbon units in the side chain of the molecule. These forms of vitamin K are designated menaquinone-*n* (MK-*n*), where *n* stands for the number of 5-carbon units. MK-*n* forms are collectively referred to as vitamin K_2.[2] MK-4 is not produced in significant amounts by bacteria; instead, it appears to be synthesized by animals (including humans) from phylloquinone. MK-4 is also formed from menadione, a synthetic form of vitamin K present in animal feed. It is found in a number of organs other than the liver at higher concentrations than phylloquinone.[3] This fact, together with the existence of a unique pathway for its synthesis, suggests that MK-4 has a unique biological function that has not yet been identified.[4]

Function

The only known biological role of vitamin K is as a cofactor for an enzyme that catalyzes the carboxylation of the amino acid, glutamic acid, resulting in its conversion to γ-carboxyglutamic acid (Gla).[5] Although vitamin K-dependent γ-carboxylation occurs only on specific glutamic acid residues in a small number of vitamin K-dependent proteins, it is critical to the calcium-binding function of those proteins.[6,7]

Coagulation

The ability to bind calcium ions (Ca^{2+}) is required for the activation of the seven vitamin K-dependent clotting factors, or proteins, in the coagulation cascade. The term *coagulation cascade* refers to a series of events, each dependent on the other, that stop bleeding through clot formation. Vitamin K-dependent γ-carboxylation of specific glutamic acid residues in those proteins makes it possible for them to bind calcium. Factors II (prothrombin), VII, IX, and X make up the core of the coagulation cascade. Protein Z appears to enhance the action of thrombin (the activated form of prothrombin) by promoting its association with phospholipids in cell membranes. Protein C and protein S are anticoagulant proteins that provide control and balance in the coagulation cascade; protein Z also has an anticoagulatory function. Control mechanisms for the coagulation cascade exist, because uncontrolled clotting may be as life threatening as uncontrolled bleeding. Vitamin K-dependent coagulation factors are synthesized in the liver. Consequently, severe liver disease results in lower blood levels of vitamin K-dependent clotting factors and an increased risk of uncontrolled bleeding (hemorrhage).[8]

Some people are at risk of forming clots, which could block the flow of blood in the arteries of the heart, brain, or lungs, resulting in heart attack, stroke, or pulmonary embolism, respectively. Some oral anticoagulants, such as warfarin, inhibit coagulation through antagonism of the action of vitamin K. Although vitamin K is a fat-soluble vitamin, the body stores very little of it, and its stores are rapidly depleted without regular dietary intake. Perhaps, because of its limited ability to store vitamin K, the body recycles it through a process called the *vitamin K cycle*. This cycle allows a small amount of vitamin K to function in the γ-carboxylation of proteins many times, decreasing the dietary requirement. Warfarin prevents the recycling of vitamin K by inhibiting two important reactions and creating a functional vitamin K deficiency (**Fig. 13.1**). Inadequate γ-carboxylation of vitamin K-dependent coagulation proteins interferes with the coagulation cascade, which inhibits blood clot formation. Large quantities of dietary or supplemental vitamin K can overcome the anticoagulant effect of vitamin K antagonists, so patients taking these drugs are cautioned against consuming very large or highly variable quantities of vita-

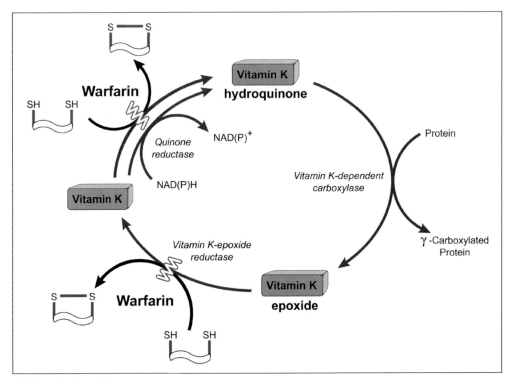

Fig. 13.1 The vitamin K cycle. Warfarin is a vitamin K antagonist that inhibits the recycling of vitamin K at two dithiol-dependent steps.

min K in their diets. Experts now advise a reasonably constant dietary intake of vitamin K that meets current dietary recommendations (90–120 µg/day) for patients on vitamin K antagonists such as warfarin.[9]

Bone Mineralization

Three vitamin-K dependent proteins have been isolated in bone: osteocalcin, matrix Gla protein (MGP), and protein S. Osteocalcin (also called bone Gla protein) is a protein synthesized by osteoblasts (bone-forming cells). The synthesis of osteocalcin by osteoblasts is regulated by the active form of vitamin D, 1,25-dihydroxyvitamin D_3 or calcitriol. The mineral-binding capacity of osteocalcin requires vitamin K-dependent γ-carboxylation of three glutamic acid residues. The function of osteocalcin is unclear but is thought to be related to bone mineralization. MGP has been found in bone, cartilage, and soft tissue, including blood vessels. The results of animal studies suggest that MGP prevents the calcification of soft tissue and cartilage, while facili-

tating normal bone growth and development. The vitamin K-dependent anticoagulant protein S is also synthesized by osteoblasts, but its role in bone metabolism is unclear. Children with inherited protein S deficiency suffer complications related to increased blood clotting as well as decreased bone density.[7,10,11]

Cell Growth

Gas6 is a vitamin K-dependent protein that was identified in 1993. It has been found throughout the nervous system, as well in the heart, lungs, stomach, kidneys, and cartilage. Although the exact mechanism of its action has not been determined, Gas6 appears to be a cellular growth regulation factor with cell-signaling activities. Gas6 appears to be important in diverse cellular functions, including cell adhesion, cell proliferation, and protection against apoptosis.[6] It may also play important roles in the developing and aging nervous system.[12,13] Further, Gas6 appears to regulate platelet signaling and vascular homeostasis.[14]

Deficiency

Overt vitamin K deficiency results in impaired blood clotting, usually demonstrated by laboratory tests that measure clotting time. Symptoms include easy bruising and bleeding that may manifest as nosebleeds, bleeding gums, blood in the urine, blood in the stool, tarry black stools, or extremely heavy menstrual bleeding. In infants, vitamin K deficiency may result in life-threatening bleeding within the skull (intracranial hemorrhage).[8]

Adults. Vitamin K deficiency is uncommon in healthy adults for a number of reasons:
• Vitamin K is widespread in foods.
• The vitamin K cycle conserves vitamin K.
• Bacteria that normally inhabit the large intestine synthesize menaquinones (vitamin K_2), although it is unclear whether significant amounts are absorbed and utilized.

Adults at risk of vitamin K deficiency include those taking vitamin K antagonist anticoagulant drugs and individuals with significant liver damage or disease.[8] In addition, individuals with disorders of fat malabsorption may be at increased risk of vitamin K deficiency.[6]

Infants. Newborn babies who are exclusively breast-fed are at increased risk of vitamin K deficiency, because human milk is relatively low in vitamin K compared with formula. Newborn infants, in general, have low vitamin K status for the following reasons:
• Vitamin K is not easily transported across the placental barrier.
• The newborn's intestines are not yet colonized with bacteria that synthesize menaquinones.
• The vitamin K cycle may not be fully functional in newborn infants, especially premature infants.[6]

Infants whose mothers are on anticonvulsant medication to prevent seizures are also at risk of vitamin K deficiency. Vitamin K deficiency in newborn infants may result in a bleeding disorder called *vitamin K deficiency bleeding* (VKDB). As VKDB is life threatening and easily prevented, the American Academy of Pediatrics and a number of similar international organizations recommend that an injection of phylloquinone (vitamin K_1) be administered to all newborns.[15]

Controversy Surrounding Vitamin K Administration and Newborn Infants

Vitamin K and childhood leukemia. In the early 1990s, two retrospective studies were published suggesting a possible association between vitamin K injections in newborn infants and the development of childhood leukemia and other forms of childhood cancer. However, two large retrospective studies in the United States and Sweden that reviewed the medical records of 54 000 and 1.3 million children, respectively, found no evidence of a relationship between childhood cancers and vitamin K injections at birth.[16,17] Moreover, a pooled analysis of six case–control studies, including 2431 children diagnosed with childhood cancer and 6338 cancer-free children, found no evidence that vitamin K injections for newborn infants increased the risk of childhood leukemia.[18] In a policy statement, the American Academy of Pediatrics recommended that routine vitamin K prophylaxis for newborn infants be continued because VKDB is life threatening and the risks of cancer are unproven and unlikely.[19]

Lower doses of vitamin K_1 for premature infants. The results of two studies of vitamin K levels in premature infants suggest that the standard initial dose of vitamin K_1 for full-term infants (1.0 mg) may be too high for premature infants.[20,21] These findings have led some experts to suggest the use of an initial vitamin K_1 dose of 0.3 mg/kg for infants with birth weights less than 1000 g (2 lb 3 oz), and an initial dose of 0.5 mg would probably prevent hemorrhagic disease in newborn infants.[20]

Adequate Intake

In January 2001, the Food and Nutrition Board (FNB) of the Institute of Medicine established the adequate intake (AI) level for vitamin K in the United States based on consumption levels of healthy individuals (**Table 13.1**). The AI for infants was based on estimated intake of vitamin K from breast milk.[22]

Table 13.1 Adequate intake for vitamin K

Life stage	Age	Males (µg/day)	Females (µg/day)
Infants	0–6 months	2.0	2.0
Infants	7–12 months	2.5	2.5
Children	1–3 years	30	30
Children	4–8 years	55	55
Children	9–13 years	60	60
Adolescents	14–18 years	75	75
Adults	≥19	120	90
Pregnancy	≤18	–	75
Pregnancy	≥19	–	90
Breast-feeding	≤18	–	75
Breast-feeding	≥19	–	90

Disease Prevention

Osteoporosis

The discovery of vitamin K-dependent proteins in bone has led to research on the role of vitamin K in maintaining bone health.

Dietary vitamin K and osteoporotic fracture. Epidemiological studies have demonstrated a relationship between vitamin K and age-related bone loss (osteoporosis). The Nurses' Health Study followed more than 72000 women for 10 years. In an analysis of this cohort, women whose vitamin K intakes were in the lowest quintile (one-fifth) had a 30% higher risk of hip fracture than women with vitamin K intakes in the highest four quintiles.[23] A study in over 800 elderly men and women, followed in the Framingham Heart Study for 7 years, found that men and women with dietary vitamin K intakes in the highest quartile (one-fourth) had a 65% lower risk of hip fracture than those with dietary vitamin K intakes in the lowest quartile (approximately 250 µg/day vs. 50 µg/day of vitamin K). However, the investigators found no association between dietary vitamin K intake and bone mineral density (BMD) in the Framingham participants.[24] Other studies have not observed a relationship between dietary vitamin K intake and measures of bone strength, BMD, or fracture incidence.[25,26] As the primary dietary source of vitamin K is generally green leafy vegetables, high vitamin K intake could just be a marker for a healthy diet that is high in vegetables.[27]

Vitamin K-dependent carboxylation of osteocalcin and osteoporotic fracture. Osteocalcin, a bone-related protein that circulates in the blood, has been shown to be a sensitive marker of bone formation. Vitamin K is required for the γ-carboxylation of osteocalcin. Undercarboxylation of osteocalcin adversely affects its capacity to bind to bone mineral, and the degree of osteocalcin γ-carboxylation has been found to be a sensitive indicator of vitamin K nutritional status.[4] Circulating levels of undercarboxylated osteocalcin (ucOC) were found to be higher in postmenopausal women than premenopausal women and markedly higher in women over the age of 70. In a study of 195 institutionalized elderly women, the relative risk of hip fracture was six times higher in those who had elevated ucOC levels at the beginning of the study.[28] In a much larger sample of 7500 elderly women living independently, circulating ucOC was also predictive of fracture risk.[29] Although vitamin K deficiency would seem the most likely cause of elevated blood ucOC, investigators have also documented an inverse relationship between measures of vitamin D nutritional status and ucOC levels, as well as a significant lowering of ucOC by vitamin D supplementation.[7] It is also possible that an increased ucOC level is a marker for poor overall nutritional status, including vitamin D or protein.

Vitamin K antagonists and osteoporotic fracture. Certain oral anticoagulants, such as warfarin, are known to be antagonists of vitamin K. At least two studies have examined the chronic use of warfarin and risk of fracture in older women. One study reported no association between long-term warfarin treatment and fracture risk,[30] whereas the other found a significantly higher risk of rib and vertebral fractures in warfarin users compared with nonusers.[31] In addition, a study in elderly patients with atrial fibrillation reported that long-term warfarin treatment was associated with a significantly higher risk of osteoporotic fracture in men but not in women.[32] A meta-analysis of the results of 11 published studies found that oral anticoagulation therapy was associated with a very modest reduction in bone density at the wrist and no change in bone density at the hip or spine.[33]

Vitamin K supplementation studies and osteoporosis. Vitamin K supplementation of 1000 µg (1 mg)/day of phylloquinone (vitamin K_1) for 2 weeks (more than 10 times the AI for vitamin K) resulted in a decrease of ucOC levels in postmenopausal women, as well as increases in several biochemical markers of bone formation. In Japan, intervention trials in hemodialysis patients and osteoporotic women using very high pharmacological doses (45 mg/day) of menatetrenone (MK-4) have reported significant reductions in the rate of bone loss.[34,35] MK-4 is not found in significant amounts in the diet, but it can be synthesized in small amounts by humans from phylloquinone. A recent meta-analysis of seven Japanese randomized controlled trials associated MK-4 supplementation with increased BMD and reduced fracture incidence,[36] but this meta-analysis did not include data from an unpublished study that reported no effect on fracture risk.[37] Nevertheless, the meta-analysis[36] reported that MK-4 supplementation lowered risk for vertebral fractures by 60%, hip fractures by 77%, and nonvertebral fractures by 81%; all associations were statistically significant. Six of the individual trials employed 45 mg MK-4 daily, whereas one trial used 15 mg MK-4 daily[36] The 45 mg/day dose of MK-4 was also used in a more recent 3-year placebo-controlled intervention trial in 325 postmenopausal women. This study found that supplemental MK-4 improved measures of bone strength compared with placebo.[38]

The doses used in most of the cited studies are about 500 times higher than the AI for vitamin K. Some experts are not sure whether the effects of such high doses of MK-4 represent a true vitamin K effect.

Long-term clinical trials of phylloquinone supplementation at doses attainable by dietary intake (200–1000 µg/day) have reported mixed results with respect to effects on BMD.[39-41] Phylloquinone supplementation at these levels does not appear to benefit older individuals who are also taking vitamin D and calcium supplements.[41] Thus, evidence of a relationship between vitamin K nutritional status and bone health in adults is considered weak. Further investigation is required to determine the physiological function of vitamin K-dependent proteins in bone and the mechanisms by which vitamin K affects bone health and osteoporotic fracture risk.[7]

Vascular Calcification and Cardiovascular Disease

One of the hallmarks of cardiovascular disease is the formation of atherosclerotic plaques in arterial walls. Calcification of atherosclerotic plaques occurs as the condition progresses, resulting in decreased elasticity of the affected vessels and increased risk of clot formation, the usual cause of a heart attack or stroke. A prospective cohort study in 807 men and women, aged 39–45 years, did not find a correlation between dietary vitamin K_1 intake and coronary artery calcification, as measured by electron-beam computed tomography.[42] In addition, vitamin K_1 intake was not associated with calcification of breast arteries in a cross-sectional study of 1689 women, aged 49–70 years.[43] A population-based study of postmenopausal women, aged 60–79 years, found that women aged 60–69 with aortic calcifications had lower vitamin K intakes than those without aortic calcifications, but this was not true for older women.[44] The mechanism by which vitamin K may promote mineralization of bone, while inhibiting mineralization (calcification) of vessels, is not entirely clear. One hypothesis is based on the function of MGP, which has been found to inhibit the calcification of cartilage and bone during early embryonic development. Some investigators have hypothesized that high levels of MGP found in calcified vessels may represent a defense against vessel calcification, but that inadequate vitamin K nutritional status results in inadequate carboxylation and, presumably, inactive MGP.

Thus, insufficient dietary vitamin K may increase the risk of vascular calcification.[45] Support for this hypothesis comes from a small human study that employed conformation-specific antibodies against MGP to examine whether impaired carboxylation of this protein possibly contributes to arterial calcification. In healthy individuals, undercarboxylated MGP (uc MGP) was not detected in the innermost lining of the carotid artery; in contrast, most MGP in the carotid arterial lining of patients with atherosclerosis was undercarboxylated.[46] Serum ucMGP may be decreased in those at risk of cardiovascular calcification due to deposition of ucMGP in local areas of vascular calcification.[47] Further investigations are necessary to establish the nature of the role of bone proteins such as MGP in human atherosclerotic plaque calcification.

Sources

Food Sources

Phylloquinone (vitamin K_1) is the major dietary form of vitamin K. Green leafy vegetables and some vegetable oils (soybean, cottonseed, canola, and olive) are major contributors of dietary vitamin K. Hydrogenation of vegetable oils may de-

Table 13.2 Food sources of vitamin K

Food	Serving	Vitamin K (µg)
Kale, raw	1 cup, chopped	547
Swiss chard, raw	1 cup	299
Parsley, raw	¼ cup	246
Broccoli, cooked	1 cup, chopped	220
Spinach, raw	1 cup	145
Watercress, raw	1 cup, chopped	85
Leaf lettuce, green, raw	1 cup, shredded	62.5
Soybean oil	1 tablespoon	25
Canola oil	1 tablespoon	16.6
Olive oil	1 tablespoon	8.1
Mayonnaise	1 tablespoon	3.7

crease the absorption and biological effect of dietary vitamin K.[48] A number of good sources of vitamin K are listed in **Table 13.2**.

Intestinal Bacteria

Bacteria that normally colonize the large intestine synthesize menaquinones (vitamin K_2), which are an active form of vitamin K. Until recently it was thought that up to 50% of the human vitamin K requirement might be met by bacterial synthesis. However, research indicates that the contribution of bacterial synthesis is much less than previously thought, although the exact contribution remains unclear.[49]

Supplements. In the United States, vitamin K_1 is available without a prescription in multivitamin and other supplements in doses that generally range from 10 µg to 120 µg per supplement.[50] A form of vitamin K_2, menatetrenone (MK-4), has been used to treat osteoporosis in Japan and is currently under study in the United States.[51]

Safety

Toxicity

Although allergic reaction is possible, there is no known toxicity associated with high doses of the phylloquinone (vitamin K_1) or menaquinone (vitamin K_2) forms of vitamin K.[22] The same is not true for synthetic menadione (vitamin K_3) and its derivatives. Menadione can interfere with the function of glutathione, one of the body's natural antioxidants, resulting in oxidative damage to cell membranes. Menadione given by injection has induced liver toxicity, jaundice, and hemolytic anemia (due to the rupture of red blood cells) in infants; therefore, menadione is no longer used for treatment of vitamin K deficiency.[6,8] No tolerable upper intake level has been established for vitamin K.[22]

Nutrient Interactions

Large doses of vitamin A and vitamin E have been found to antagonize vitamin K.[8] Excess vitamin A appears to interfere with vitamin K absorption, whereas a form of vitamin E (tocopherol quinone) may inhibit vitamin K-dependent carboxylase enzymes. One study in adults with normal coagulation status found that supplementation with 1000 IU vitamin E for 12 weeks decreased γ-carboxylation of prothrombin, a vitamin K-dependent protein.[52] A vitamin E–vitamin K interaction has also been reported in patients taking anticoagulatory drugs such as warfarin. Hemorrhage (excessive bleeding) was reported in a man taking 5 mg warfarin and 1200 IU vitamin E daily.[53]

Drug Interactions

The anticoagulant effect of vitamin K antagonists (e.g., warfarin) may be inhibited by very high dietary or supplemental vitamin K intake. It is generally recommended that individuals using warfarin try to consume the AI for vitamin K (90–120 µg), while avoiding large fluctuations in vitamin K intake that might interfere with the adjustment of their anticoagulant dose.[9] When given to pregnant women, warfarin, anticonvulsants, rifampin, and isoniazid can interfere with fetal vitamin K synthesis and place the newborn infant at increased risk of vitamin K deficiency.[15] Other drugs can interfere with endogenous synthesis of vitamin K or with vitamin K recycling. Prolonged use of broad-spectrum antibiotics may decrease vitamin K synthesis by intestinal bacteria. Cephalosporins and salicylates may decrease vitamin K recycling by inhibiting vitamin K epoxide reductase. Further, cholestyramine, colestipol, orlistat, mineral oil, and the fat substitute olestra may decrease vitamin K absorption.[50]

LPI Recommendation

Although the AI for vitamin K was recently increased, it is not clear if it will be enough to optimize the γ-carboxylation of vitamin K-dependent proteins in bone. Multivitamins generally contain 10–25 µg vitamin K, whereas vitamin K or "bone" supplements may contain 100–120 µg vitamin K. To consume the amount of vitamin K associated with a decreased risk of hip fracture in the Framingham Heart Study (about 250 µg/day), an individual would need to eat a little more than half a cup of chopped broccoli or a large salad of mixed greens every day. Although the dietary intake of vitamin K required for optimal function of all vitamin K-dependent proteins is not yet known, the Linus Pauling Institute recommends taking a multivitamin/mineral supplement and eating at least one cup of dark-green leafy vegetables daily. Replacing dietary saturated fats such as butter and cheese with monounsaturated fats

found in olive oil and canola oil will also increase dietary vitamin K intake and may also decrease the risk of cardiovascular diseases.

Older Adults

As older adults are at increased risk of osteoporosis and hip fracture, the above recommendation for a multivitamin/mineral supplement and at least one cup of dark-green leafy vegetables per day is especially relevant.

References

1. Brody T. Nutritional Biochemistry. 2nd ed. San Diego: Academic Press; 1999
2. Shearer MJ. Vitamin K. Lancet 1995;345(8944): 229–234
3. Okano T, Shimomura Y, Yamane M, et al. Conversion of phylloquinone (Vitamin K1) into menaquinone-4 (Vitamin K2) in mice: two possible routes for menaquinone-4 accumulation in cerebra of mice. J Biol Chem 2008;283(17):11270–11279
4. Booth SL, Suttie JW. Dietary intake and adequacy of vitamin K. J Nutr 1998;128(5):785–788
5. Furie B, Bouchard BA, Furie BC. Vitamin K-dependent biosynthesis of gamma-carboxyglutamic acid. Blood 1999;93(6):1798–1808
6. Ferland G. Vitamin K. In: Bowman BA, Russell RM, eds. Present Knowledge in Nutrition. 9th ed. Vol 1. Washington, DC: ILSI Press; 2006:220–230
7. Shearer MJ. The roles of vitamins D and K in bone health and osteoporosis prevention. Proc Nutr Soc 1997;56(3):915–937
8. Olson RE. Vitamin K. In: Shils M, Olson JA, Shike M, Ross AC, eds. Modern Nutrition in Health and Disease. 9th ed. Baltimore, MD: Lippincott Williams & Wilkins; 1999:363–380
9. Booth SL, Centurelli MA. Vitamin K: a practical guide to the dietary management of patients on warfarin. Nutr Rev 1999;57(9 Pt 1):288–296
10. Booth SL. Skeletal functions of vitamin K-dependent proteins: not just for clotting anymore. Nutr Rev 1997;55(7):282–284
11. Suttie JW. Vitamin K. In: Shils ME, Shike M, Ross AC, Caballero B, Cousins RJ, eds. Modern Nutrition in Health and Disease. 10th ed. Baltimore, MD: Lippincott Williams & Wilkins; 2006:412–425
12. Ferland G. The vitamin K-dependent proteins: an update. Nutr Rev 1998;56(8):223–230
13. Tsaioun KI. Vitamin K-dependent proteins in the developing and aging nervous system. Nutr Rev 1999;57(8):231–240
14. Maree AO, Jneid H, Palacios IF, Rosenfield K, MacRae CA, Fitzgerald DJ. Growth arrest specific gene (GAS) 6 modulates platelet thrombus formation and vascular wall homeostasis and represents an attractive drug target. Curr Pharm Des 2007;13(26):2656–2661
15. Thorp JA, Gaston L, Caspers DR, Pal ML. Current concepts and controversies in the use of vitamin K. Drugs 1995;49(3):376–387
16. Klebanoff MA, Read JS, Mills JL, Shiono PH. The risk of childhood cancer after neonatal exposure to vitamin K. N Engl J Med 1993;329(13):905–908
17. Ekelund H, Finnström O, Gunnarskog J, Källén B, Larsson Y. Administration of vitamin K to newborn in-

fants and childhood cancer. BMJ 1993;307(6896): 89–91

18. Roman E, Fear NT, Ansell P, et al. Vitamin K and childhood cancer: analysis of individual patient data from six case-control studies. Br J Cancer 2002;86(1): 63–69

19. American Academy of Pediatrics Committee on Fetus and Newborn. Controversies concerning vitamin K and the newborn. Pediatrics 2003;112(1 Pt 1):191–192

20. Costakos DT, Greer FR, Love LA, Dahlen LR, Suttie JW. Vitamin K prophylaxis for premature infants: 1 mg versus 0.5 mg. Am J Perinatol 2003;20(8):485–490

21. Kumar D, Greer FR, Super DM, Suttie JW, Moore JJ. Vitamin K status of premature infants: implications for current recommendations. Pediatrics 2001;108(5): 1117–1122

22. Food and Nutrition Board, Institute of Medicine. Vitamin K. In: Dietary Reference Intakes for Vitamin A, Vitamin K, Arsenic, Boron, Chromium, Copper, Iodine, Iron, Manganese, Molybdenum, Nickel, Silicon, Vanadium, and Zinc. Washington, DC: National Academy Press; 2001:162–196

23. Feskanich D, Weber P, Willett WC, Rockett H, Booth SL, Colditz GA. Vitamin K intake and hip fractures in women: a prospective study. Am J Clin Nutr 1999;69(1):74–79

24. Booth SL, Tucker KL, Chen H, et al. Dietary vitamin K intakes are associated with hip fracture but not with bone mineral density in elderly men and women. Am J Clin Nutr 2000;71(5):1201–1208

25. Rejnmark L, Vestergaard P, Charles P, et al. No effect of vitamin K1 intake on bone mineral density and fracture risk in perimenopausal women. Osteoporos Int 2006;17(8):1122–1132

26. McLean RR, Booth SL, Kiel DP, et al. Association of dietary and biochemical measures of vitamin K with quantitative ultrasound of the heel in men and women. Osteoporos Int 2006;17(4):600–607

27. Booth SL, Mayer J. Warfarin use and fracture risk. Nutr Rev 2000;58(1):20–22

28. Szulc P, Chapuy MC, Meunier PJ, Delmas PD. Serum undercarboxylated osteocalcin is a marker of the risk of hip fracture in elderly women. J Clin Invest 1993;91(4):1769–1774

29. Vergnaud P, Garnero P, Meunier PJ, Bréart G, Kamihagi K, Delmas PD. Undercarboxylated osteocalcin measured with a specific immunoassay predicts hip fracture in elderly women: the EPIDOS Study. J Clin Endocrinol Metab 1997;82(3):719–724

30. Jamal SA, Browner WS, Bauer DC, Cummings SR; Study of Osteoporotic Fractures Research Group. Warfarin use and risk for osteoporosis in elderly women. Ann Intern Med 1998;128(10):829–832

31. Caraballo PJ, Heit JA, Atkinson EJ, et al. Long-term use of oral anticoagulants and the risk of fracture. Arch Intern Med 1999;159(15):1750–1756

32. Gage BF, Birman-Deych E, Radford MJ, Nilasena DS, Binder EF. Risk of osteoporotic fracture in elderly patients taking warfarin: results from the National Registry of Atrial Fibrillation 2. Arch Intern Med 2006;166(2):241–246

33. Caraballo PJ, Gabriel SE, Castro MR, Atkinson EJ, Melton LJ III. Changes in bone density after exposure to oral anticoagulants: a meta-analysis. Osteoporos Int 1999;9(5):441–448

34. Iwamoto J, Takeda T, Ichimura S. Effect of menatetrenone on bone mineral density and incidence of vertebral fractures in postmenopausal women with osteoporosis: a comparison with the effect of etidronate. J Orthop Sci 2001;6(6):487–492

35. Vermeer C, Jie KS, Knapen MH. Role of vitamin K in bone metabolism. Annu Rev Nutr 1995;15:1–22

36. Cockayne S, Adamson J, Lanham-New S, Shearer MJ, Gilbody S, Torgerson DJ. Vitamin K and the prevention of fractures: systematic review and meta-analysis of randomized controlled trials. Arch Intern Med 2006;166(12):1256–1261

37. Tamura T, Morgan SL, Takimoto H. Vitamin K and the prevention of fractures. Arch Intern Med 2007;167(1):94, author reply 94–95

38. Knapen MH, Schurgers LJ, Vermeer C. Vitamin K2 supplementation improves hip bone geometry and bone strength indices in postmenopausal women. Osteoporos Int 2007;18(7):963–972

39. Braam LA, Knapen MH, Geusens P, et al. Vitamin K1 supplementation retards bone loss in postmenopausal women between 50 and 60 years of age. Calcif Tissue Int 2003;73(1):21–26

40. Bolton-Smith C, McMurdo ME, Paterson CR, et al. Two-year randomized controlled trial of vitamin K1 (phylloquinone) and vitamin D 3 plus calcium on the bone health of older women. J Bone Miner Res 2007;22(4):509–519

41. Booth SL, Dallal G, Shea MK, Gundberg C, Peterson JW, Dawson-Hughes B. Effect of vitamin K supplementation on bone loss in elderly men and women. J Clin Endocrinol Metab 2008;93(4):1217–1223

42. Villines TC, Hatzigeorgiou C, Feuerstein IM, O'Malley PG, Taylor AJ. Vitamin K1 intake and coronary calcification. Coron Artery Dis 2005;16(3):199–203

43. Maas AH, van der Schouw YT, Beijerinck D, et al. Vitamin K intake and calcifications in breast arteries. Maturitas 2007;56(3):273–279

44. Jie KS, Bots ML, Vermeer C, Witteman JC, Grobbee DE. Vitamin K intake and osteocalcin levels in women with and without aortic atherosclerosis: a population-based study. Atherosclerosis 1995;116(1): 117–123

45. Schurgers LJ, Dissel PE, Spronk HM, et al. Role of vitamin K and vitamin K-dependent proteins in vascular calcification. Z Kardiol 2001;90(Suppl 3):57–63

46. Schurgers LJ, Teunissen KJ, Knapen MH, et al. Novel conformation-specific antibodies against matrix gamma-carboxyglutamic acid (Gla) protein: undercarboxylated matrix Gla protein as marker for vascular calcification. Arterioscler Thromb Vasc Biol 2005; 25(8):1629–1633

47. Cranenburg EC, Vermeer C, Koos R, et al. The circulating inactive form of matrix Gla Protein (ucMGP) as a biomarker for cardiovascular calcification. J Vasc Res 2008;45(5):427–436

48. Booth SL, Lichtenstein AH, O'Brien-Morse M, et al. Effects of a hydrogenated form of vitamin K on bone formation and resorption. Am J Clin Nutr 2001; 74(6):783–790

49. Suttie JW. The importance of menaquinones in human nutrition. Annu Rev Nutr 1995;15:399–417

50. Hendler SS, Rorvik DR, eds. PDR for Nutritional Supplements. Montvale: Medical Economics Co., Inc.; 2001

51. National Institutes of Health. Vitamin K and Bone Turnover in Postmenopausal Women. ClinicalTrials. gov [Web page]. Available at: http://www.clinicaltrials.gov/ct/show/NCT00062595?order=11 Accessed 4 Jan 2011

52. Booth SL, Golly I, Sacheck JM, et al. Effect of vitamin E supplementation on vitamin K status in adults with normal coagulation status. Am J Clin Nutr 2004; 80(1):143–148

53. Corrigan JJ Jr, Marcus FI. Coagulopathy associated with vitamin E ingestion. JAMA 1974;230(9):1300–1301

14   Calcium

Calcium is the most common mineral in the human body. About 99% of the calcium in the body is found in bones and teeth, whereas the other 1% is found in the blood and soft tissues. Calcium levels in the blood and fluid surrounding the cells (extracellular fluid) must be maintained within a very narrow concentration range for normal physiological functioning. The physiological functions of calcium are so vital to survival that the body will demineralize bone to maintain normal blood calcium levels when calcium intake is inadequate. Thus, adequate dietary calcium is a critical factor in maintaining a healthy skeleton.[1]

Function

Structure

Calcium is a major structural element in bones and teeth. The mineral component of bone consists mainly of hydroxyapatite [$Ca_{10}(PO_4)_6(OH)_2$] crystals, which contain large amounts of calcium and phosphate.[2] Bone is a dynamic tissue that is remodeled throughout life. Bone cells called *osteoclasts* begin the process of remodeling by dissolving or resorbing bone. Bone-forming cells called *osteoblasts* then synthesize new bone to replace the bone that was resorbed. During normal growth, bone formation exceeds bone resorption. Osteoporosis may result when bone resorption chronically exceeds formation.[1]

Cell Signaling

Calcium plays a role in mediating the constriction and relaxation of blood vessels (vasoconstriction and vasodilation), nerve impulse transmission, muscle contraction, and secretion of hormones such as insulin.[3] Excitable cells, such as skeletal muscle and nerve cells, contain voltage-dependent calcium channels in their cell membranes that allow for rapid changes in calcium concentrations. For example, when a muscle fiber receives a nerve impulse that stimulates it to contract, calcium channels in the cell membrane open to allow a few calcium ions into the muscle cell. These calcium ions bind to activator proteins within the cell, which release a flood of calcium ions from storage vesicles inside the cell. The binding of calcium to the protein troponin C initiates a series of steps that lead to muscle contraction. The binding of calcium to the protein calmodulin activates enzymes that break down muscle glycogen to provide energy for muscle contraction.[1]

Cofactor for Enzymes and Proteins

Calcium is necessary to stabilize a number of proteins and enzymes, optimizing their activities. The binding of calcium ions is required for the activation of the seven "vitamin K-dependent" clotting factors in the coagulation cascade. The term *coagulation cascade* refers to a series of events, dependent on each other, that stops bleeding through clot formation.[4]

Regulation of Calcium Levels

Calcium concentrations in the blood and fluid that surrounds cells are tightly controlled in order to preserve normal physiological function (**Fig. 14.1**). When blood calcium decreases (e.g., in the case of inadequate calcium intake), calcium-sensing proteins in the parathyroid glands send signals that result in the secretion of parathyroid hormone (PTH).[5] PTH stimulates the conversion of vitamin D to its active form, calcitriol, in the kidneys. Calcitriol increases the absorption of calcium from the small intestine. Together with PTH, calcitriol stimulates the release of calcium from bone by activating osteoclasts and decreases the urinary excretion of calcium by increasing its reabsorption in the kidneys. When blood calcium rises to normal levels, the parathyroid glands stop secreting PTH and the kidneys begin to excrete any excess calcium in the urine. Although this complex system allows for rapid and tight control of blood calcium levels, it does so at the expense of the skeleton.[1]

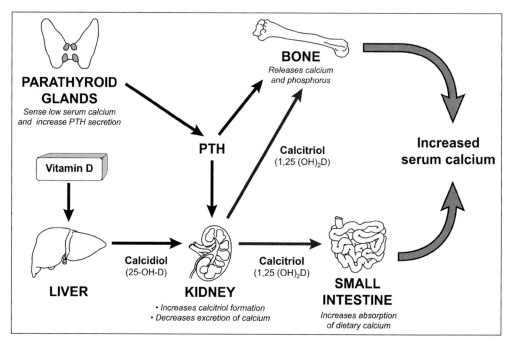

Fig. 14.1 Regulation of serum calcium. Calcium-sensing proteins in the parathyroid glands sense serum calcium levels. In response to slight declines in serum calcium, the parathyroid glands secrete parathyroid hormone (PTH). PTH stimulates the activity of the 1-hydroxylase enzyme in the kidney, resulting in increased production of calcitriol, the biologically active form of vitamin D. Calcitriol acts to restore normal serum calcium levels in three ways: (1) by activating the vitamin D-dependent transport system in the small intestine, increasing the absorption of dietary calcium; (2) by increasing the mobilization of calcium from bone into the circulation; and (3) by increasing the reabsorption of calcium by the kidneys. PTH is also required to increase bone calcium mobilization and calcium reabsorption by the kidneys.

Deficiency

A low blood calcium level usually implies abnormal parathyroid function and is rarely due to low dietary calcium intake because the skeleton provides a large reserve of calcium for maintaining normal blood levels. Other causes of abnormally low blood calcium levels include chronic kidney failure, vitamin D deficiency, and low blood magnesium levels which occur mainly in cases of severe alcoholism. Magnesium deficiency results in a decrease in the responsiveness of osteoclasts to PTH. A chronically low calcium intake in growing individuals may prevent the attainment of optimal peak bone mass. Once peak bone mass is achieved, inadequate calcium intake may contribute to accelerated bone loss and ultimately to the development of osteoporosis.[1]

Nutrient Interactions

Vitamin D. Vitamin D is required for optimal calcium absorption. Several other nutrients (and non-nutrients) influence the retention of calcium by the body and may affect calcium nutritional status.

Sodium. High sodium intake results in increased loss of calcium in the urine, possibly due to competition between sodium and calcium for reabsorption in the kidney or by an effect of sodium on PTH secretion. Each 2.3 g increment of sodium (5.8 g salt or NaCl) excreted by the kidney has been found to draw about 24–40 mg calcium into the urine. As urinary losses account for about half the difference in calcium retention among individuals, dietary sodium has a large potential to influence bone loss. In women, each extra gram of sodium consumed per day is projected to produce an additional rate of bone loss of 1% per year if all the calcium loss comes from the skeleton.

Although animal studies have shown bone loss to be greater with high-salt intakes, no controlled clinical trials have been conducted to confirm the relationship between salt intake and bone loss in humans.[1,6] However, a 2-year study of postmenopausal women found increased urinary sodium excretion (an indicator of increased sodium intake) to be associated with decreased bone mineral density (BMD) at the hip.[7] In addition, a longitudinal study in 40 postmenopausal women found that adherence to a low-sodium diet (2 g/day) for 6 months was associated with significant reductions in sodium excretion, calcium excretion, and amino-terminal propeptide of type I collagen, a biomarker of bone resorption. However, these associations were observed only in women with baseline urinary sodium excretion of 3.4 g/day or more (i. e., the mean sodium intake for the US adult population).[8] Racial differences for the effect of dietary sodium on urinary sodium and calcium excretion and retention have been reported in adolescent girls. White girls excreted the extra sodium on a high-salt diet, but black girls went into positive sodium balance, which resulted in reduced urinary calcium loss compared with white girls.[9]

Protein. As dietary protein intake increases, the urinary excretion of calcium also increases. Recommended calcium intakes for the US population are higher than those for populations of less industrialized nations because protein intake in the United States is generally higher. The US recommended dietary allowance (RDA) for protein is 46 g/day for women and 56 g/day for men; however, the average intake of protein in the United States tends to be higher (65–70 g/day in women and 90–110 g/day in men).[3] Recently, the overall calcium economy has not been demonstrated to be affected by dietary protein, partly due to offsetting changes in calcium absorption.[10] Inadequate protein intakes have been associated with poor recovery from osteoporotic fractures and serum albumin values (an indicator of protein nutritional status) have been found to be inversely related to hip fracture risk.[3]

Phosphorus. Phosphorus, which is typically found in protein-rich foods, tends to decrease the excretion of calcium in the urine. However, phos-phorus-rich foods also tend to increase the calcium content of digestive secretions, resulting in increased calcium loss in the feces. Thus, phosphorus does not offset the net loss of calcium associated with increased protein intake.[1] Increasing intakes of phosphates from soft drinks and food additives have caused concern among some researchers regarding the implications for bone health. Diets high in phosphorus and low in calcium have been found to increase PTH secretion, as have diets low in calcium.[3,6] Although the effect of high phosphorus intakes on calcium balance and bone health is currently unclear, the substitution of large quantities of soft drinks for milk or other sources of dietary calcium is cause for concern with respect to bone health in adolescents and adults.

Caffeine. Caffeine in large amounts increases urinary calcium content for a short time. However, caffeine intakes of 400 mg/day did not significantly change urinary calcium excretion over 24 hours in premenopausal women when compared with a placebo.[11] Although one observational study found accelerated bone loss in postmenopausal women who consumed less than 744 mg of calcium per day and reported that they drank 2 to 3 cups of coffee per day,[12] a more recent study that measured caffeine intake found no association between caffeine intake and bone loss in postmenopausal women.[13] On average, one 8-oz (224 g) cup of coffee decreases calcium retention by only 2–3 mg.[1]

Recommended Dietary Allowance

Updated recommendations for calcium intake based on the optimization of bone health were released by the Food and Nutrition Board (FNB) of the Institute of Medicine in 2010. The Recommended Dietary Allowance (RDA) for calcium is listed in **Table 14.1** by life stage and gender.

Table 14.1 Recommended dietary intake (RDA) for calcium

Life stage	Age	Males (mg/day)	Females (mg/day)
Infants	0–6 months	200 (AI)	200 (AI)
Infants	6–12 months	260 (AI)	260 (AI)
Children	1–3 years	700	700
Children	4–8 years	1000	1000
Children	9–13 years	1300	1300
Adolescents	14–18 years	1300	1300
Adults	19–50 years	1000	1000
Adults	51–70 years	1000	1200
Adults	≥71 years	1200	1200
Pregnancy	≤18 years	–	1300
Pregnancy	≥19 years	–	1000
Breast-feeding	≤18 years	–	1300
Breast-feeding	≥19 years	–	1000

AI, adequate intake.

Disease Prevention

Colorectal Cancer

Colorectal cancer is the most common gastrointestinal cancer and the second leading cause of cancer deaths in the United States. Colorectal cancer is caused by a combination of genetic and environmental factors, but the degree to which these two types of factors influence the risk of colon cancer in individuals varies widely. In individuals with familial adenomatous polyposis, the cause of colon cancer is thought to be almost entirely genetic, whereas dietary factors appear to influence the risk for other types of colon cancer. Animal studies are strongly supportive of a protective role for calcium in preventing intestinal cancers.[14] In humans, controlled clinical trials have found modest decreases in the recurrence of colorectal adenomas (precancerous polyps) with calcium supplementation of 1200–2000 mg/day,[15,16] and a recent study found that the protective effect extended up to 5 years after the intervention ended.[17] A pooled analysis of 10 prospective cohort studies, including 534 536 men and women, found that those in the highest quintile (one-fifth) of calcium intake (from food) had a 14% lower risk of colorectal cancer compared with those in the lowest quintile; dietary intakes of calcium ranged from 674 mg/day to 1051 mg/day in the 10 cohorts.[18] In this pooled analysis, participants in the highest quintile of total calcium intake (from food and supplements) had a 22% lower risk of colorectal cancer. Total daily intake of calcium ranged from 732 mg to 1087 mg in the examined studies. However, most large prospective studies, individually, have reported that increased calcium intakes are only weakly associated with a decreased risk of colorectal cancer.

These weak associations might be explained by the presence of groups within the population that differ in their response to calcium. For instance, there is some evidence that individuals with increased circulating levels of insulin-like growth factor-1 (IGF-1) are at increased risk of colorectal cancer, and increased calcium intake may benefit this subgroup more than others. A case–control study of 511 men found that increased calcium intake was more strongly associated with decreased colorectal cancer risk in men with higher circulating levels of IGF-1.[19] Before conclusions can be drawn, more research is needed to clarify whether specific subgroups in the larger population have different calcium requirements with respect to decreasing the risk of colorectal cancer.

Osteoporosis

Osteoporosis is a skeletal disorder in which bone strength is compromised, resulting in an increased risk of fracture. Sustaining a hip fracture is one of the most serious consequences of osteoporosis. Nearly one-third of those who sustain osteoporotic hip fractures enter nursing homes within the year following the fracture, and one person in five dies within 1 year of experiencing an osteoporotic hip fracture. Although osteoporosis is most commonly diagnosed in white postmenopausal women, women of other racial groups and ages, men, and children may also develop osteoporosis.[20]

Osteoporosis is a multifactorial disorder, and nutrition is only one factor contributing to its development and progression.[2] Other factors that increase the risk of developing osteoporosis include, but are not limited to, increased age, female gender, estrogen deficiency, smoking, metabolic disease (e.g., hyperthyroidism), and the use of certain medications (e.g., corticosteroids and anticonvulsants). A predisposition to osteoporotic fracture is related to one's peak bone mass and to the rate of bone loss after peak bone mass has been attained. After adult height has been reached, the skeleton continues to accumulate bone until the third decade of life. Genetic factors exert a strong influence on peak bone mass, but lifestyle factors can also play a significant role. Strategies for reducing the risk of osteoporotic fracture include the attainment of maximal peak bone mass and the reduction of bone loss later in life. Although calcium is the nutrient consistently found to be most important for attaining peak bone mass and preventing osteoporosis, adequate vitamin D intake is also required for optimal calcium absorption.[20]

Physical exercise is another lifestyle factor of benefit in the prevention of osteoporosis and osteoporotic fracture. There is evidence to suggest that physical activity early in life contributes to the attainment of higher peak bone mass. Exercise in the presence of adequate calcium and vitamin D intake probably has a modest effect on slowing the rate of bone loss later in life. One compilation of published calcium trials indicated that the beneficial skeletal effect of increased physical activity was achievable only at calcium intakes above 1000 mg/day.[21] High impact exercise and resistance exercise (weights) are likely the most beneficial for preventing bone loss. Lower impact exercise such as walking, swimming, and cycling have beneficial effects on other aspects of health and function, but their effects on bone loss are minimal. However, exercise later in life, even beyond 90 years of age, can still increase strength and reduce the likelihood of a fall, another important risk factor for hip fracture.[20] Supplemental calcium alone cannot usually restore lost bone in individuals with osteoporosis. However, optimal treatment of osteoporosis with any drug therapy also requires adequate intake of calcium (1200 mg/day) and vitamin D (600 IU/day).[2,20]

Kidney Stones

Approximately 12% of the US population will have a kidney stone at some time. Most kidney stones are composed of calcium oxalate or calcium phosphate. Although their cause is usually unknown, abnormally elevated urinary calcium (hypercalciuria) increases the risk of developing calcium stones. Increasing dietary calcium increases urinary calcium slightly, and the rise is more pronounced in those with hypercalciuria. However, other dietary factors such as sodium and protein are also known to increase urinary calcium.[22,23] A large prospective study that followed men over a period of 12 years found the incidence of symptomatic kidney stones to be 44% lower in men in the highest quintile of calcium intake, averaging 1326 mg/day, compared with men in the lowest quintile of calcium intake, averaging 516 mg/day.[24] Similar results were observed in a large prospective study of women followed over 12 years.[25]

A 14-year follow-up analysis of the study in men reported that calcium intake was related to a lower risk of kidney stones in those aged less than 60 years but not in older men.[26] In addition, a prospective study in a cohort of 96 245 younger women, aged 27–44 years, found that higher dietary calcium intakes were associated with a lower risk of kidney stones.[27] The authors of these two studies suggest that increased dietary calcium might inhibit the absorption of dietary oxalate and reduce urinary oxalate, a risk factor for calcium oxalate stones. Support for this idea comes from a study in which people ingested oxalate with or without supplemental calcium.[28] Providing 200 mg elemental calcium along with oxalate significantly reduced both oxalate absorption and excretion.

Although people who form calcium stones have been advised to restrict calcium intake in the past, a cross-sectional study of 282 patients with calcium oxalate stones found that dietary salt, as measured by urinary sodium excretion, was the dietary factor most strongly associated with urinary calcium excretion.[29] A study of 85 calcium stone-forming patients found that those with low BMD were significantly more likely to have a high salt intake and high urinary sodium excretion, leading the authors to suggest that reduced salt intake should be recommended for such patients.[30] Findings that calcium stone-forming patients with lower calcium intakes are more likely to have decreased BMD also call into question the therapeutic use of dietary calcium restriction. At present, the only dietary change proven effective in reducing kidney stone recurrence is increasing fluid intake. However, a recent randomized, double-blind, placebo-controlled trial in 36 282 postmenopausal women reported that a combination of supplemental calcium (1000 mg/day) and vitamin D (400 IU/day) was associated with a significantly increased risk for kidney stones. More controlled trials are necessary to determine whether supplemental calcium affects the development of kidney stones.[31]

Pregnancy-induced Hypertension

Pregnancy-induced hypertension (PIH) occurs in 10% of pregnancies and is a major health risk for pregnant women and their offspring. PIH is a term that includes gestational hypertension, pre-eclampsia, and eclampsia. Gestational hypertension is defined as an abnormally high blood pressure that usually develops after week 20 of pregnancy. In addition to gestational hypertension, pre-eclampsia includes the development of edema (severe swelling) and proteinuria (protein in the urine). Pre-eclampsia may progress to eclampsia (also called *toxemia*) in which life-threatening convulsions and coma may occur.[32] Although the cause of PIH is not entirely understood, calcium metabolism appears to play a role.

Risk factors for PIH include first pregnancies, multiple gestations (e.g., twins or triplets), chronic high blood pressure, diabetes, and some autoimmune diseases. Data from epidemiological studies suggest an inverse relationship between calcium intake and the incidence of PIH, but the results of experimental research on calcium supplementation and PIH have been less clear. A systematic review of randomized placebo-controlled studies found that calcium supplementation reduced the incidence of high blood pressure in pregnant women at high risk of PIH, as well as in pregnant women with low dietary calcium intake. However, in women at low risk of PIH and with adequate calcium intake the benefit of calcium supplementation was judged small and unlikely to be clinically significant.[33] A large multicenter clinical trial, Calcium for Pre-eclampsia Prevention (CPEP), in over 4500 pregnant women found no effect of 2000 mg supplemental calcium on PIH. However, women in the placebo group had a mean intake of 980 mg/day, whereas those in the supplemental group had a mean intake of 2300 mg/day.[34] For the general population, meeting current recommendations for calcium intake during pregnancy may help prevent PIH. Further research is required to determine whether women at high risk for PIH would benefit from calcium supplementation above the current recommendations.

Lead Toxicity

Children who are chronically exposed to lead, even in small amounts, are more likely to develop learning disabilities and behavioral problems, and to have low IQs. Abnormal growth and neurological development may occur in the infants of women exposed to lead during pregnancy. In adults, lead toxicity may result in kidney damage and high blood pressure. Although the use of lead paint and leaded gasoline has been discontinued in the United States, lead toxicity continues to be a significant health problem, especially in children living in urban areas. A study of over 300 children in an urban neighborhood found that 49% of children aged 1–8 years had blood lead levels above current guidelines, indicating excessive lead exposure. In this study, only 59% of children aged 1–3 years and 41% of children aged 4–8 years had calcium intakes meeting the recommended levels.[35]

Adequate calcium intake could protect against lead toxicity in at least two ways. Increased dietary intake of calcium is known to decrease the gastrointestinal absorption of lead. Once lead enters the body it tends to accumulate in the skeleton, where it may remain for more than 20 years. Adequate calcium intake also prevents exposure to lead mobilized from the skeleton during bone demineralization. A study of blood lead levels during pregnancy found that women with inadequate calcium intake during the second half of pregnancy were more likely to have elevated blood lead levels, probably related to increased bone demineralization, with the release of accumulated lead into the blood.[36] Lead in the blood of a pregnant woman is readily transported across the placenta, resulting in fetal lead exposure at a time when the developing nervous system is highly vulnerable. In addition, in postmenopausal women, increased calcium intake has been associated with decreased blood lead levels. Other factors known to decrease bone demineralization, including estrogen replacement therapy and physical activity, have also been inversely associated with blood lead levels.[37]

Disease Treatment

Hypertension

The relationship between calcium intake and blood pressure has been investigated extensively over the past two decades. An analysis of 23 large observational studies found a reduction in systolic blood pressure of 0.34 mmHg per 100 mg calcium consumed daily and a reduction in diastolic blood pressure of 0.15 mmHg per 100 mg calcium.[38] A large systematic review of 42 randomized controlled trials examining the effect of calcium supplementation on blood pressure compared with placebo found an overall reduction of 1.44 mmHg in systolic blood pressure and of 0.84 mmHg in diastolic blood pressure.[39] Calcium supplementation in these randomized controlled trials ranged from 500 mg/day to 2000 mg/day, with 1000–1500 mg/day being the most common dose. In the Dietary Approaches to Stop Hypertension (DASH) study, 549 people were randomized to one of three diets for 8 weeks:

1. A control diet that was low in fruit, vegetables, and dairy products
2. A diet rich in fruit (about five servings per day) and vegetables (about three servings per day)
3. A combination diet rich in fruit and vegetables as well as low-fat dairy products (about three servings per day).[40]

The combination diet represented an increase of about 800 mg calcium/day over the control and fruit-/vegetable-rich diets for a total of about 1200 mg calcium/day. The combination diet re-duced systolic blood pressure by 5.5 mmHg and diastolic blood pressure by 3.0 mmHg more than the control diet, whereas the fruit/vegetable diet reduced systolic blood pressure by 2.8 mmHg and diastolic blood pressure by 1.1 mmHg more than the control diet. Among those participants diagnosed with hypertension, the combination diet reduced systolic blood pressure by 11.4 mmHg and diastolic pressure by 5.5 mmHg more than the control diet, whereas the reduction for the fruit/vegetable diet was 7.2 mmHg systolic and 2.8 mmHg diastolic compared with the control diet.[41] This research indicates that a calcium intake at the recommended level (1000–1200 mg/day) may be helpful in preventing and treating moderate hypertension.[42]

Premenstrual Syndrome

Premenstrual syndrome (PMS) refers to a cluster of symptoms, including but not limited to fatigue, irritability, moodiness/depression, fluid retention, and breast tenderness, that begins sometime after ovulation (midcycle) and subsides with the onset of menstruation (the monthly period).[43] Low dietary calcium intakes have been linked to PMS in several studies, and supplemental calcium has been shown to decrease symptom severity.[44] In a randomized, double-blind, placebo-controlled clinical trial of 466 women, supplemental calcium (1200 mg/day) for three menstrual cycles was associated with a 48% reduction in total symptom scores, compared with a 30% reduction observed in the placebo group.[45] Similar positive effects were reported in two double-blind, placebo-controlled, crossover trials that administered 1000 mg calcium daily.[46,47] A case–control study in women participating in the Nurses' Health Study II found that those who consumed the most calcium (median of 1283 mg/day) from food had a 30% lower risk of developing PMS compared with those with the lowest calcium intake (median of 529 mg/day from food).[48] However, calcium intake from supplements had no effect on PMS in this study. Large-scale clinical trials are needed to determine whether increasing dietary calcium intake or taking calcium supplements has therapeutic benefits in treating and preventing PMS.

Sources

Food Sources

Average dietary intakes of calcium in the United States are well below the RDA for every age and gender group, especially in females. Only about 25% of boys and 10% of girls aged 9–17 are estimated to meet the recommendations. Dairy foods provide 75% of the calcium in the American diet. However, it is typically during the most critical period for peak bone mass development that adolescents tend to replace milk with soft drinks.[1,3] Dairy products represent rich and absorbable sources of calcium, but certain vegetables and grains also provide calcium. However, the bioavailability of the calcium must be taken into consideration. Although the calcium-rich plants in the kale family (broccoli, bok choy, cabbage, mustard, and turnip greens) contain calcium that is as bioavailable as that in milk, some food components have been found to inhibit the absorption of calcium. Oxalic acid, also known as *oxalate*, is the most potent inhibitor of calcium absorption and is found at high concentrations in spinach and rhubarb and somewhat lower concentrations in sweet potatoes and dried beans. Phytic acid is a less potent inhibitor of calcium absorption than oxalate. Yeast possesses an enzyme (phytase) that breaks down phytic acid in grains during fermentation, lowering the phytic acid content of breads and other fermented foods. Only concentrated sources of phytate, such as wheat bran or dried beans, substantially reduce calcium absorption.[1] **Table 14.2** lists a number of calcium-rich foods, along with their calcium content and the number of servings of that food required to equal the absorbable calcium from one glass of milk.[49]

Supplements

Most experts recommend obtaining as much calcium as possible from food because calcium in food is accompanied by other important nutrients that help the body utilize the calcium. However, calcium supplements may be necessary for those who have difficulty consuming enough calcium from food. No multivitamin/mineral tablet contains 100% of the recommended daily value for calcium because it is too bulky, and the resulting pill would be too large to swallow. The "Supplement Facts" label, now required on all supplements marketed in the United States, lists the calcium content of the supplement as elemental calcium. Calcium preparations used as supplements include calcium carbonate, calcium lactate, calcium gluconate, calcium citrate, and

Table 14.2 Food sources and relative absorbability of calcium

Food	Serving	Elemental calcium (mg)	Percentage calcium absorbed	Estimated absorbable calcium (mg)	Servings needed to equal 8 oz milk[a]
Milk	8 ounces	300	32	96	1.0
Cheddar cheese	1.5 ounces	303	32	97	1.0
Yogurt	8 ounces	300	32	96	1.0
Tofu, calcium set	½ cup	258	31	80	1.2
Rhubarb	½ cup, cooked	174	9	10	9.5
Spinach	½ cup, cooked	115	5	6	16.3
White beans	½ cup, cooked	113	22	25	3.9
Bok choy	½ cup, cooked	79	54	43	2.3
Kale	½ cup, cooked	61	49	30	3.2
Pinto beans	½ cup, cooked	45	27	12	8.1
Red beans	½ cup, cooked	41	24	10	9.7
Broccoli	½ cup, cooked	35	61	22	4.5

Reproduced with permission by the *American Journal of Clinical Nutrition*, American Society for Clinical Nutrition.[71]
[a]All other foods are compared with milk in terms of calcium availability.

calcium citrate malate. To determine which calcium preparation is in your supplement, you may have to look at the ingredient list. Calcium carbonate is generally the most economical calcium supplement. To maximize absorption, take no more than 500 mg elemental calcium at one time. Most calcium supplements should be taken with meals, although calcium citrate and calcium citrate malate can be taken anytime.[50]

Lead in Calcium Supplements

Several years ago concern was raised about the lead levels in calcium supplements obtained from natural sources (oyster shell, bone meal, dolomite). In 1993, investigators found measurable quantities of lead in most of the 70 different preparations that they tested.[51] Since then, manufacturers have made an effort to reduce the amount of lead in calcium supplements to less than 0.5 µg/1000 mg elemental calcium. The federal limit is 7.5 µg/1000 mg elemental calcium. As lead is so widespread and long lasting, no one can guarantee entirely lead-free food or supplements. One study found measurable lead in eight of 21 supplements, in amounts averaging between 1 and 2 µg/1000 mg elemental calcium.[52] Calcium inhibits intestinal absorption of lead, and adequate calcium intake is protective against lead toxicity, so trace amounts of lead in calcium supplementation may pose less of a risk of excessive lead exposure than inadequate calcium consumption. Although most calcium sources today are relatively safe, look for supplements that are labeled "lead-free" and avoid large doses of supplemental calcium (more than 1500 mg/day).

Safety

Toxicity

Abnormally elevated blood calcium (hypercalcemia) resulting from the over-consumption of calcium has never been documented to occur from food, only from calcium supplements. Mild hypercalcemia may be without symptoms or may result in loss of appetite, nausea, vomiting, constipation, abdominal pain, dry mouth, thirst, and frequent urination. More severe hypercalcemia may result in confusion, delirium, coma, and, if not treated, death. Hypercalcemia has been reported only with the consumption of large quantities of calcium supplements, usually in combination with antacids, particularly in the days when peptic ulcers were treated with large quantities of milk, calcium carbonate (antacid), and sodium bicarbonate (absorbable alkali).[1] This condition was termed *milk alkali syndrome* and has been reported at calcium supplement levels from 1.5 g/day to 16.5 g/day for 2 days to 30 years. As the treatment for peptic ulcers has changed, the incidence of this syndrome has decreased considerably.[3]

Although the risk of forming kidney stones is increased in individuals with abnormally elevated urinary calcium (hypercalciuria), this condition is not usually related to calcium intake, rather to increased excretion of calcium by the kidneys. Overall, increased dietary calcium has been associated with a decreased risk of kidney stones. However, in a large prospective study, the risk of developing kidney stones in women taking supplemental calcium was 20% higher than in those who did not take supplements.[25] This effect may be related to the fact that calcium supplements can be taken without food, eliminating their beneficial effect of decreasing intestinal oxalate absorption.

In 2010 the FNB of the Institute of Medicine updated the tolerable upper intake level (UL) for calcium. The UL is listed in **Table 14.3** by age group.

Table 14.3 Tolerable upper intake level (UL) for calcium

Life stage	Age	UL (mg/day)
Infants	0–6 months	1000
Infants	6–12 months	1500
Children	1–8 years	2500
Children	9–13 years	3000
Adolescents	14–18 years	3000
Adults	19–50 years	2500
Adults	≥51 years	2000

Do High Calcium Intakes Increase the Risk of Prostate Cancer?

Some epidemiological studies have raised concern that high calcium intakes are associated with increased risk of prostate cancer. A large prospective cohort study in the United States followed more than 50000 male health professionals for 8 years and found that men whose calcium intake was 2000 mg/day or more had a risk of developing advanced prostate cancer that was three times higher than men whose calcium intake was less than 500 mg/day, and a risk of developing metastasized prostate cancer that was more than four times greater.[53] Similar results were observed in a case–control study in Sweden, which compared the calcium consumption of 526 men diagnosed with prostate cancer with that of 536 controls.[54] Neither study found calcium intake to be associated with an increased risk of total prostate cancer or nonadvanced prostate cancer. More recently, another prospective study of US physicians found that increased intake of calcium from dairy foods was associated with an increased risk of prostate cancer.[55] Although this study did not examine supplement use, each 500 mg/day increase in calcium intake from dairy foods was associated with a 16% increase in the risk of prostate cancer (advanced and nonadvanced, combined). Most recently, a prospective study in a cohort of 29133 men who smoked, followed for 17 years, found that high calcium consumption (> 1000 mg/day) was associated with an increased risk for prostate cancer.[56]

The physiological mechanisms underlying the relationship between calcium intake and prostate cancer are not yet clear. High levels of dietary calcium may lead to decreased circulating levels of calcitriol, the active form of vitamin D. In experimental studies conducted in prostate cancer cell lines and animal models, calcitriol was found to have protective effects. However, the findings of studies conducted in humans on serum calcitriol levels and prostate cancer risk have been much less consistent.

Not all epidemiological studies have demonstrated an association between calcium intake and prostate cancer. One review reported that 7 of 14 case–control studies and 5 of 9 prospective cohort studies found statistically significant positive associations between prostate cancer and some measure of dairy product consumption. Of those studies that examined calcium intake, three of six case–control studies and two of four cohort studies reported statistically significant associations between prostate cancer and calcium intake.[57] However, one Serbian case–control study found increased calcium intake to be associated with a decreased risk of prostate cancer.[58] In a meta-analysis of six prospective studies, Gao et al. reported that men with higher daily calcium intakes had a 39% increased risk of developing prostate cancer compared with those with lower intakes; men with higher dairy product intakes had an 11% higher risk of prostate cancer compared with those with lower dairy product intakes.[59] However, only half the distinct studies included in this meta-analysis reported an association between higher calcium intakes and prostate cancer.

More recently, a prospective study in 14642 men participating in the Melbourne Collaborative Cohort Study found that calcium intake was not associated with prostate cancer risk.[60] Gao et al. repeated their meta-analysis[59] to include this most recently published study. They found that those with higher calcium intakes had a 32% increased risk of prostate cancer; however, meta-analysis of all seven studies revealed that dairy intake was no longer associated with a significantly increased risk of prostate cancer.[60] The lack of agreement in the studies suggests complex interactions among the risk factors for prostate cancer and may also reflect the difficulties associated with assessing calcium intake in free-living humans. Until the relationship between calcium and prostate cancer is clarified, it is reasonable for men to consume a total of 1000–1200 mg/day of calcium (diet and supplements combined), which is the RDA.

Drug Interactions

Taking calcium supplements in combination with thiazide diuretics (e.g., hydrochlorthiazide) increases the risk of developing hypercalcemia due to increased reabsorption of calcium in the kidneys. High doses of supplemental calcium could increase the likelihood of abnormal heart rhythms in people taking digitalis (digoxin) for heart failure.[61] Calcium, when provided intravenously, may decrease the efficacy of calcium channel blockers.[62] However, dietary and oral supplemental calcium do not appear to affect the action of calcium channel blockers.[63] Calcium may decrease the absorption of tetracycline, quinolone class antibiotics, bisphosphonates, and levothyroxine; therefore, it is advisable to separate doses of these medications and calcium-rich foods or supplements by 2 hours. Use of H_2-receptor blockers (e.g., cimetidine) and proton pump inhibitors (e.g., omeprazole) may decrease the absorption of calcium carbonate and calcium phosphate.[50,64]

Nutrient Interactions

The presence of calcium decreases iron absorption from nonheme sources (i.e., most supplements and food sources other than meat). However, calcium supplementation up to 12 weeks has not been found to change iron nutritional status, probably due to a compensatory increase in iron absorption. Individuals taking iron supplements should take them 2 hours apart from calcium-rich foods or supplements to maximize iron absorption. High calcium intakes in rats have produced relative magnesium deficiencies, but calcium intake was not found to affect magnesium retention in humans.[1] Although a number of studies did not find high calcium intakes to affect zinc absorption or zinc nutritional status, a study in 10 men and women indicated that 600 mg calcium consumed with a meal decreased the absorption of zinc from that meal by 50%.[65]

Recent Research

Calcium and Weight Loss

Diets with higher calcium density (calcium per total calories) have been associated with a reduced incidence of being overweight or obese in some studies. These studies were not designed to examine the effect of calcium on obesity or body fat, and their significance was unclear until recent studies in cell culture and animal models indicated that low calcium intakes could result in hormonal and metabolic changes that increase the tendency of fat cells to accumulate fat.[66] In a 2-year exercise trial, higher dietary calcium intakes were associated with weight loss whether participants were in the exercise group or the control group.[67] A placebo-controlled calcium supplementation trial found significantly greater weight loss in elderly women supplemented with 1200 mg calcium/day compared with a control group.[68] More recently, a 1-year dairy product intervention (1000–1400 mg calcium/day) in healthy young women did not alter body weight or fat mass compared with the control group (< 800 mg calcium/day);[69] however, a slight reduction in body fat mass was observed in the high-dairy group (1300–1400 mg calcium/day) at the 6-month follow-up.[70] Controlled feeding studies in which calories remain fixed are needed to quantify the likely small effect of calcium, if any, on body fat and body weight. Such studies are currently under way.

LPI Recommendation

The Linus Pauling Institute supports the RDA set by the FNB. Following these recommendations should provide adequate calcium to promote skeletal health and may also decrease the risks of some chronic diseases.

Children and Adolescents
To promote the attainment of maximal peak bone mass, children and adolescents (9–18 years) should consume a total (diet plus supplements) of 1300 mg/day of calcium.

Adults
After adult height has been reached, the skeleton continues to accumulate bone until the third decade of life when peak bone mass is attained. To promote the attainment of maximal peak bone mass and to minimize bone loss later in life, adult women (aged 50 years and younger) and adult men (aged 70 years and younger) should consume a total (diet plus supplements) of 1000 mg/day of calcium.

Older Women
To minimize bone loss, postmenopausal women should consume a total (diet plus supplements) of 1200 mg/day of calcium. Taking a multivitamin/mineral supplement containing at least 10 µg (400 IU)/day of vitamin D will help to ensure adequate calcium absorption (see Chapter 11, Vitamin D).

Older Men
To minimize bone loss, men aged 71 years and older should consume a total (diet plus supplements) of 1200 mg/day of calcium. Taking a multivitamin/mineral supplement containing at least 10 µg (400 IU)/day of vitamin D will help to ensure adequate calcium absorption (see Chapter 11, Vitamin D).

Pregnant and Breast-feeding Women
Pregnant and breast-feeding adolescents (under 19 years of age) should consume a total of 1300 mg/day of calcium, while pregnant and breastfeeding adults (19–50 years) should consume a total of 1000 mg/day of calcium.

References

1. Weaver CM, Heaney RP. Calcium. In: Shils M, Olson JA, Shike M, Ross AC, eds. Modern Nutrition in Health and Disease, 9th ed. Baltimore, MD: Lippincott Williams & Wilkins; 1999:141–155
2. Heaney RP. Calcium, dairy products and osteoporosis. J Am Coll Nutr 2000; 19(2, Suppl):83S–99S
3. Food and Nutrition Board, Institute of Medicine. Calcium. In: Dietary Reference Intakes for Calcium, Phosphorus, Magnesium, Vitamin D, and Fluoride. Washington, DC: National Academy Press; 1997:71–145
4. Brody T. Nutritional Biochemistry, 2nd ed. San Diego, CA: Academic Press; 1999
5. Pearce SH, Thakker RV. The calcium-sensing receptor: insights into extracellular calcium homeostasis in health and disease. J Endocrinol 1997;154(3):371–378
6. Calvo MS. Dietary considerations to prevent loss of bone and renal function. Nutrition 2000;16(7-8):564–566
7. Devine A, Criddle RA, Dick IM, Kerr DA, Prince RL. A longitudinal study of the effect of sodium and calcium intakes on regional bone density in postmenopausal women. Am J Clin Nutr 1995;62(4):740–745
8. Carbone LD, Barrow KD, Bush AJ, et al. Effects of a low sodium diet on bone metabolism. J Bone Miner Metab 2005;23(6):506–513
9. Wigertz K, Palacios C, Jackman LA, et al. Racial differences in calcium retention in response to dietary salt in adolescent girls. Am J Clin Nutr 2005;81(4):845–850
10. Bonjour JP. Dietary protein: an essential nutrient for bone health. J Am Coll Nutr 2005;24(6, Suppl):526S–536S
11. Barger-Lux MJ, Heaney RP, Stegman MR. Effects of moderate caffeine intake on the calcium economy of premenopausal women. Am J Clin Nutr 1990;52(4):722–725
12. Harris SS, Dawson-Hughes B. Caffeine and bone loss in healthy postmenopausal women. Am J Clin Nutr 1994;60(4):573–578
13. Lloyd T, Johnson-Rollings N, Eggli DF, Kieselhorst K, Mauger EA, Cusatis DC. Bone status among postmenopausal women with different habitual caffeine intakes: a longitudinal investigation. J Am Coll Nutr 2000;19(2):256–261
14. Bostick R. Diet and nutrition in the prevention of colon cancer. In: Bendich A, Deckelbaum RJ, eds. Preventive Nutrition: The Comprehensive Guide for Health Professionals, 2nd ed. Totowa, NJ: Humana Press, Inc.; 2001:57–95
15. Bonithon-Kopp C, Kronborg O, Giacosa A, Räth U, Faivre J. European Cancer Prevention Organisation Study Group. Calcium and fibre supplementation in prevention of colorectal adenoma recurrence: a randomised intervention trial. Lancet 2000;356(9238):1300–1306
16. Baron JA, Beach M, Mandel JS, et al. Polyp Prevention Study Group. Calcium supplements and colorectal adenomas. Ann N Y Acad Sci 1999;889:138–145
17. Grau MV, Baron JA, Sandler RS, et al. Prolonged effect of calcium supplementation on risk of colorectal adenomas in a randomized trial. J Natl Cancer Inst 2007;99(2):129–136
18. Cho E, Smith-Warner SA, Spiegelman D, et al. Dairy foods, calcium, and colorectal cancer: a pooled analysis of 10 cohort studies. J Natl Cancer Inst 2004;96(13):1015–1022
19. Ma J, Giovannucci E, Pollak M, et al. Milk intake, circulating levels of insulin-like growth factor-I, and risk of colorectal cancer in men. J Natl Cancer Inst 2001;93(17):1330–1336
20. National Institutes of Health. Osteoporosis prevention, diagnosis, and therapy. NIH Consensus Statement 2000;17(1):1–45 http://consensus.nih.gov/2000/2000Osteoporosis111html.htm
21. Specker BL. Evidence for an interaction between calcium intake and physical activity on changes in bone mineral density. J Bone Miner Res 1996;11(10):1539–1544
22. Heller HJ. The role of calcium in the prevention of kidney stones. J Am Coll Nutr 1999;18(5, Suppl):373S–378S
23. Martini LA, Wood RJ. Should dietary calcium and protein be restricted in patients with nephrolithiasis? Nutr Rev 2000;58(4):111–117
24. Curhan GC, Willett WC, Rimm EB, Stampfer MJ. A prospective study of dietary calcium and other nutrients and the risk of symptomatic kidney stones. N Engl J Med 1993;328(12):833–838
25. Curhan GC, Willett WC, Speizer FE, Spiegelman D, Stampfer MJ. Comparison of dietary calcium with supplemental calcium and other nutrients as factors affecting the risk for kidney stones in women. Ann Intern Med 1997;126(7):497–504
26. Taylor EN, Stampfer MJ, Curhan GC. Dietary factors and the risk of incident kidney stones in men: new insights after 14 years of follow-up. J Am Soc Nephrol 2004;15(12):3225–3232
27. Curhan GC, Willett WC, Knight EL, Stampfer MJ. Dietary factors and the risk of incident kidney stones in younger women: Nurses' Health Study II. Arch Intern Med 2004;164(8):885–891
28. Liebman M, Chai W. Effect of dietary calcium on urinary oxalate excretion after oxalate loads. Am J Clin Nutr 1997;65(5):1453–1459
29. Burtis WJ, Gay L, Insogna KL, Ellison A, Broadus AE. Dietary hypercalciuria in patients with calcium oxalate kidney stones. Am J Clin Nutr 1994;60(3):424–429
30. Martini LA, Cuppari L, Colugnati FA, et al. High sodium chloride intake is associated with low bone density in calcium stone-forming patients. Clin Nephrol 2000;54(2):85–93
31. Jackson RD, LaCroix AZ, Gass M, et al. Women's Health Initiative Investigators. Calcium plus vitamin D supplementation and the risk of fractures. N Engl J Med 2006;354(7):669–683
32. Ritchie LD, King JC. Dietary calcium and pregnancy-induced hypertension: is there a relation? Am J Clin Nutr 2000; 71(5, Suppl):1371S–1374S
33. Kulier R, de Onis M, Gülmezoglu AM, Villar J. Nutritional interventions for the prevention of maternal morbidity. Int J Gynaecol Obstet 1998;63(3):231–246
34. Levine RJ, Hauth JC, Curet LB, et al. Trial of calcium to prevent preeclampsia. N Engl J Med 1997;337(2):69–76
35. Bruening K, Kemp FW, Simone N, Holding Y, Louria DB, Bogden JD. Dietary calcium intakes of urban children at risk of lead poisoning. Environ Health Perspect 1999;107(6):431–435
36. Hertz-Picciotto I, Schramm M, Watt-Morse M, Chantala K, Anderson J, Osterloh J. Patterns and determi-

nants of blood lead during pregnancy. Am J Epidemiol 2000;152(9):829–837

37. Muldoon SB, Cauley JA, Kuller LH, Scott J, Rohay J. Lifestyle and sociodemographic factors as determinants of blood lead levels in elderly women. Am J Epidemiol 1994;139(6):599–608

38. Birkett NJ. Comments on a meta-analysis of the relation between dietary calcium intake and blood pressure. Am J Epidemiol 1998;148(3):223–228; discussion 232–233

39. Griffith LE, Guyatt GH, Cook RJ, Bucher HC, Cook DJ. The influence of dietary and nondietary calcium supplementation on blood pressure: an updated meta-analysis of randomized controlled trials. Am J Hypertens 1999;12(1 Pt 1):84–92

40. Appel LJ, Moore TJ, Obarzanek E, et al; DASH Collaborative Research Group. A clinical trial of the effects of dietary patterns on blood pressure. N Engl J Med 1997;336(16):1117–1124

41. Conlin PR, Chow D, Miller ER III, et al. The effect of dietary patterns on blood pressure control in hypertensive patients: results from the Dietary Approaches to Stop Hypertension (DASH) trial. Am J Hypertens 2000;13(9):949–955

42. Miller GD, DiRienzo DD, Reusser ME, McCarron DA. Benefits of dairy product consumption on blood pressure in humans: a summary of the biomedical literature. J Am Coll Nutr 2000; 19(2, Suppl):147S–164S

43. Brown JE. Preconception Nutrition: Conditions and Interventions. In: Brown JE, ed. Nutrition through the Life Cycle. Belmont, CA: Wadsworth/Thomson Learning; 2002:53–60

44. Bendich A. The potential for dietary supplements to reduce premenstrual syndrome (PMS) symptoms. J Am Coll Nutr 2000;19(1):3–12

45. Thys-Jacobs S, Starkey P, Bernstein D, Tian J. Premenstrual Syndrome Study Group. Calcium carbonate and the premenstrual syndrome: effects on premenstrual and menstrual symptoms. Am J Obstet Gynecol 1998;179(2):444–452

46. Thys-Jacobs S, Ceccarelli S, Bierman A, Weisman H, Cohen MA, Alvir J. Calcium supplementation in premenstrual syndrome: a randomized crossover trial. J Gen Intern Med 1989;4(3):183–189

47. Alvir JM, Thys-Jacobs S. Premenstrual and menstrual symptom clusters and response to calcium treatment. Psychopharmacol Bull 1991;27(2):145–148

48. Bertone-Johnson ER, Hankinson SE, Bendich A, Johnson SR, Willett WC, Manson JE. Calcium and vitamin D intake and risk of incident premenstrual syndrome. Arch Intern Med 2005;165(11):1246–1252

49. Weaver CM, Proulx WR, Heaney R. Choices for achieving adequate dietary calcium with a vegetarian diet. Am J Clin Nutr 1999; 70(3, Suppl):543S–548S

50. Hendler SS, Rorvik DR, eds. PDR for Nutritional Supplements. Montvale, NJ: Medical Economics Co., Inc.; 2001

51. Bourgoin BP, Evans DR, Cornett JR, Lingard SM, Quattrone AJ. Lead content in 70 brands of dietary calcium supplements. Am J Public Health 1993;83(8): 1155–1160

52. Ross EA, Szabo NJ, Tebbett IR. Lead content of calcium supplements. JAMA 2000;284(11):1425–1429

53. Giovannucci E, Rimm EB, Wolk A, et al. Calcium and fructose intake in relation to risk of prostate cancer. Cancer Res 1998;58(3):442–447

54. Chan JM, Giovannucci E, Andersson SO, Yuen J, Adami HO, Wolk A. Dairy products, calcium, phosphorous, vitamin D, and risk of prostate cancer (Sweden). Cancer Causes Control 1998;9(6):559–566

55. Chan JM, Stampfer MJ, Ma J, Gann PH, Gaziano JM, Giovannucci EL. Dairy products, calcium, and prostate cancer risk in the Physicians' Health Study. Am J Clin Nutr 2001;74(4):549–554

56. Mitrou PN, Albanes D, Weinstein SJ, et al. A prospective study of dietary calcium, dairy products and prostate cancer risk (Finland). Int J Cancer 2007;120(11):2466–2473

57. Chan JM, Giovannucci EL. Dairy products, calcium, and vitamin D and risk of prostate cancer. Epidemiol Rev 2001;23(1):87–92

58. Vlajinac HD, Marinković JM, Ilić MD, Kocev NI. Diet and prostate cancer: a case-control study. Eur J Cancer 1997;33(1):101–107

59. Gao X, LaValley MP, Tucker KL. Prospective studies of dairy product and calcium intakes and prostate cancer risk: a meta-analysis. J Natl Cancer Inst 2005;97(23):1768–1777

60. Severi G, English DR, Hopper JL, Giles GG. Re: Prospective studies of dairy product and calcium intakes and prostate cancer risk: a meta-analysis. J Natl Cancer Inst 2006;98(11):794–795, author reply 795

61. Vella A, Gerber TC, Hayes DL, Reeder GS. Digoxin, hypercalcaemia, and cardiac conduction. Postgrad Med J 1999;75(887):554–556

62. Moser LR, Smythe MA, Tisdale JE. The use of calcium salts in the prevention and management of verapamil-induced hypotension. Ann Pharmacother 2000;34(5):622–629

63. Bania TC, Blaufeux B, Hughes S, Almond GL, Homel P. Calcium and digoxin vs. calcium alone for severe verapamil toxicity. Acad Emerg Med 2000; 7(10):1089–1096

64. Minerals. Drug Facts and Comparisons, 54th ed. St. Louis: Facts and Comparisons; 2000: 27–28

65. Wood RJ, Zheng JJ. High dietary calcium intakes reduce zinc absorption and balance in humans. Am J Clin Nutr 1997;65(6):1803–1809

66. Zemel MB, Shi H, Greer B, Dirienzo D, Zemel PC. Regulation of adiposity by dietary calcium. FASEB J 2000;14(9):1132–1138

67. Lin YC, Lyle RM, McCabe LD, McCabe GP, Weaver CM, Teegarden D. Dairy calcium is related to changes in body composition during a two-year exercise intervention in young women. J Am Coll Nutr 2000;19(6):754–760

68. Davies KM, Heaney RP, Recker RR, et al. Calcium intake and body weight. J Clin Endocrinol Metab 2000;85(12):4635–4638

69. Gunther CW, Legowski PA, Lyle RM, et al. Dairy products do not lead to alterations in body weight or fat mass in young women in a 1-y intervention. Am J Clin Nutr 2005;81(4):751–756

70. Eagan MS, Lyle RM, Gunther CW, Peacock M, Teegarden D. Effect of 1-year dairy product intervention on fat mass in young women: 6-month follow-up. Obesity (Silver Spring) 2006;14(12):2242–2248

71. Weaver CM, Proulx WR, Heaney R. Choices for achieving adequate dietary calcium with a vegetarian diet. Am J Clin Nutr 1999;70(Suppl):5435–5485

15 Chromium

Although trivalent chromium is recognized as a nutritionally essential mineral, scientists are not yet certain exactly how it functions in the body. The two most common forms of chromium are trivalent chromium (III) and the hexavalent chromium (VI). Chromium (III) is the principal form in food as well as the form used by the body. Chromium (VI) is derived from chromium (III) by heating at alkaline pH and is used as a source of chromium for industrial purposes. It is a strong irritant and is recognized as a carcinogen when inhaled. At low levels, chromium (VI) is readily reduced to chromium (III) by reducing substances in food and the acidic environment of the stomach, which serve to prevent the ingestion of chromium (VI).[1–3]

Function

A biologically active form of chromium participates in glucose metabolism by enhancing the effects of insulin. Insulin is secreted by specialized cells in the pancreas in response to increased blood glucose levels, such as after a meal. Insulin binds to insulin receptors on the surface of cells, which activates the receptors and stimulates glucose uptake by cells. Through its interaction with insulin receptors, insulin provides cells with glucose for energy and prevents blood glucose levels from becoming elevated. In addition to its effects on carbohydrate (glucose) metabolism, insulin also influences the metabolism of fat and protein. A decreased response to insulin or decreased insulin sensitivity may result in impaired glucose tolerance or type 2 diabetes. Type 2 diabetes is characterized by elevated blood glucose levels and insulin resistance.[1]

The precise structure of the biologically active form of chromium is not known. Recent research suggests that a low-molecular-weight chromium-binding substance (LMWCr) may enhance the response of the insulin receptor to insulin. **Figure 15.1** is a proposed model for the effect of chromium on insulin action. First, the inactive form of the insulin receptor is converted to the active

form by binding insulin. This stimulates the movement of chromium into the cell and results in binding of chromium to apo-LMWCr, a form of the LMWCr that lacks chromium. Once it binds chromium, the LMWCr binds to the insulin receptor and enhances its tyrosine kinase activity. The ability of the LMWCr to activate the insulin receptor is dependent on its chromium content. When insulin levels drop due to normalization of blood glucose levels, the LMWCr may be released from the cell in order to terminate its effects.[4] More recent studies have indicated that chromium enhances insulin action by increasing the insulin-stimulated translocation of glucose transporters to the cell membrane.[5] The mechanism for the effect of chromium on insulin action is currently under investigation.[5–7]

Nutrient Interactions

Iron. Chromium competes for one of the binding sites on the iron transport protein, transferrin. However, supplementation of older men with 925 µg chromium per day for 12 weeks did not significantly affect measures of iron nutritional status.[8] A study of younger men found an insignificant decrease in transferrin saturation with iron after supplementation of 200 µg chromium per day for 8 weeks, but no long-term studies have addressed this issue.[9] Iron overload in hereditary hemochromatosis may interfere with chromium transport by competing for transferrin binding. This has led to the hypothesis that decreased chromium transport might contribute to the diabetes associated with hereditary hemochromatosis.[1]

Vitamin C. Chromium uptake is enhanced in animals when given at the same time as vitamin C.[3] In a study of three women, administration of 100 mg vitamin C together with 1 mg chromium resulted in higher plasma levels of chromium than 1 mg chromium without vitamin C.[1]

Carbohydrates. Compared with diets rich in complex carbohydrates (e.g., whole grains), diets

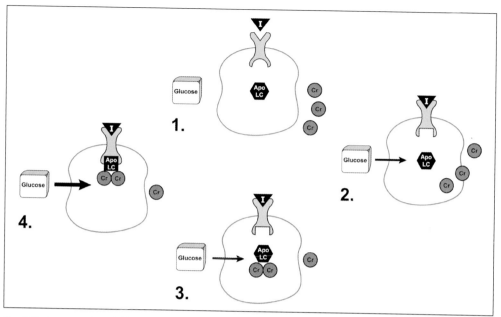

Fig. 15.1 A proposed model for the enhancing effects of chromium on insulin activity: (1) insulin binds to and activates the insulin receptor; (2) insulin receptor activation stimulates the movement of chromium into the cell; (3) chromium binds to a peptide known as apo-low-molecular-weight chromium-binding substance (apo-LMWCr; Apo-LC); (4) functional LMWCr (LC) binds to the insulin receptor and enhances its activity. (Adapted from Vincent JB. Quest for the molecular mechanism of chromium action and its relationship to diabetes. *Nutr Rev* 2000;58:67–72, with permission from John Wiley and Sons, Inc.)

high in simple sugars (e.g., sucrose) result in increased urinary chromium excretion in adults. This effect may be related to increased insulin secretion in response to the consumption of simple sugars compared with complex carbohydrates.[1]

Deficiency

Chromium deficiency was reported in three patients on long-term intravenous feeding who did not receive supplemental chromium in their intravenous solutions. These patients developed abnormal glucose utilization and increased insulin requirements that responded to chromium supplementation. In addition, impaired glucose tolerance in malnourished infants responded to an oral dose of chromium chloride. As chromium appears to enhance the action of insulin and chromium deficiency has resulted in impaired glucose tolerance, chromium insufficiency has been hypothesized to be a contributing factor to the development of type 2 diabetes.[1,10]

Several studies of male runners indicated that urinary chromium loss was increased by endurance exercise, suggesting that chromium needs may be greater in individuals who exercise regularly.[11] In a more recent study, resistive exercise (weight lifting) was found to increase urinary excretion of chromium in older men. However, chromium absorption was also increased, leading to little or no net loss of chromium as a result of resistive exercise.[12]

At present, research on the effects of inadequate chromium intake and risk factors for chromium insufficiency are limited by the lack of sensitive and accurate tests for determining chromium nutritional status.[1,3]

Adequate Intake

As there was not enough information on chromium requirements to set a recommended dietary allowance, the Food and Nutrition Board (FNB) of the Institute of Medicine set an adequate intake (AI) based on the chromium content in normal diets (**Table 15.1**).[1]

Table 15.1 Adequate intake for chromium

Life stage	Age	Males (µg/day)	Females (µg/day)
Infants	0–6 months	0.2	0.2
Infants	7–12 months	5.5	5.5
Children	1–3 years	11	11
Children	4–8 years	15	15
Children	9–13 years	25	21
Adolescents	14–18 years	35	24
Adults	19–50 years	35	25
Adults	≥51 years	30	20
Pregnancy	≤18 years	–	29
Pregnancy	≥19 years	–	30
Breast-feeding	≤18 years	–	44
Breast-feeding	≥19 years	–	45

Disease Prevention

Impaired Glucose Tolerance and Type 2 Diabetes Mellitus

In 12 of 15 controlled studies of people with impaired glucose tolerance, chromium supplementation was found to improve some measure of glucose utilization or to have beneficial effects on blood lipid profiles.[13] Impaired glucose tolerance refers to a metabolic state between normal glucose regulation and overt diabetes. Commonly, blood glucose levels are higher than normal but lower than those accepted as diagnostic for diabetes. Impaired glucose tolerance is associated with increased risk for cardiovascular diseases but is not associated with the other classic complications of diabetes. About 25%–30% of individuals with impaired glucose tolerance eventually develop type 2 diabetes.[14] Generally, chromium supplementation in a variety of forms, at doses of about 200 µg/day for 2–3 months, has been found to be beneficial. The reasons for the variation or lack of effect in some studies are not clear, but chromium depletion is not the only known cause of impaired glucose tolerance. In addition, the lack of an accurate measure of chromium nutritional status prevents researchers from identifying those individuals who are most likely to benefit from chromium supplementation.[3,15] A meta-analysis of 15 randomized clinical trials reported that chromium had no effect on glucose or insulin concentrations in nondiabetic individuals.[16]

Cardiovascular Diseases

Impaired glucose tolerance and type 2 diabetes are associated with adverse changes in lipid profiles and increased risk of cardiovascular diseases. Studies examining the effects of chromium supplementation on lipid profiles have been notable for their inconsistent results. Although some studies have observed reductions in serum total cholesterol, low-density lipoprotein (LDL)-cholesterol, and triglyceride levels or increases in high-density lipoprotein (HDL)-cholesterol levels, others have observed no effect. Such inconsistent responses of lipid and lipoprotein levels to chromium supplementation may reflect differences in chromium nutritional status. It is possible that only those individuals with insufficient dietary intake of chromium will experience beneficial effects on lipid profiles after chromium supplementation.[2,3,17]

Health Claims

Increases muscle mass. Claims that chromium supplementation increases lean body mass and decreases body fat are based on the relationship between chromium and insulin action. In addition to affecting glucose metabolism, insulin is known to affect fat and protein metabolism. At least 12 placebo-controlled studies have compared the effect of chromium supplementation (200–1000 µg/day as chromium picolinate) with or without an exercise program on lean body mass and measures of body fat. In general, those studies that have used the most sensitive and accurate methods of measuring body fat and lean mass (dual energy X-ray absorptiometry or DXA and hydrodensitometry or underwater weighing) do not indicate a beneficial effect of chromium supplementation on body composition.[2,17]

Promotes weight loss. Controlled studies of chromium supplementation (200–400 µg/day as chromium picolinate) have demonstrated little if any beneficial effect on weight or fat loss,[18] and claims of weight loss in humans appear to be exaggerated. In 1997, the US Federal Trade Commission ruled that there is no basis for claims that chromium picolinate promotes weight loss and fat loss in humans.[2,15,17] More recently, a meta-analysis of 10 randomized, double-blind, placebo-controlled trials of chromium picolinate supplementation found that chromium picolinate was associated with a 1.1 kg (2.4 lb) reduction in body weight; however, such a small change may not be clinically relevant.[19] In addition, a recent study reported that chromium picolinate supplementation attenuated body weight gain in type 2 diabetic patients taking sulfonylurea drugs.[20]

Disease Treatment

Type 2 Diabetes Mellitus

Type 2 diabetes is characterized by elevated blood glucose levels and insulin resistance. Although insulin levels in people with type 2 diabetes may be higher than in healthy individuals, the physiological effects of insulin are reduced. As chromium is known to enhance the action of insulin, the relationship between chromium nutritional status and type 2 diabetes has generated considerable scientific interest. Individuals with type 2 diabetes have been found to have higher rates of urinary chromium loss than healthy individuals, especially those with diabetes of more than 2 years' duration.[21] Before 1997, well-designed studies of chromium supplementation in individuals with type 2 diabetes showed no improvement in blood glucose control, although they provided some evidence of reduced insulin levels and improved blood lipid profiles.[22] In 1997, the results of a placebo-controlled trial conducted in China indicated that chro-

mium supplementation might be beneficial in the treatment of type 2 diabetes;[23] 180 participants took either a placebo or chromium in the form of chromium picolinate at doses of 200 µg/day and 1000 µg/day. At the end of 4 months, blood glucose levels were 15%–19% lower in those who took 1000 µg/day compared with those who took the placebo. Blood glucose levels in those taking 200 µg/day did not differ significantly from those who took placebo. Insulin levels were lower in those who took either 200 µg/day or 1000 µg/day of chromium picolinate. Glycated hemoglobin levels, a measure of long-term control of blood glucose, were also lower in both chromium-supplemented groups, especially in the group taking 1000 µg/day. As the chromium nutritional status of the Chinese participants had not been evaluated and the prevalence of obesity was much lower than is typically associated with type 2 diabetics in the United States, extrapolation of these results to a US population is difficult. There have been subsequent studies investigating the utility of chromium picolinate for the treatment of type 2 diabetes.

A recent review reported that 13 of 15 clinical studies, including the study conducted in China, found that chromium picolinate improved at least one measure of glycemic control in diabetic patients.[24] Chromium picolinate is more bioavailable than other supplemental forms of chromium and therefore may be more efficacious. However, large-scale randomized controlled trials of chromium supplementation for type 2 diabetes are needed to determine if chromium is effective in its treatment.

Gestational Diabetes

Few studies have examined the effects of chromium supplementation on gestational diabetes. Gestational diabetes occurs in about 2% of pregnant women and usually appears in the second or third trimester of pregnancy. Blood glucose levels must be tightly controlled to prevent adverse effects on the developing fetus. After delivery, glucose tolerance generally reverts to normal. However, 30%–40% of women who have had gestational diabetes develop type 2 diabetes within 5–10 years. An observational study in pregnant women did not find serum chromium levels to be associated with measures of glucose tolerance or insulin resistance in late pregnancy, although serum chromium levels may not reflect tissue chromium levels.[25] Women with gestational diabetes whose diets were supplemented with 4 µg chromium/kg body weight daily as chromium picolinate for 8 weeks had decreased fasting blood glucose and insulin levels compared with those who took a placebo. However, insulin therapy rather than chromium picolinate was required to normalize severely elevated blood glucose levels.[2,26]

Sources

Food Sources

The amount of chromium in foods is variable and has been measured accurately in relatively few foods. Currently, there is no large database for the chromium content of foods. Processed meats, whole-grain products, ready-to-eat bran cereals, green beans, broccoli, and spices are relatively rich in chromium. Foods high in simple sugars, such as sucrose and fructose, are not only low in chromium but have been found to promote chromium loss.[2] Estimated average chromium intakes in the US range from 23 µg/day to 29 µg/day for women and from 39 µg/day to 54 µg/day for men.[1] The chromium content of some foods is listed in **Table 15.2**.[27] As chromium content in different batches of the same food has been found to vary significantly, the information in **Table**

15.2 should serve only as a guide to the chromium content of foods.

Supplements

Chromium (III) is available as a supplement in several forms: chromium chloride, chromium nicotinate, chromium picolinate, and high-chromium yeast. These are available as stand-alone supplements or in combination products. Doses typically range from 50 µg to 200 µg elemental chromium.[28] Chromium nicotinate and chromium picolinate may be more bioavailable than chromium chloride.[17] In much of the research on impaired glucose tolerance and type 2 diabetes, chromium picolinate was the source of chromium. However, some concerns have been raised over the long-term safety of chromium picolinate supplementation.

Safety

Toxicity

Hexavalent chromium or chromium (VI) is a recognized carcinogen. Exposure to chromium (VI) in dust is associated with increased incidence of lung cancer and is known to cause inflammation of the skin (dermatitis). In contrast, there is little evidence that trivalent chromium or chromium (III) is toxic to humans. Because no adverse effects have been convincingly associated with excess intake of chromium (III) from food or supplements, the FNB did not set a tolerable upper intake level for chromium. As information is limited, the FNB acknowledged a potential for adverse effects of high intakes of supplemental chromium (III) and advised caution.[1]

Most of the concerns about the long-term safety of chromium (III) supplementation arise from several studies in cell culture, suggesting that chromium (III), especially in the form of chromium picolinate, may increase DNA damage.[29–31] Currently, there is no evidence that chromium (III) increases DNA damage in living organisms,[1] and a study in 10 women taking 400 µg/day of chromium as chromium picolinate found no evidence of increased oxidative damage to DNA as measured by antibodies to an oxidized DNA base.[32]

Several studies have demonstrated the safety of daily doses of up to 1000 µg chromium for sev-

Table 15.2 Food sources of chromium

Food	Serving	Chromium (µg)
Broccoli	½ cup	11.0
Turkey ham (processed)	3 ounces	10.4
Grape juice	8 fluid ounces	7.5
Waffle	1 (~2.5 ounces)	6.7
English muffin	1	3.6
Potatoes	1 cup, mashed	2.7
Bagel	1	2.5
Orange juice	8 fluid ounces	2.2
Beef	3 ounces[a]	2.0
Turkey breast	3 ounces[a]	1.7
Apple with peel	1 medium	1.4
Green beans	½ cup	1.1
Banana	1 medium	1.0

[a]A 3-ounce serving of meat is about the size of a deck of cards.

eral months.[23,33] However, there have been a few isolated reports of serious adverse reactions to chromium picolinate. Kidney failure was reported 5 months after a 6-week course of 600 µg chromium/day in the form of chromium picolinate,[34] whereas kidney failure and impaired liver function were reported after the use of 1200–2400 µg/day of chromium in the form of chromium picolinate over a period of 4–5 months.[35] In addition, a 24-year-old healthy man reportedly developed reversible, acute renal failure after taking chromium picolinate-containing supplements for 2 weeks.[36] Individuals with pre-existing kidney or liver disease may be at increased risk of adverse effects and should limit supplemental chromium intake.[1]

Drug Interactions

Little is known about drug interactions with chromium in humans. Large doses of calcium carbonate- or magnesium hydroxide-containing antacids decreased chromium absorption in rats. In contrast, aspirin and indometacin (a nonsteroidal anti-inflammatory drug) both increased chromium absorption in rats.[3]

LPI Recommendation

The lack of sensitive indicators of chromium nutritional status in humans makes it difficult to determine the level of chromium intake most likely to promote optimum health. Following the Linus Pauling Institute recommendation to take a multivitamin/mineral supplement containing 100% of the daily values (DVs) of most nutrients will generally provide 60–120 µg/day of chromium, well above the adequate intake of 20–25 µg/day for women and 30–35 µg for men.

Older Adults

Although the requirement for chromium is not known to be higher for older adults, one study found that chromium concentrations in hair, sweat, and urine decreased with age.[37] Following the Linus Pauling Institute recommendation to take a multivitamin/mineral supplement containing 100% of the DVs of most nutrients should provide sufficient chromium for most older adults.

As impaired glucose tolerance and type 2 diabetes are associated with potentially serious health problems, individuals considering high-dose chromium supplementation to treat either condition should do so in collaboration with a qualified health-care provider.

References

1. Food and Nutrition Board, Institute of Medicine. Chromium. In: Dietary Reference Intakes for Vitamin A, Vitamin K, Boron, Chromium, Copper, Iodine, Iron, Manganese, Molybdenum, Nickel, Silicon, Vanadium, and Zinc. Washington, DC: National Academy Press; 2001:197–223
2. Lukaski HC. Chromium as a supplement. Annu Rev Nutr 1999;19:279–302
3. Stoecker BJ. Chromium. In: Shils M, Olson JA, Shike M, Ross AC, eds. Modern Nutrition in Health and Disease. 9th ed. Baltimore, MD: Lippincott Williams & Wilkins; 1999:277–282
4. Vincent JB. Elucidating a biological role for chromium at a molecular level. Acc Chem Res 2000;33(7): 503–510
5. Chen G, Liu P, Pattar GR, et al. Chromium activates glucose transporter 4 trafficking and enhances insulin-stimulated glucose transport in 3T3-L1 adipocytes via a cholesterol-dependent mechanism. Mol Endocrinol 2006;20(4):857–870
6. Pattar GR, Tackett L, Liu P, Elmendorf JS. Chromium picolinate positively influences the glucose transporter system via affecting cholesterol homeostasis in adipocytes cultured under hyperglycemic diabetic conditions. Mutat Res 2006;610(1-2):93–100
7. Wang H, Kruszewski A, Brautigan DL. Cellular chromium enhances activation of insulin receptor kinase. Biochemistry 2005;44(22):8167–8175
8. Campbell WW, Beard JL, Joseph LJ, Davey SL, Evans WJ. Chromium picolinate supplementation and resistive training by older men: effects on iron-status and hematologic indexes. Am J Clin Nutr 1997;66(4): 944–949
9. Lukaski HC, Bolonchuk WW, Siders WA, Milne DB. Chromium supplementation and resistance training: effects on body composition, strength, and trace element status of men. Am J Clin Nutr 1996;63(6): 954–965
10. Jeejeebhoy KN. The role of chromium in nutrition and therapeutics and as a potential toxin. Nutr Rev 1999;57(11):329–335
11. Lukaski HC. Magnesium, zinc, and chromium nutriture and physical activity. Am J Clin Nutr 2000; 72(2, Suppl):585S–593S
12. Rubin MA, Miller JP, Ryan AS, et al. Acute and chronic resistive exercise increase urinary chromium excretion in men as measured with an enriched chromium stable isotope. J Nutr 1998;128(1):73–78
13. Mertz W. Chromium in human nutrition: a review. J Nutr 1993;123(4):626–633
14. Goldman L, Bennett JC. Cecil Textbook of Medicine, 21st ed. Philadelphia, PA: WB Saunders Co.; 2000
15. Anderson RA. Effects of chromium on body composition and weight loss. Nutr Rev 1998;56(9):266–270
16. Althuis MD, Jordan NE, Ludington EA, Wittes JT. Glucose and insulin responses to dietary chromium supplements: a meta-analysis. Am J Clin Nutr 2002; 76(1):148–155
17. Kobla HV, Volpe SL. Chromium, exercise, and body composition. Crit Rev Food Sci Nutr 2000;40(4): 291–308
18. Volpe SL, Huang HW, Larpadisorn K, Lesser II. Effect of chromium supplementation and exercise on body composition, resting metabolic rate and selected biochemical parameters in moderately obese women

following an exercise program. J Am Coll Nutr 2001; 20(4):293–306

19. Pittler MH, Stevinson C, Ernst E. Chromium picolinate for reducing body weight: meta-analysis of random-ized trials. Int J Obes Relat Metab Disord 2003;27 (4):522–529

20. Martin J, Wang ZQ, Zhang XH, et al. Chromium pico-linate supplementation attenuates body weight gain and increases insulin sensitivity in subjects with type 2 diabetes. Diabetes Care 2006;29(8):1826–1832

21. Morris BW, MacNeil S, Hardisty CA, Heller S, Burgin C, Gray TA. Chromium homeostasis in patients with type II (NIDDM) diabetes. J Trace Elem Med Biol 1999; 13(1-2):57–61

22. Hellerstein MK. Is chromium supplementation effec-tive in managing type II diabetes? Nutr Rev 1998; 56(10):302–306

23. Anderson RA, Cheng N, Bryden NA, et al. Elevated in-takes of supplemental chromium improve glucose and insulin variables in individuals with type 2 dia-betes. Diabetes 1997;46(11):1786–1791

24. Broadhurst CL, Domenico P. Clinical studies on chro-mium picolinate supplementation in diabetes melli-tus—a review. Diabetes Technol Ther 2006;8(6): 677–687

25. Gunton JE, Hams G, Hitchman R, McElduff A. Serum chromium does not predict glucose tolerance in late pregnancy. Am J Clin Nutr 2001;73(1):99–104

26. Jovanovic-Peterson L, Peterson CM. Vitamin and min-eral deficiencies which may predispose to glucose intolerance of pregnancy. J Am Coll Nutr 1996;15(1): 14–20

27. Anderson RA, Bryden NA, Polansky MM. Dietary chromium intake. Freely chosen diets, institutional diet, and individual foods. Biol Trace Elem Res 1992; 32:117–121

28. Hendler SS, Rorvik DR, eds. PDR for Nutritional Sup-plements. Montvale, NJ: Medical Economics Co., Inc.; 2001

29. Blasiak J, Kowalik J. A comparison of the in vitro geno-toxicity of tri- and hexavalent chromium. Mutat Res 2000;469(1):135–145

30. Speetjens JK, Collins RA, Vincent JB, Woski SA. The nutritional supplement chromium(III) tris(picolinate) cleaves DNA. Chem Res Toxicol 1999;12(6):483–487

31. Stearns DM, Wise JP Sr, Patierno SR, Wetterhahn KE. Chromium(III) picolinate produces chromosome damage in Chinese hamster ovary cells. FASEB J 1995; 9(15):1643–1648

32. Kato I, Vogelman JH, Dilman V, et al. Effect of supple-mentation with chromium picolinate on antibody ti-ters to 5-hydroxymethyl uracil. Eur J Epidemiol 1998;14(6):621–626

33. Hathcock JN. Vitamins and minerals: efficacy and safety. Am J Clin Nutr 1997;66(2):427–437

34. Wasser WG, Feldman NS, D'Agati VD. Chronic renal failure after ingestion of over-the-counter chromium picolinate. Ann Intern Med 1997;126(5):410

35. Cerulli J, Grabe DW, Gauthier I, Malone M, McGold-rick MD. Chromium picolinate toxicity. Ann Pharma-cother 1998;32(4):428–431

36. Wani S, Weskamp C, Marple J, Spry L. Acute tubular necrosis associated with chromium picolinate-con-taining dietary supplement. Ann Pharmacother 2006;40(3):563–566

37. Davies S, McLaren Howard J, Hunnisett A, Howard M. Age-related decreases in chromium levels in 51,665 hair, sweat, and serum samples from 40,872 pa-tients—implications for the prevention of cardiovas-cular disease and type II diabetes mellitus. Metabo-lism 1997;46(5):469–473

16   Copper

Copper (Cu) is an essential trace element for humans and animals. In the body, copper shifts between the cuprous (Cu^+) and cupric (Cu^{2+}) forms, although most of the body's copper is in the Cu^{2+} form. The ability of copper to easily accept and donate electrons explains its important role in oxidation–reduction (redox) reactions and in scavenging free radicals.[1] Although Hippocrates is said to have prescribed copper compounds to treat diseases as early as 400 BC,[2] scientists are still uncovering new information about the functions of copper in the human body.

Function

Copper is a critical functional component of a number of essential enzymes known as *cuproenzymes*. Some of the physiological functions known to be copper dependent are discussed below.

Energy Production

The copper-dependent enzyme, cytochrome *c* oxidase, plays a critical role in cellular energy production. By catalyzing the reduction of molecular oxygen (O_2) to water (H_2O), cytochrome *c* oxidase generates an electrical gradient used by the mitochondria to create the vital energy-storing molecule, ATP.[3]

Connective Tissue Formation

Another cuproenzyme, lysyl oxidase, is required for the cross-linking of collagen and elastin, which is essential for the formation of strong and flexible connective tissue. The action of lysyl oxidase helps maintain the integrity of connective tissue in the heart and blood vessels, and also plays a role in bone formation.[2]

Iron Metabolism

Two copper-containing enzymes, ceruloplasmin (ferroxidase I) and ferroxidase II, have the capacity to oxidize ferrous iron (Fe^{2+}) to ferric iron (Fe^{3+}), the form of iron that can be loaded on to the protein transferrin for transport to the site of red blood cell formation. Although the ferroxidase activity of these two cuproenzymes has not yet been proven to be physiologically significant, the fact that iron mobilization from storage sites is impaired in copper deficiency supports their role in iron metabolism.[2,4]

Central Nervous System

A number of reactions essential to normal function of the brain and nervous system are catalyzed by cuproenzymes:
- *Neurotransmitter synthesis*: dopamine-β-mono-oxygenase catalyzes the conversion of dopamine to the neurotransmitter norepinephrine.[4]
- *Metabolism of neurotransmitters*: monoamine oxidase (MAO) plays a role in the metabolism of the neurotransmitters norepinephrine, epinephrine, and dopamine. MAO also functions in the degradation of the neurotransmitter serotonin, which is the basis for the use of MAO inhibitors as antidepressants.[5]
- *Formation and maintenance of myelin*: the myelin sheath is made of phospholipids, the synthesis of which depends on cytochrome *c* oxidase activity.[2]

Melanin Formation

The cuproenzyme, tyrosinase, is required for the formation of the pigment melanin. Melanin is formed in cells called *melanocytes* and plays a role in the pigmentation of the hair, skin, and eyes.[2]

Antioxidant Functions

Superoxide dismutase (SOD) functions as an antioxidant by catalyzing the conversion of superoxide radicals (free radicals or reactive oxygen species [ROS]) to hydrogen peroxide, which can subsequently be reduced to water by other antioxidant enzymes.[6] Two forms of SOD contain copper:

1. Copper/zinc SOD is found within most cells of the body, including red blood cells.
2. Extracellular SOD is a copper-containing enzyme found at high levels in the lungs and at low levels in blood plasma.[2]

Ceruloplasmin may function as an antioxidant in two different ways. Free copper and iron ions are powerful catalysts of free radical damage. By binding copper, ceruloplasmin prevents free copper ions from catalyzing oxidative damage. The ferroxidase activity of ceruloplasmin (oxidation of ferrous iron) facilitates iron loading onto its transport protein, transferrin, and may prevent free ferrous ions (Fe^{2+}) from participating in harmful free radical-generating reactions.[6]

Regulation of Gene Expression

Copper-dependent transcription factors regulate transcription of specific genes. Thus, cellular copper levels may affect the synthesis of proteins by enhancing or inhibiting the transcription of specific genes. Genes regulated by copper-dependent transcription factors include genes for Cu/ZnSOD, catalase (another antioxidant enzyme), and proteins related to the cellular storage of copper.[3]

Nutrient Interactions

Iron. Adequate copper nutritional status appears to be necessary for normal iron metabolism and red blood cell formation. Anemia is a clinical sign of copper deficiency, and iron has been found to accumulate in the livers of copper-deficient animals, indicating that copper (probably in the form of ceruloplasmin) is required for iron transport to the bone marrow for red blood cell formation.[2] Infants fed a high-iron formula absorbed less copper than infants fed a low-iron formula, suggesting that high iron intakes may interfere with copper absorption in infants.[5]

Zinc. High supplemental zinc intakes of 50 mg/day or more for extended periods of time may result in copper deficiency. High dietary zinc increases the synthesis of an intestinal cell protein called *metallothionein*, which binds certain metals and prevents their absorption by trapping them in intestinal cells. Metallothionein has a stronger affinity for copper than zinc, so high levels of metallothionein induced by excess zinc cause a decrease in copper absorption. In contrast, high copper intakes have not been found to affect zinc nutritional status.[2,5]

Fructose. High fructose diets have exacerbated copper deficiency in rats but not in pigs which have gastrointestinal systems more like those of humans. Very high levels of dietary fructose (20% of total calories) did not result in copper depletion in humans, suggesting that fructose intake does not result in copper depletion at levels relevant to normal diets.[2,5]

Vitamin C. Although vitamin C supplements have produced copper deficiency in guinea pigs,[7] the effect of vitamin C supplements on copper nutritional status in humans is less clear. Two small studies in healthy young men indicate that the oxidase activity of ceruloplasmin may be impaired by relatively high doses of supplemental vitamin C. In one study, vitamin C supplementation of 1500 mg/day for 2 months resulted in a significant decline in ceruloplasmin oxidase activity.[8] In the other study, supplements of 605 mg vitamin C/day for 3 weeks resulted in decreased ceruloplasmin oxidase activity, although copper absorption did not decline.[9] Neither of these studies found vitamin C supplementation to adversely affect copper nutritional status.

Deficiency

Clinically evident or frank copper deficiency is relatively uncommon. Serum copper and ceruloplasmin levels may fall to 30% of normal in cases of severe copper deficiency. One of the most common clinical signs of copper deficiency is an anemia that is unresponsive to iron therapy but corrected by copper supplementation. The anemia is thought to result from defective iron mobilization due to decreased ceruloplasmin activity. Copper deficiency may also result in abnormally low numbers of white blood cells, known as *neutrophils* (neutropenia), a condition that may be accompanied by increased susceptibility to infection. Osteoporosis and other abnormalities of bone development related to copper deficiency are most common in copper-deficient low-birth-

Table 16.1 Recommended dietary allowance for copper

Life stage	Age	Males (µg/day)	Females (µg/day)
Infants	0–6 months	200 (AI)	200 (AI)
Infants	7–12 months	220 (AI)	220 (AI)
Children	1–3 years	340	340
Children	4–8 years	440	440
Children	9–13 years	700	700
Adolescents	14–18 years	890	890
Adults	≥19 years	900	900
Pregnancy	All ages	–	1000
Breast-feeding	All ages	–	1300

AI, adequate intake.

weight infants and young children. Less common features of copper deficiency may include loss of pigmentation, neurological symptoms, and impaired growth.[2,3]

Individuals at Risk of Deficiency

Cow's milk is relatively low in copper, and cases of copper deficiency have been reported in high-risk infants and children fed only cow's milk formula. High-risk individuals include: premature infants (especially those with low birth weight), infants with prolonged diarrhea, infants and children recovering from malnutrition, and individuals with malabsorption syndromes, including celiac disease, sprue, and short bowel syndrome resulting from surgical removal of a large portion of the intestine. Individuals receiving intravenous total parenteral nutrition or other restricted diets may also require supplementation with copper and other trace elements.[2,3] Recent research indicates that cystic fibrosis patients may also be at increased risk of copper insufficiency.[10]

Recommended Dietary Allowance

A variety of indicators were used to establish the recommended dietary allowance (RDA) for copper, including plasma copper concentration, serum ceruloplasmin activity, SOD activity in red blood cells, and platelet copper concentration.[5] The RDA for copper reflects the results of depletion–repletion studies and is based on the prevention of deficiency (**Table 16.1**).

Disease Prevention

Cardiovascular Diseases

Although it is clear that severe copper deficiency results in heart abnormalities and damage (cardiomyopathy) in some animal species, the pathology differs from the atherosclerotic cardiovascular disease prevalent in humans.[5] Studies in humans have produced inconsistent results, and their interpretation is hindered by the lack of a reliable marker of copper nutritional status. Outside the body, free copper is known to be a pro-oxidant and is frequently used to produce oxidation of low-density lipoprotein (LDL) in the test tube. The copper-containing protein ceruloplasmin has been found to stimulate LDL oxidation in the test tube,[11] leading some scientists to propose that increased copper levels could increase the risk of atherosclerosis by promoting the oxidation of LDLs. However, there is little evidence that copper or ceruloplasmin promotes LDL oxidation in the human body. In addition, the cuproenzymes, SOD and ceruloplasmin, are known to have antioxidant properties, leading some experts to propose that copper deficiency rather than excess copper increases the risk of cardiovascular diseases.[12]

Epidemiological studies. Several epidemiological studies have found increased serum copper levels to be associated with increased risk of cardiovascular disease. A prospective study in the United States examined serum copper levels in more than 4500 men and women aged 30 years and older.[13] During the following 16 years, 151 participants died from coronary heart disease (CHD). After adjusting for other risk factors for heart disease, those with serum copper levels in the two highest quartiles (one-fourth) had a significantly greater risk of dying from CHD. Three other case–control studies conducted in Europe had similar findings. One small study in 60 patients with chronic heart failure or ischemic heart disease reported that serum copper was a predictor of short-term outcome.[14] A recent prospective study in 4035 middle-aged men reported that high serum copper levels were significantly related to a 50% increase in all-cause mortality; however, serum copper was not significantly associated with cardiovascular mortality in this study.[15] It is important to note that serum copper largely reflects serum ceruloplasmin and is not a sensitive indicator of copper nutritional status. Serum ceruloplasmin levels are known to increase by 50% or more under certain conditions of physical stress, such as trauma, inflammation, or disease. As over 90% of serum copper is carried in ceruloplasmin, which is increased in many inflammatory conditions, elevated serum copper may simply be a marker of inflammation that accompanies atherosclerosis. In fact, serum copper was recently found to be elevated in patients with rheumatic heart disease.[16] In contrast to the epidemiological findings linking serum copper to heart disease, two autopsy studies found that copper levels in heart muscle were actually lower in patients who died of CHD than those who died of other causes.[17] In addition, the copper content of white blood cells has been positively correlated with the degree of patency of coronary arteries in CHD patients.[18,19] Further, patients with a history of myocardial infarction (MI) had lower concentrations of extracellular SOD than those without a history of MI.[20] Thus, due to a lack of a reliable biomarker of copper nutritional status, it is not clear whether copper is related to cardiovascular disease.

Experimental studies. Although studies in very small numbers of adults fed experimental diets low in copper have demonstrated adverse changes in blood cholesterol levels, including increased total and LDL-cholesterol levels and decreased high-density lipoprotein (HDL)-cholesterol levels,[21] other studies have not confirmed those results.[22] Copper supplementation of 2–3 mg/day for 4–6 weeks did not result in clinically signifi-

cant changes in cholesterol levels.[12,23] More recent research has also failed to find evidence that increased copper intake increases oxidative stress. In a multicenter placebo-controlled study, copper supplementation of 3 and 6 mg/day for 6 weeks did not result in increased susceptibility of LDL to oxidation induced outside the body (ex vivo) by copper or peroxynitrite (a reactive nitrogen species).[24] Moreover, supplementation with 3 and 6 mg/day of copper decreased the in vitro oxidizability of red blood cells,[25] indicating that relatively high intakes of copper do not increase the susceptibility of LDL or red blood cells to oxidation.

Summary. Although free copper and ceruloplasmin can promote LDL oxidation in the test tube, there is little evidence that increased dietary copper increases oxidative stress in the human body. Increased serum copper levels have been associated with increased cardiovascular disease risk, but the significance of these findings is unclear due to the association between serum ceruloplasmin levels and inflammatory conditions. Clarification of the relationships of copper nutritional status, ceruloplasmin levels, and cardiovascular disease risk requires further research.

Immune System Function

Copper is known to play an important role in the development and maintenance of immune system function, but its exact mechanism of action is not yet known. Neutropenia (abnormally low numbers of *neutrophils*) is a clinical sign of copper deficiency in humans. Adverse effects of insufficient copper on immune function appear most pronounced in infants. Infants with Menkes disease, a genetic disorder that results in severe copper deficiency, have frequent and severe infections.[26,27] In a study of 11 malnourished infants with evidence of copper deficiency, the ability of certain white blood cells to engulf pathogens increased significantly after 1 month of copper supplementation.[28] More recently, 11 men on a low-copper diet (0.66 mg/day for 24 days and 0.38 mg/day for another 40 days) showed a decreased proliferation response when white blood cells, called *mononuclear cells*, were isolated from their blood and presented with an immune challenge in cell culture.[29] Although severe copper deficiency has adverse effects on immune function, the effects of marginal copper insufficiency in humans are not yet clear.

Osteoporosis

The copper-dependent enzyme, lysyl oxidase, is required for the maturation (cross-linking) of collagen, a key element in the organic matrix of bone. Osteoporosis has been observed in infants and adults with severe copper deficiency, but it is not clear whether marginal copper deficiency contributes to osteoporosis. Research regarding the role of copper nutritional status in age-related osteoporosis is limited. Serum copper levels of 46 elderly patients with hip fractures were reported to be significantly lower than those of matched controls.[30] A small study in perimenopausal women, who consumed an average of 1 mg dietary copper daily, reported decreased loss of bone mineral density (BMD) from the lumbar spine after copper supplementation of 3 mg/day for 2 years.[31] In addition, a 2-year double-blind, placebo-controlled trial in 59 postmenopausal women found that a combination of supplemental calcium and trace minerals, including 2.5 mg copper daily, resulted in maintenance of spinal bone density, whereas supplemental calcium or trace minerals, alone, were not effective in preventing loss of bone density.[32] A study in 11 healthy men found that marginal copper intake of 0.7 mg/day for 6 weeks significantly increased a measurement of bone resorption (breakdown) in healthy men.[33] However, copper supplementation of 3–6 mg/day for 6 weeks had no effect on biochemical markers of bone resorption or bone formation in a study of healthy men and women.[34] Although severe copper deficiency is known to adversely affect bone health, the effects of marginal copper deficiency and copper supplementation on bone metabolism and age-related osteoporosis require further research before conclusions can be drawn.

Sources

Food Sources

Copper is found in a wide variety of foods and is most plentiful in organ meats, shellfish, nuts, and seeds. Wheat bran cereals and whole-grain products are also good sources of copper. According to national surveys, the average dietary intake of

Table 16.2 Food sources of copper

Food	Serving	Copper (µg)
Liver (beef), cooked	1 ounce	4049
Oysters, cooked	1 medium oyster	670
Cashews	1 ounce	629
Crab meat, cooked	3 ounces	624
Clams, cooked	3 ounces	585
Sunflower seeds	1 ounce	519
Lentils, cooked	1 cup	497
Hazelnuts	1 ounce	496
Mushrooms, raw	1 cup (sliced)	344
Almonds	1 ounce	332
Chocolate, semisweet	1 ounce	198
Peanut butter, chunky	2 tablespoons	185
Shredded wheat cereal	2 biscuits	167
Hot cocoa mix	1 ounce (1-cup sachet)	93

copper in the United States is approximately 1.0–1.1 mg (1000–1100 µg)/day for women and 1.2–1.6 mg (1200–1600 µg)/day for men.[5] The copper content of some foods that are relatively rich in copper is listed in **Table 16.2**.

Supplements

Copper supplements are available as cupric oxide, copper gluconate, copper sulfate, and copper amino acid chelates.[35]

Safety

Toxicity

Copper toxicity is rare in the general population. Acute copper poisoning has occurred through the contamination of beverages by storage in copper-containing containers as well as from contaminated water supplies.[36] In the United States, the health-based guideline for a maximum water copper concentration of 1.3 mg/L is enforced by the Environmental Protection Agency.[37] Symptoms of acute copper toxicity include abdominal pain, nausea, vomiting, and diarrhea, which help

Table 16.3 Tolerable upper intake level (UL) for copper

Life stage	Age	UL (μg/day)
Infants	0–12 months	Not possible to establish[a]
Children	1–3 years	1000
Children	4–8 years	3000
Children	9–13 years	5000
Adolescents	14–18 years	8000
Adults	≥19 years	10 000

[a]Source of intake should be from food and formula only.

prevent additional ingestion and absorption of copper. More serious signs of acute copper toxicity include severe liver damage, kidney failure, coma, and death. Of more concern from a nutritional standpoint is the possibility of liver damage resulting from long-term exposure to lower doses of copper. In generally healthy individuals, doses of up to 10 mg (10 000 μg) daily have not resulted in liver damage. For this reason, the US Food and Nutrition Board (FNB) of the Institute of Medicine set the tolerable upper intake level (UL) for copper at 10 mg/day from food and supplements (**Table 16.3**).[5] It should be noted that individuals with genetic disorders affecting copper metabolism (e.g., Wilson disease, Indian childhood cirrhosis, and idiopathic copper toxicosis) may be at risk for adverse effects of chronic copper toxicity at significantly lower intake levels. Recent evidence suggests that the UL of 10 mg/day may be too high. Specifically, men in a research study consumed 7.8 mg/day of copper for 147 days. They accumulated copper during that time, and some indices of immune function and antioxidant status suggested that these functions may have been adversely affected by the high copper intake.[38,39]

Drug Interactions

Relatively little is known about the interaction of copper with drugs. Penicillamine is used to bind copper and enhance its elimination in Wilson disease, a genetic disorder resulting in copper overload. Because penicillamine dramatically increases the urinary excretion of copper, individuals taking the medication for reasons other than copper overload may have an increased copper requirement. In addition, antacids may interfere with copper absorption when used in very high amounts.[2]

LPI Recommendation

The RDA for copper (900 μg/day for adults) is sufficient to prevent deficiency, but the lack of clear indicators of copper nutritional status in humans makes it difficult to determine the level of copper intake most likely to promote optimum health or prevent chronic disease. A varied diet should provide enough copper for most people. For those who are concerned that their diet may not provide adequate copper, a multivitamin/mineral supplement will generally provide at least the RDA for copper.

Older Adults

Because aging has not been associated with significant changes in the requirement for copper,[40] our recommendation for copper is the same for adults aged over 50 (900 μg/day).

References

1. Linder MC, Hazegh-Azam M. Copper biochemistry and molecular biology. Am J Clin Nutr 1996;63(5):797S–811S
2. Turnlund JR. Copper. In: Shils ME, Shike M, Ross AC, Caballero B, Cousins RJ, eds. Modern Nutrition in Health and Disease. 10th ed. Philadelphia, PA: Lippincott Williams & Wilkins; 2006:286–299
3. Uauy R, Olivares M, Gonzalez M. Essentiality of copper in humans. Am J Clin Nutr 1998; 67(5, Suppl) 952S–959S
4. Harris ED. Copper. In: O'Dell BL, Sunde RA, eds. Handbook of Nutritionally Essential Minerals. New York: Marcel Dekker, Inc.; 1997:231–273
5. Food and Nutrition Board, Institute of Medicine. Copper. In: Dietary Reference Intakes for Vitamin A, Vitamin K, Boron, Chromium, Copper, Iodine, Iron, Manganese, Molybdenum, Nickel, Silicon, Vanadium, and Zinc. Washington, DC: National Academy Press; 2001: 224–257
6. Johnson MA, Fischer JG, Kays SE. Is copper an antioxidant nutrient? Crit Rev Food Sci Nutr 1992;32(1): 1–31
7. Milne DB, Omaye ST. Effect of vitamin C on copper and iron metabolism in the guinea pig. Int J Vitam Nutr Res 1980;50(3):301–308
8. Finley EB, Cerklewski FL. Influence of ascorbic acid supplementation on copper status in young adult men. Am J Clin Nutr 1983;37(4):553–556
9. Jacob RA, Skala JH, Omaye ST, Turnlund JR. Effect of varying ascorbic acid intakes on copper absorption and ceruloplasmin levels of young men. J Nutr 1987;117(12):2109–2115
10. Percival SS, Kauwell GP, Bowser E, Wagner M. Altered copper status in adult men with cystic fibrosis. J Am Coll Nutr 1999;18(6):614–619
11. Fox PL, Mazumder B, Ehrenwald E, Mukhopadhyay CK. Ceruloplasmin and cardiovascular disease. Free Radic Biol Med 2000;28(12):1735–1744
12. Jones AA, DiSilvestro RA, Coleman M, Wagner TL. Copper supplementation of adult men: effects on blood copper enzyme activities and indicators of cardiovascular disease risk. Metabolism 1997;46(12): 1380–1383

13. Ford ES. Serum copper concentration and coronary heart disease among US adults. Am J Epidemiol 2000;151(12):1182–1188

14. Malek F, Jiresova E, Dohnalova A, Koprivova H, Spacek R. Serum copper as a marker of inflammation in prediction of short term outcome in high risk patients with chronic heart failure. Int J Cardiol 2006;113(2):e51–e53

15. Leone N, Courbon D, Ducimetiere P, Zureik M. Zinc, copper, and magnesium and risks for all-cause, cancer, and cardiovascular mortality. Epidemiology 2006; 17(3):308–314

16. Kosar F, Sahin I, Acikgöz N, Aksoy Y, Kucukbay Z, Cehreli S. Significance of serum trace element status in patients with rheumatic heart disease: a prospective study. Biol Trace Elem Res 2005;107(1):1–10

17. Klevay LM. Cardiovascular disease from copper deficiency—a history. J Nutr 2000;130(2S, Suppl) 489S–492S

18. Mielcarz G, Howard AN, Mielcarz B, et al. Leucocyte copper, a marker of copper body status is low in coronary artery disease. J Trace Elem Med Biol 2001; 15(1):31–35

19. Kinsman GD, Howard AN, Stone DL, Mullins PA. Studies in copper status and atherosclerosis. Biochem Soc Trans 1990;18(6):1186–1188

20. Wang XL, Adachi T, Sim AS, Wilcken DE. Plasma extracellular superoxide dismutase levels in an Australian population with coronary artery disease. Arterioscler Thromb Vasc Biol 1998;18(12):1915–1921

21. Klevay LM. Lack of a recommended dietary allowance for copper may be hazardous to your health. J Am Coll Nutr 1998;17(4):322–326

22. Milne DB, Nielsen FH. Effects of a diet low in copper on copper-status indicators in postmenopausal women. Am J Clin Nutr 1996;63(3):358–364

23. Medeiros DM, Milton A, Brunett E, Stacy L. Copper supplementation effects on indicators of copper status and serum cholesterol in adult males. Biol Trace Elem Res 1991;30(1):19–35

24. Turley E, McKeown A, Bonham MP, et al. Copper supplementation in humans does not affect the susceptibility of low density lipoprotein to in vitro induced oxidation (FOODCUE project). Free Radic Biol Med 2000;29(11):1129–1134

25. Rock E, Mazur A, O'Connor JM, Bonham MP, Rayssiguier Y, Strain JJ. The effect of copper supplementation on red blood cell oxidizability and plasma antioxidants in middle-aged healthy volunteers. Free Radic Biol Med 2000;28(3):324–329

26. Failla ML, Hopkins RG. Is low copper status immunosuppressive? Nutr Rev 1998;56(1 Pt 2):S59–S64

27. Percival SS. Copper and immunity. Am J Clin Nutr 1998;67(5, Suppl):1064S–1068S

28. Heresi G, Castillo-Duran C, Muñoz C, Arévalo M, Schlesinger L. Phagocytosis and immunoglobulin levels in hypocupremic children. Nutr Res 1985;5: 1327–1334

29. Kelley DS, Daudu PA, Taylor PC, Mackey BE, Turnlund JR. Effects of low-copper diets on human immune response. Am J Clin Nutr 1995;62(2):412–416

30. Conlan D, Korula R, Tallentire D. Serum copper levels in elderly patients with femoral-neck fractures. Age Ageing 1990;19(3):212–214

31. Eaton-Evans J, Mellwrath EM, Jackson WE, McCartney H, Strain JJ. Copper supplementation and the maintenance of bone mineral density in middle-aged women. J Trace Elem Exp Med 1996;9(3):87–94

32. Strause L, Saltman P, Smith KT, Bracker M, Andon MB. Spinal bone loss in postmenopausal women supplemented with calcium and trace minerals. J Nutr 1994;124(7):1060–1064

33. Baker A, Harvey L, Majask-Newman G, Fairweather-Tait S, Flynn A, Cashman K. Effect of dietary copper intakes on biochemical markers of bone metabolism in healthy adult males. Eur J Clin Nutr 1999;53(5): 408–412

34. Baker A, Turley E, Bonham MP, et al. No effect of copper supplementation on biochemical markers of bone metabolism in healthy adults. Br J Nutr 1999;82(4): 283–290

35. Hendler SS, Rorvik DR, eds. PDR for Nutritional Supplements. Montvale, NJ: Medical Economics Co., Inc.; 2001

36. Bremner I. Manifestations of copper excess. Am J Clin Nutr 1998;67(5, Suppl):1069S–1073S

37. Fitzgerald DJ. Safety guidelines for copper in water. Am J Clin Nutr 1998;67(5, Suppl):1098S–1102S

38. Turnlund JR, Jacob RA, Keen CL, et al. Long-term high copper intake: effects on indexes of copper status, antioxidant status, and immune function in young men. Am J Clin Nutr 2004;79(6):1037–1044

39. Turnlund JR, Keyes WR, Kim SK, Domek JM. Long-term high copper intake: effects on copper absorption, retention, and homeostasis in men. Am J Clin Nutr 2005;81(4):822–828

40. Wood RJ, Suter PM, Russell RM. Mineral requirements of elderly people. Am J Clin Nutr 1995;62(3):493–505

17 Fluoride (Fluorine)

Fluorine occurs naturally as the negatively charged ion, fluoride (F⁻). Fluoride is considered a trace element because only small amounts are present in the body (about 2.6 g in adults), and because the daily requirement for maintaining dental health is only a few milligrams a day. About 95% of the total body fluoride is found in bones and teeth.[1] Although its role in the prevention of dental caries (tooth decay) is well established, fluoride is not generally considered an essential mineral element because humans do not require it for growth or to sustain life.[2] However, if one considers the prevention of chronic disease (dental caries) an important criterion in determining essentiality, then fluoride might well be considered an essential trace element.[3]

Function

Fluoride is absorbed in the stomach and small intestine. Once in the bloodstream it rapidly enters mineralized tissue (bones and developing teeth). At usual intake levels, fluoride does not accumulate in soft tissue. The predominant mineral elements in bone are crystals of calcium and phosphate, known as *hydroxyapatite crystals*. Fluoride's high chemical reactivity and small radius allow it to either displace the larger hydroxyl ion in the hydroxyapatite crystal, forming fluoroapatite, or to increase crystal density by entering spaces within the hydroxyapatite crystal. Fluoroapatite hardens tooth enamel and stabilizes bone mineral.[4]

Nutrient Interactions

Both calcium and magnesium form insoluble complexes with fluoride and are capable of significantly decreasing fluoride absorption when present in the same meal. However, the absorption of fluoride in the form of monofluorophosphate, unlike sodium fluoride, is unaffected by calcium. Also, a diet low in chloride (i.e., salt) has been found to increase fluoride retention by reducing urinary excretion of fluoride.[1]

Deficiency

In humans, the only clear effect of inadequate fluoride intake is an increased risk of dental caries (tooth decay) for individuals of all ages. Epidemiological investigations of patterns of water consumption and the prevalence of dental caries across various US regions with different water fluoride concentrations led to the development of a recommended optimum range of fluoride concentration of 0.7–1.2 mg/L or parts per million (ppm); the lower concentration was recommended for warmer climates where water consumption is higher, and the higher concentration was recommended for colder climates. A number of studies conducted before the introduction of fluoride-containing toothpastes demonstrated that the prevalence of dental caries was 40%–60% lower in communities with optimal water fluoride concentrations than in communities with low water fluoride concentrations.[5]

Adequate Intake

The Food and Nutrition Board (FNB) of the Institute of Medicine updated its recommendations for fluoride intake in 1997 (**Table 17.1**). The FNB felt that there were inadequate data to set a recommended dietary allowance (RDA); instead, adequate intake (AI) was set based on estimated intakes (0.05 mg/kg body weight) that have been shown to reduce the occurrence of dental caries most effectively without causing the unwanted side effect of tooth enamel mottling known as dental fluorosis.[5] See "Safety," p. 46, for a discussion of dental fluorosis.

Table 17.1 Adequate intake for fluoride

Life stage	Age	Males (mg/day)	Females (mg/day)
Infants	0–6 months	0.01	0.01
Infants	7–12 months	0.5	0.5
Children	1–3 years	0.7	0.7
Children	4–8 years	1.0	1.0
Children	9–13 years	2.0	2.0
Adolescents	14–18 years	3.0	3.0
Adults	≥19 years	4.0	3.0
Pregnancy	All ages	–	3.0
Breast-feeding	All ages	–	3.0

Disease Prevention

Dental Caries

Specific cariogenic (cavity-causing) bacteria found in dental plaque are capable of metabolizing certain carbohydrates (sugars) and converting them to organic acids that can dissolve susceptible tooth enamel. If unchecked, the bacteria may penetrate deeper layers of the tooth and progress into the soft pulp tissue at the center. Untreated caries can lead to severe pain, local infection, tooth loss or extraction, nutritional problems, and serious systemic infections in susceptible individuals.[6] Increased fluoride exposure, most commonly through water fluoridation, has been found to decrease dental caries in children and adults.[7] Fluoride consumed in water appears to have a systemic effect in children before teeth erupt, as well as a topical (surface) effect in adults and children after teeth have erupted. Between 1950 and 1980, clinical studies in 20 different countries demonstrated that the addition of fluoride to community water supplies (0.7–1.2 ppm) reduced caries by 40%–50% in primary (baby) teeth and 50%–60% in permanent teeth.[7]

Although the role of fluoride in preventing dental caries is well established, the mechanisms for its effects are not entirely understood. Originally, it was believed that fluoride incorporated into the enamel during tooth development resulted in a more acid-resistant enamel. More recent research indicates that the primary action of fluoride occurs topically after the teeth erupt into the mouth. When enamel is partially demineralized by organic acids, fluoride in the saliva can enhance the remineralization of enamel through its interactions with calcium and phosphate. In the presence of fluoride, remineralized enamel contains more fluoride and is more resistant to demineralization. In salivary concentrations associated with optimum fluoride intake, fluoride has been found to inhibit bacterial enzymes, resulting in reduced acid production by cariogenic bacteria.[6,7]

Osteoporosis

Although fluoride in pharmacological doses has been shown to be a potent therapeutic agent for increasing spinal bone mass, there is little evidence that water fluoridation at optimum levels for the prevention of dental caries is helpful in the prevention of osteoporosis. Most studies conducted to date have failed to find clinically significant differences in bone mineral density (BMD) or fracture incidence when comparing residents of areas with fluoridated water supplies with residents in areas without fluoridated water supplies.[8] However, two studies found that drinking water fluoridation was associated with decreased incidence of hip fracture in elderly people. In addition, one study in Italy found a significantly greater risk of femoral (hip) fractures in men and women residing in an area with low water fluoridation (0.05 ppm) compared with the risk in a similar population where the water supply was naturally fluoridated (1.45 ppm) at higher than optimum levels for prevention of dental caries.[9] Another study in Germany found no significant difference in BMD between residents of a community whose water supply had been optimally fluoridated for 30 years (1 ppm) compared with those who resided in a community without fluoridated water. However, this study reported that the incidence of hip fracture in men and women, aged 85 years or older, was significantly lower in the community with fluoridated water compared with the community with nonfluoridated water, despite higher calcium levels in the nonfluoridated water supply.[10] More recently, a community-based study in 1300 women found that elevated serum fluoride concentrations were not related to BMD or to osteoporotic fracture incidence.[11]

Disease Treatment

Osteoporosis

Osteoporosis is characterized by decreased BMD and increased bone fragility and susceptibility to fracture. In general, decreased BMD is associated with increased risk of fracture. However, the usual relationship between BMD and fracture risk does not always hold true when very high (pharmacological) doses of fluoride are used to treat osteoporosis. Most available therapies for osteoporosis (e.g., estrogen, calcitonin, and bisphosphonates) decrease bone loss (resorption), resulting in very small increases in BMD. Pharmacological doses of fluoride are capable of producing large increases in the BMD of the lumbar spine. Overall, therapeutic trials of fluoride in patients with osteoporosis have not consistently demonstrated significant decreases in the occurrence of vertebral fracture despite dramatic increases in lumbar spine BMD.[12] A meta-analysis of 11 controlled studies, including 1429 participants, found that fluoride treatment resulted in increased BMD at the lumbar spine but was not associated with a lower risk of vertebral fractures.[13] This meta-analysis also found that higher concentrations of fluoride were associated with increased risk of nonvertebral fractures. Early studies using high doses of sodium fluoride (75 mg/day) may have induced rapid bone mineralization in the absence of adequate calcium and vitamin D, resulting in denser bones that were not mechanically stronger.[14] Some controlled studies using lower doses, intermittent dosage schedules, or slow-release formulations (enteric-coated sodium fluoride) have demonstrated a decreased incidence of vertebral frac-

ture along with increased bone density of the lumbar spine.[15-17]

Analysis of bone architecture has also shed some light on the inconsistent effect of fluoride therapy in reducing vertebral fractures. Recent research indicates that osteoporosis may be associated with an irreversible change in the architecture of bone known as *decreased trabecular connectivity*. Normal bone consists of a series of plates interconnected by thick rods. Severely osteoporotic bone has fewer plates, and the rods may be fractured or disconnected (decreased trabecular connectivity). Despite fluoride therapy increasing bone density, it probably cannot restore connectivity in patients with severe bone loss. Thus, fluoride therapy may be less effective in osteoporotic individuals who have already lost substantial trabecular connectivity.[12,18]

Serious side effects have been associated with the high doses of fluoride used to treat osteoporosis. They include gastrointestinal irritation, joint pain in the lower extremities, and the development of calcium deficiency as well as stress fractures. The reasons for the occurrence of lower extremity joint pain and stress fractures in patients taking fluoride for osteoporosis remain unclear, but they may be related to rapid increases in bone formation without sufficient calcium to support such an increase.[12] Currently, enteric-coated sodium fluoride or monofluorophosphate preparations offer a lower side-effect profile than the high-dose sodium fluoride used in earlier trials. In addition, sufficient calcium and vitamin D must be provided to support fluoride-induced bone formation. Although fluoride therapy may be beneficial for the treatment of osteoporosis in appropriately selected and closely monitored individuals, uncertainty about its safety and benefit in reducing fractures has kept the US Food and Drug Administration from approving fluoride therapy for osteoporosis.[19] Combinations of lower doses of fluoride with antiresorptive agents, such as estrogen or bisphosphonates, may improve therapeutic results while minimizing side effects, and thus these therapies are considered worthy of further study.[20,21]

Sources

Water Fluoridation

The major source of dietary fluoride in the US diet is drinking water. When water is fluoridated, it is adjusted to between 0.7 and 1.2 mg fluoride/liter, which is 0.7–1.2 ppm. This concentration has been found to decrease the incidence of dental caries while minimizing the risk of dental fluorosis and other adverse effects. Approximately 62% of the US population consumes water with sufficient fluoride for the prevention of dental caries. The average fluoride intake for adults living in fluoridated communities ranges from 1.4 mg/day to 3.4 mg/day. As well water can vary greatly in its fluoride content, people who consume water from wells should have the fluoride content of their water tested by their local water district or health department. Water fluoride testing may also be warranted in households that use home water treatment systems. Although water softeners are not thought to change water fluoride levels, reverse osmosis systems, distillation units, and some water filters have been found to remove significant amounts of fluoride from water. However, Brita-type filters do not remove fluoride.[5,19]

Bottled water sales have grown exponentially in the United States in recent years, and studies have found that most bottled waters contain suboptimal levels of fluoride, although there is considerable variation. For example, a study of 78 different bottled water products in Iowa found that over 80% had fluoride concentrations of less than 0.3 ppm; however, 10% of the tested products had fluoride concentrations of 0.7 ppm or greater.[22] Several other studies have reported similar findings, with most bottled waters relatively low in fluoride, but a few in the optimal range or higher.[23,24]

Although consumption of fluoride from water presents very little risk of adverse effects in adults except in extreme circumstances, consumption of relatively large amounts of water mixed with formula concentrates appears to increase the risk for the development of dental fluorosis in infants.[25,26] One study found that, on average, at least half of all fluoride ingested by infants aged 6 months and younger was from water mixed with formula concentrates.[27]

Table 17.2 Food sources of fluoride

Food	Serving	Fluoride (mg)
Canned sardines, with bones	100 g (3.5 ounces)	0.2–0.4
Tea	100 mL (3.5 fluid ounces)	0.1–0.6
Fish, without bones	100 g (3.5 ounces)	0.01–0.17
Chicken	100 g (3.5 ounces)	0.06–0.10

Food and Beverage Sources

The fluoride content of most foods is low (<0.05 mg/100 g). Rich sources of fluoride include tea, which concentrates fluoride in its leaves, and marine fish that are consumed with their bones (e.g., sardines). Foods made with mechanically separated (boned) chicken, such as canned meats, hot dogs, and infant foods, also add fluoride to the diet.[28] In addition, certain fruit juices, particularly grape juices, often have relatively high fluoride concentrations.[29] Foods generally contribute only 0.3–0.6 mg of the daily intake of fluoride. An adult male residing in a community with fluoridated water has an intake range from 1 mg/day to 3 mg/day. Intake is less than 1 mg/day in nonfluoridated areas.[2] **Table 17.2** provides a range of fluoride content for a few fluoride-rich foods and beverages.[5]

Supplements

Fluoride supplements, available only by prescription, are intended for children living in areas with low water fluoride concentrations for the purpose of bringing their intake to approximately 1 mg/day.[5] The American Dental Association recommends fluoride supplements for those children living in areas with suboptimal water fluoridation.[30] The supplemental fluoride dosage schedule in **Table 17.3** was recommended by the American Dental Association, the American Academy of Pediatric Dentistry, and the American Academy of Pediatrics.[31] It requires knowledge of the fluoride concentration of local drinking water as well as other possible sources of fluoride intake.

Table 17.3 Fluoride Supplement Schedule Recommended by the American Dental Association, the American Academy of Pediatric Dentistry, and the American Academy of Pediatrics

Age	Quantity needed if fluoride ion level in drinking water (ppm)[a]		
	<0.3	0.3–0.6	>0.6
Birth–6 months	None	None	None
6 months–3 years	0.25 mg/day[b]	None	None
3 years–6 years	0.50 mg/day	0.25 mg/day	None
6 years–16 years	1.0 mg/day	0.50 mg/day	None

[a] 1.0 part per million (ppm) = 1 mg/L.
[b] 2.2 mg sodium fluoride contains 1 mg fluoride ion.

Toothpaste

Fluoridated toothpastes are very effective in preventing dental caries but also add considerably to fluoride intake of children, especially young children who are more likely to swallow toothpaste. Researchers estimate that children under 6 years of age ingest an average of 0.3 mg fluoride from toothpaste with each brushing. Children under the age of 6 years who ingest more than two or three times the recommended fluoride intake are at increased risk of a white speckling or mottling of the permanent teeth, known as *dental fluorosis*. A major source of excess fluoride intake in this age group comes from swallowing fluoride-containing toothpaste. To prevent dental fluorosis while providing optimum protection from tooth decay, it is recommended that parents supervise children aged under 6 years while brushing with fluoridated toothpaste. In addition to discouraging the swallowing of toothpaste, children should be encouraged to use no more than a pea-size application of toothpaste and to rinse their mouths with water after brushing.[1,5]

Safety

Adverse Effects

Fluoridation of public drinking water in the United States was initiated over 50 years ago. Since then, a number of adverse effects have been attributed to water fluoridation. However, extensive scientific research has uncovered no evidence of increased risks of cancer, heart disease, kidney disease, liver disease, Alzheimer disease, birth defects, or Down syndrome.[32,33] The use of high doses of fluoride to treat osteoporosis has been associated with some adverse effects, which are discussed under "Disease Treatment," p. 144.

Acute toxicity. Fluoride is toxic when consumed in excessive amounts, so concentrated fluoride products should be used and stored with caution to prevent the possibility of acute fluoride poisoning, especially in children and other vulnerable individuals. The lowest dose that could trigger adverse symptoms is considered to be 5 mg/kg body weight, with the lowest potentially fatal dose considered to be 15 mg/kg body weight. Nausea, abdominal pain, and vomiting almost always accompany acute fluoride toxicity. Other symptoms such as diarrhea, excessive salivation and tearing, sweating, and generalized weakness may also occur.[32] To prevent acute fluoride poisoning, the American Dental Association has recommended that no more than 120 mg fluoride (224 mg sodium fluoride) be dispensed at one time.[19]

Dental fluorosis. The mildest form of dental fluorosis is detectable only to the trained observer and is characterized by small opaque white flecks or spots on the enamel of the teeth. Moderate dental fluorosis is characterized by mottling and mild staining of the teeth, and severe dental fluorosis results in marked staining and pitting of the teeth. In its moderate-to-severe forms, dental fluorosis becomes a cosmetic concern when it affects the incisors and canines (front teeth). Dental fluorosis is a result of excess fluoride intake before the eruption of the first permanent teeth (generally before 8 years of age). It is also a dose-dependent condition, with higher fluoride intakes being associated with more pronounced effects on the teeth. The risk of mild-to-moderate dental fluorosis appears to increase significantly at an intake two to three times that recommended for children of a susceptible age, while severe dental fluorosis has been seen in the United

Table 17.4 Tolerable upper intake level (UL) for fluoride

Life stage	Age	UL (mg/day)
Infants	0–6 months	0.7
Infants	7–12 months	0.9
Children	1–3 years	1.3
Children	4–8 years	2.2
Children	9–13 years	10.0
Adolescents	14–18 years	10.0
Adults	≥19 years	10.0

States only at fluoride intakes about five times the recommended level.[33] The incidence of mild and moderate dental fluorosis has increased over the past 50 years, mainly due to increasing fluoride intake from toothpaste, although inappropriate use of fluoride supplements may also contribute. In 1997, the FNB based the tolerable upper intake levels (ULs) for fluoride on the prevention of moderate enamel fluorosis.[5] The UL for each life stage is presented in **Table 17.4**.

Skeletal fluorosis. Intake of fluoride at excessive levels for long periods of time may lead to changes in bone structure known as *skeletal fluorosis*. The early stages of skeletal fluorosis are characterized by increased bone mass, detectable on a radiograph. If very high fluoride intake persists over many years, joint pain and stiffness may result from the skeletal changes. The most severe form of skeletal fluorosis is known as *crippling skeletal fluorosis*, which may result in calcification of ligaments, immobility, muscle wasting, and neurological problems related to spinal cord compression. Most estimates indicate that crippling skeletal fluorosis occurs only when fluoride intakes exceed 10–25 mg/day for at least 10 years. Crippling skeletal fluorosis is extremely rare in the United States; in fact, only five cases have been confirmed in the last 35 years. Interestingly, studies of communities in the United States where water fluoride concentrations were as high as 20 mg/L (ppm), allowing for fluoride intakes as high as 20 mg/day, did not find evidence of crippling skeletal fluorosis. Such water fluoride concentrations are higher than those known to have resulted in crippling skeletal fluorosis in other countries, suggesting that metabolic or dietary factors might render some populations more susceptible.[5,32]

Drug Interactions

Calcium supplements, as well as calcium- and aluminum-containing antacids, can decrease the absorption of fluoride. It is best to take these products 2 hours before or after fluoride supplements.[34]

LPI Recommendation

The safety and public health benefits of optimally fluoridated water for prevention of tooth decay in people of all ages have been well established. The Linus Pauling Institute supports the recommendations of the American Dental Association and the Centers for Disease Control and Prevention, which include optimally fluoridated water as well as the use of fluoride toothpaste, fluoride mouthrinse, fluoride varnish, and, when necessary, fluoride supplementation. Due to the risk of fluorosis, any fluoride supplementation should be prescribed and closely monitored by a dentist or physician.

Older Adults

Available evidence does not support a need for fluoride supplementation in generally healthy older adults (50 years), even in communities without optimally fluoridated water supplies.

References

1. Cerklewski FL. Fluoride bioavailability—nutritional and clinical aspects. Nutr Res 1997;17:(5)907–929
2. Nielsen FH. Ultratrace minerals. In: Shils M, Olson JA, Shike M, Ross AC, eds. Modern Nutrition in Health and Disease. 9th ed. Baltimore, MD: Lippincott Williams & Wilkins; 1999:283–303
3. Cerklewski FL. Fluoride—essential or just beneficial. Nutrition 1998;14(5):475–476
4. Cerklewski FL. Fluorine. In: O'Dell BL, Sunde RA, eds. Handbook of Nutritionally Essential Minerals. New York: Marcel Dekker, Inc.; 1997:583–602
5. Food and Nutrition Board, Institute of Medicine. Fluoride. In: Dietary Reference Intakes for Calcium, Phosphorus, Magnesium, Vitamin D, and Fluoride. Washington, DC: National Academy Press; 1997:288–313
6. Centers for Disease Control. Achievements in public health, 1900–1999: fluoridation of drinking water to prevent dental caries. MMWR weekly 1999; 48:(41)933–940
7. DePaola DP. Nutrition in relation to dental medicine. In: Shils M, Olson JA, Shike M, Ross AC, eds. Modern Nutrition in Health and Disease, 9th ed. Baltimore, MD: Lippincott Williams & Wilkins;1999:1099–1124
8. Krall EA, Dawson-Hughes B. Osteoporosis. In: Shils M, Olson JA, Shike M, Ross AC, eds. Modern Nutrition in Health and Disease. 9th ed. Baltimore, MD: Lippincott Williams & Wilkins; 1999:1353–1364
9. Fabiani L, Leoni V, Vitali M. Bone-fracture incidence rate in two Italian regions with different fluoride concentration levels in drinking water. J Trace Elem Med Biol 1999;13(4):232–237

10. Lehmann R, Wapniarz M, Hofmann B, Pieper B, Haubitz I, Allolio B. Drinking water fluoridation: bone mineral density and hip fracture incidence. Bone 1998; 22(3):273–278
11. Sowers M, Whitford GM, Clark MK, Jannausch ML. Elevated serum fluoride concentrations in women are not related to fractures and bone mineral density. J Nutr 2005;135(9):2247–2252
12. Cesar Libanati K-H. Fluoride therapy for osteoporosis. In: Marcus R, ed. Osteoporosis. San Diego, CA: Academic Press; 1996:1259–1277
13. Haguenauer D, Welch V, Shea B, Tugwell P, Adachi JD, Wells G. Fluoride for the treatment of postmenopausal osteoporotic fractures: a meta-analysis. Osteoporos Int 2000;11(9):727–738
14. Riggs BL, Hodgson SF, O'Fallon WM, et al. Effect of fluoride treatment on the fracture rate in postmenopausal women with osteoporosis. N Engl J Med 1990;322(12):802–809
15. Ringe JD, Kipshoven C, Cöster A, Umbach R. Therapy of established postmenopausal osteoporosis with monofluorophosphate plus calcium: dose-related effects on bone density and fracture rate. Osteoporos Int 1999;9(2):171–178
16. Reginster JY, Meurmans L, Zegels B, et al. The effect of sodium monofluorophosphate plus calcium on vertebral fracture rate in postmenopausal women with moderate osteoporosis. A randomized, controlled trial. Ann Intern Med 1998;129(1):1–8
17. Pak CY, Sakhaee K, Adams-Huet B, Piziak V, Peterson RD, Poindexter JR. Treatment of postmenopausal osteoporosis with slow-release sodium fluoride. Final report of a randomized controlled trial. Ann Intern Med 1995;123(6):401–408
18. Balena R, Kleerekoper M, Foldes JA, et al. Effects of different regimens of sodium fluoride treatment for osteoporosis on the structure, remodeling and mineralization of bone. Osteoporos Int 1998;8(5):428–435
19. American Dietetic Association. Position of the American Dietetic Association: the impact of fluoride on health. J Am Diet Assoc 2001;101(1):126–132
20. Murray TM, Ste-Marie LG. Prevention and management of osteoporosis: consensus statements from the Scientific Advisory Board of the Osteoporosis Society of Canada. 7. Fluoride therapy for osteoporosis. CMAJ 1996;155(7):949–954
21. Alexandersen P, Riis BJ, Christiansen C. Monofluorophosphate combined with hormone replacement therapy induces a synergistic effect on bone mass by dissociating bone formation and resorption in postmenopausal women: a randomized study. J Clin Endocrinol Metab 1999;84(9):3013–3020
22. Van Winkle S, Levy SM, Kiritsy MC, Heilman JR, Wefel JS, Marshall T. Water and formula fluoride concentrations: significance for infants fed formula. Pediatr Dent 1995;17(4):305–310
23. Tate WH, Chan JT. Fluoride concentrations in bottled and filtered waters. Gen Dent 1994;42(4):362–366
24. McGuire S. Fluoride content of bottled water. N Engl J Med 1989;321(12):836–837
25. Marshall TA, Levy SM, Warren JJ, Broffitt B, Eichenberger-Gilmore JM, Stumbo PJ. Associations between Intakes of fluoride from beverages during infancy and dental fluorosis of primary teeth. J Am Coll Nutr 2004;23(2):108–116
26. Pendrys DG. Risk of enamel fluorosis in nonfluoridated and optimally fluoridated populations: considerations for the dental professional. J Am Dent Assoc 2000;131(6):746–755
27. Levy SM, Kohout FJ, Guha-Chowdhury N, Kiritsy MC, Heilman JR, Wefel JS. Infants' fluoride intake from drinking water alone, and from water added to formula, beverages, and food. J Dent Res 1995;74(7):1399–1407
28. Fein NJ, Cerklewski FL. Fluoride content of foods made with mechanically separated chicken. J Agric Food Chem 2001;49(9):4284–4286
29. Kiritsy MC, Levy SM, Warren JJ, Guha-Chowdhury N, Heilman JR, Marshall T. Assessing fluoride concentrations of juices and juice-flavored drinks. J Am Dent Assoc 1996;127(7):895–902
30. Adair SM. Overview of the history and current status of fluoride supplementation schedules. J Public Health Dent 1999;59(4):252–258
31. Centers for Disease Control and Prevention. Recommendations for using fluoride to prevent and control dental caries in the United States. MMWR Recomm Rep 2001;50(RR-14):1–42 http://www.cdc.gov/mmwr/preview/mmwrhtml/rr5014a1.htm
32. Whitford GM. The Metabolism and Toxicity of Fluoride. Vol. 13. Basel: S Karger AG; 1996
33. National Research Council. Health Effects of Ingested Fluoride. Washington, DC: National Academy Press; 1993
34. Trace elements. Drug Facts and Comparisons, 54th ed. St. Louis: Facts and Comparisons; 2000:44

18 Iodine

Iodine, a nonmetallic trace element, is required by humans for the synthesis of thyroid hormones. Iodine deficiency is an important health problem throughout much of the world. Most of the earth's iodine is found in oceans, and the iodine content in the soil varies with the region. The older an exposed soil surface, the more likely that the iodine has been leached away by erosion. Mountainous regions, such as the Himalayas, the Andes, and the Alps, and flooded river valleys, such as the Ganges, are among the most severely iodine-deficient areas in the world.[1]

Function

Iodine is an essential component of the thyroid hormones, triiodothyronine (T_3) and thyroxine (T_4), and is therefore essential for normal thyroid function. To meet the body's demand for thyroid hormones, the thyroid gland traps iodine from the blood and incorporates it into thyroid hormones that are stored and released into the circulation when needed. In target tissues, such as the liver and the brain, T_3, the physiologically active thyroid hormone, can bind to thyroid receptors in the nuclei of cells and regulate gene expression. In target tissues, T_4, the most abundant circulating thyroid hormone, can be converted to T_3 by selenium-containing enzymes known as *deiodinases*. In this manner, thyroid hormones regulate a number of physiological processes, including growth, development, metabolism, and reproductive function.[1,2]

The regulation of thyroid function is a complex process that involves the brain (hypothalamus) and pituitary gland. In response to thyrotropin-releasing hormone (TRH) secretion by the hypothalamus, the pituitary gland secretes thyroid-stimulating hormone (TSH), which stimulates iodine trapping, thyroid hormone synthesis, and release of T_3 and T_4 by the thyroid gland. The presence of adequate circulating T_4 and T_3 levels feeds back at the level of both the hypothalamus and the pituitary, decreasing TRH and TSH production (**Fig. 18.1**). When circulating T_4 levels decrease, the pituitary increases its secretion of TSH, resulting in increased iodine trapping as well as increased production and release of both T_3 and T_4. Iodine deficiency results in inadequate production of T_4. In response to decreased blood levels of T_4, the pituitary gland increases its output of TSH. Persistently elevated TSH levels may lead to hypertrophy (enlargement) of the thyroid gland, also known as *goiter*.[3]

Deficiency

Iodine deficiency is now accepted as the most common cause of preventable brain damage in the world. The spectrum of iodine deficiency disorders includes learning disabilities, hypothyroidism, goiter, and varying degrees of other growth and developmental abnormalities.[1,4] The World Health Organization (WHO) estimated that over 30% of the world's population (2 billion people) has insufficient iodine intake as measured by urinary iodine excretion below 100 µg/L;[5] urinary iodine is an indicator of iodine status. Moreover, an estimated 31.5% of school-age children (6–12 years old) worldwide (266 million total children) have insufficient iodine intake.[5] Major international efforts have produced dramatic improvements in the correction of iodine deficiency in the 1990s, mainly through the use of iodized salt in iodine-deficient countries.[6] Today, 70% of households in the world use iodized salt.[7]

Thyroid enlargement, or goiter, is one of the earliest and most visible signs of iodine deficiency. The thyroid enlarges in response to persistent stimulation by TSH. In mild iodine deficiency, this adaptive response may be enough to provide the body with sufficient thyroid hormone. However, more severe cases of iodine deficiency result in hypothyroidism. Adequate iodine intake will generally reduce the size of goiters, but the reversibility of the effects of hypothyroidism depends on an individual's stage of development. Iodine deficiency has adverse effects in all stages of development but is most damaging to the

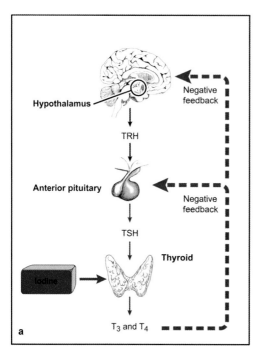
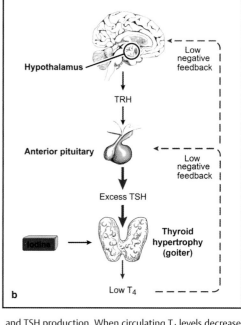

Fig. 18.1a,b Iodine intake and thyroid function. In response to thyrotropin-releasing hormone (TRH) secretion by the hypothalamus, the pituitary gland secretes thyroid-stimulating hormone (TSH), which stimulates iodine trapping, thyroid hormone synthesis, and release of T_3 (triiodothyronine) and T_4 (thyroxine) by the thyroid gland. **(a)** When dietary iodine intake is sufficient, the presence of adequate circulating T_4 and T_3 feeds back at the level of both the hypothalamus and the pituitary, decreasing TRH

and TSH production. When circulating T_4 levels decrease, the pituitary increases its secretion of TSH, resulting in increased iodine trapping as well as increased production and release of both T_3 and T_4. **(b)** Dietary iodine deficiency results in inadequate production of T_4. In response to decreased blood levels of T_4, the pituitary gland increases its output of TSH. Persistently elevated TSH levels may lead to hypertrophy of the thyroid gland, also known as *goiter*.

developing brain. In addition to regulating many aspects of growth and development, thyroid hormone is important for myelination of the central nervous system, which is most active before and shortly after birth.[2,6]

The Effects of Iodine Deficiency by Developmental Stage

Prenatal development. Fetal iodine deficiency is caused by iodine deficiency in the pregnant woman. One of the most devastating effects of maternal iodine deficiency is congenital hypothyroidism. A severe form of congenital hypothyroidism may lead to a condition that is sometimes referred to as *cretinism* and result in irreversible learning disability. Cretinism occurs in two forms, although there is considerable overlap between them. The neurological form is char-

acterized by learning disability and physical retardation and deafness, and is the result of maternal iodine deficiency that affects the fetus before its own thyroid is functional. The myxedematous or hypothyroid form is characterized by short stature and learning disability. In addition to iodine deficiency, the hypothyroid form has been associated with selenium deficiency and the presence of goitrogens in the diet which interfere with thyroid hormone production.[8]

Newborns and infants. Infant mortality is increased in areas of iodine deficiency, and several studies have demonstrated an increase in childhood survival on correction of the iodine deficiency.[9] Infancy is a period of rapid brain growth and development. Sufficient thyroid hormone, which depends on adequate iodine intake, is essential for normal brain development. Even in the absence of congenital hypothyroidism, iodine deficiency during infancy may result in abnormal brain development and, consequently, impaired intellectual development.[10]

Children and adolescents. Iodine deficiency in children and adolescents is often associated with goiter. The incidence of goiter peaks in adolescence and is more common in girls. Schoolchildren in iodine-deficient areas show poorer school performance, lower IQs, and a higher incidence of learning disabilities than matched groups from iodine-sufficient areas. A meta-analysis of 18 studies concluded that iodine deficiency alone lowered mean IQ scores in children by 13.5 points.[11,12]

Adults. Inadequate iodine intake may also result in goiter and hypothyroidism in adults. Although the effects of hypothyroidism are more subtle in the brains of adults than children, research suggests that hypothyroidism results in slower response times and impaired mental function.[1] Other symptoms of hypothyroidism include fatigue, weight gain, cold intolerance, and constipation.

Pregnancy and lactation. Iodine requirements are increased in pregnant and breast-feeding women (**Table 18.1**).[6] Iodine deficiency during pregnancy has been associated with increased incidence of miscarriage, stillbirth, and birth defects. Moreover, severe iodine deficiency during pregnancy may result in congenital hypothyroidism and neurocognitive deficits in the offspring.[6,8]

Iodine-deficient women who are breast-feeding may not be able to provide sufficient iodine to their infants who are particularly vulnerable to the effects of iodine deficiency.[1] A daily prenatal supplement providing 150 µg iodine, as recommended by the American Thyroid Association,[13] will help to ensure that US pregnant and breast-feeding women consume sufficient iodine during these critical periods.

Because iodine deficiency results in increased iodine trapping by the thyroid, iodine-deficient individuals of all ages are more susceptible to radiation-induced thyroid cancer as well as to iodine-induced hyperthyroidism.[1]

Nutrient Interactions

Selenium deficiency can exacerbate the effects of iodine deficiency. Iodine is essential for the synthesis of thyroid hormone, but selenium-dependent enzymes (iodothyronine deiodinases) are also required for the conversion of T_4 to the biologically active thyroid hormone, T_3.[6,8] In addition, deficiencies of vitamin A or iron may exacerbate the effects of iodine deficiency.[6,14]

Goitrogens

Some foods contain substances that interfere with iodine utilization or thyroid hormone production; these substances are called *goitrogens*. The occurrence of goiter in the Democratic Republic of Congo has been related to the consumption of cassava, which contains a compound that is metabolized to thiocyanate and blocks thyroi-

Table 18.1 Recommended dietary allowance for iodine

Life stage	Age	Males (µg/day)	Females (µg/day)
Infants	0–6 months	110 (AI)	110 (AI)
Infants	7–12 months	130 (AI)	130 (AI)
Children	1–3 years	90	90
Children	4–8 years	90	90
Children	9–13 years	120	120
Adolescents	14–18 years	150	150
Adults	≥19 years	150	150
Pregnancy	All ages	–	220
Breast-feeding	All ages	–	290

AI, adequate intake.

dal uptake of iodine. Some species of millet and cruciferous vegetables (e.g., cabbage, broccoli, cauliflower, and Brussels sprouts) also contain goitrogens. Further, the soybean isoflavones, genistein and daidzein, have been found to inhibit thyroid hormone synthesis.[15] Most of these goitrogens are not of clinical importance unless they are consumed in large amounts or there is coexisting iodine deficiency. Tobacco smoking may be associated with an increased risk of goiter in iodine-deficient areas.[16]

Individuals at Risk of Iodine Deficiency

Although the risk of iodine deficiency for populations living in iodine-deficient areas without adequate iodine fortification programs is well recognized, concerns have been raised that certain subpopulations may not consume adequate iodine in countries considered to be iodine sufficient. Vegetarian and nonvegetarian diets that exclude iodized salt, fish, and seaweed have been found to contain very little iodine.[1,6,17,18] Urinary iodine excretion studies suggest that iodine intakes have declined in Switzerland,[19] New Zealand,[20] and the United States,[21] possibly due to increased adherence to dietary recommendations to reduce salt intake. However, data from the latest US assessment, the National Health and Nutrition Examination Survey 2003–2004, indicate that iodine intake has stabilized,[22] and the United States is currently considered to be iodine sufficient. Also, a recent study found that the iodine status of children and pregnant women in Switzerland improved after a mandated increase in iodine concentration of iodized salt in 1998.[19] Switzerland is now considered to be iodine sufficient.[23]

Recommended Dietary Allowance

The recommended dietary allowance (RDA) for iodine was re-evaluated by the Food and Nutrition Board (FNB) of the Institute of Medicine in 2001 (see **Table 18.1**). The recommended amounts were calculated using several methods, including the measurement of iodine accumulation in the thyroid glands of individuals with normal thyroid function.[6] These recommendations are in agreement with those of the International Council for the Control of Iodine Deficiency Disorders, the WHO, and UNICEF.[2]

Disease Prevention

Radiation-induced Thyroid Cancer

Radioactive iodine, especially ^{131}I, may be released into the environment as a result of nuclear reactor accidents. Thyroid accumulation of radioactive iodine increases the risk of developing thyroid cancer, especially in children. The increased iodine trapping activity of the thyroid gland in iodine deficiency results in increased thyroid accumulation of ^{131}I. Thus, iodine-deficient individuals are at increased risk of developing radiation-induced thyroid cancer because they will accumulate greater amounts of radioactive iodine. Potassium iodide administered in pharmacological doses (50–100 mg for adults) within 48 hours before or 8 hours after radiation exposure from a nuclear reactor accident can significantly reduce thyroid uptake of ^{131}I and decrease the risk of radiation-induced thyroid cancer.[24] The prompt and widespread use of potassium iodide prophylaxis in Poland after the 1986 Chernobyl nuclear reactor accident may explain the lack of a significant increase in childhood thyroid cancer in Poland compared with fallout areas where potassium iodide prophylaxis was not widely used.[25] In the United States, the Nuclear Regulatory Commission requires that consideration be given to potassium iodide as a protective measure for the general public in the case of a major release of radioactivity from a nuclear power plant.[26]

Disease Treatment

Fibrocystic Breast Condition

Fibrocystic breast condition is a benign (noncancerous) condition of the breasts, characterized by lumpiness and discomfort in one or both breasts. In estrogen-treated rats, iodine deficiency leads to changes similar to those seen in fibrocystic breast condition, whereas iodine repletion reverses those changes.[27] An uncontrolled study of 233 women with fibrocystic breast condition found that treatment with aqueous molecular iodine (I_2) at a dose of 0.08 mg I_2/kg body weight daily over 6–18 months was associated with improvement in pain and other symptoms in over 70% of those treated.[28] About 10% of the study participants reported side effects that were described by the investigators as minor. A double-blind, placebo-controlled trial of aqueous I_2 (0.07–0.09 mg I_2/kg body weight daily for 6 months) in 56 women with fibrocystic breast condition found that 65% of the women taking I_2 reported improvement compared with 33% of those taking the placebo.[28] More recently, a double-blind, placebo-controlled, clinical trial in 111 women with documented breast pain reported that I_2 (3 or 6 mg/day) for 5 months improved overall pain.[29] In this study, more than half the women receiving the highest dosage of I_2 reported a reduction of 50% or more in self-assessed breast pain compared with 8.3% in those receiving placebo. Large-scale, controlled clinical trials are needed to determine the therapeutic value of I_2 in fibrocystic breast condition. The doses of iodine used in these studies (3–7 mg/day for a 60-kg person) are several times higher than the tolerable upper intake level (UL) recommended by the FNB and should be used only under medical supervision.

Table 18.2 Food sources of iodine

Food	Serving	Iodine (µg)
Cod	3 ounces[a]	99
Salt (iodized)	1 gram	77
Potato with peel, baked	1 medium	60
Milk (cow's)	1 cup (8 fluid ounces)	56
Shrimp	3 ounces	35
Fish sticks	2 fish sticks	35
Turkey breast, baked	3 ounces	34
Navy beans, cooked	½ cup	32
Tuna, canned in oil	3 ounces (½ can)	17
Egg, boiled	1 large	12
Seaweed	¼ ounce, dried	Variable; may be > 4500 µg (4.5 mg)

[a]A three-ounce serving of meat or seafood is about the size of a deck of cards.

Sources

Food Sources

The iodine content of most foods depends on the iodine content of the soil. Seafood is rich in iodine because marine animals can concentrate the iodine from seawater. Certain types of seaweed (e.g., wakame) are also very rich in iodine. Processed foods may contain slightly higher levels of iodine due to the addition of iodized salt or food additives, such as calcium and potassium iodate. Dairy products are relatively good sources of iodine because iodine is commonly added to animal feed in the United States. In the United Kingdom and northern Europe, iodine levels in dairy products tend to be lower in summer when cattle are allowed to graze in pastures with low soil iodine content.[6] **Table 18.2** lists the iodine content of some iodine-rich foods. Because the iodine content of foods can vary considerably, these values should be considered approximate.[30]

Supplements

Potassium iodide is available as a nutritional supplement, typically in combination products, such as multivitamin/mineral supplements. Iodine makes up approximately 77% of the total weight of potassium iodide.[15] A multivitamin/mineral supplement that contains 100% of the daily value for iodine provides 150 µg iodine. Although most people in the United States consume sufficient iodine in their diets from iodized salt and food additives, an additional 150 µg/day is unlikely to result in excessive iodine intake.

Potassium iodide as well as potassium iodate may be used to iodize salt. In the United States and Canada, iodized salt contains 77 µg iodine/g salt. In other countries, salt commonly contains 20–40 µg iodine/g salt; the iodization level depends on variables such as iodine intake from other sources and daily salt consumption. Annual doses of iodized vegetable oil are also used in some countries as an iodine source.[2,15]

Safety

Acute Toxicity

Acute iodine poisoning is rare and usually occurs only with doses of many grams. Symptoms of acute iodine poisoning include burning of the mouth, throat, and stomach; fever; nausea; vomiting; diarrhea; a weak pulse; and coma.[6]

Iodine Excess

It is rare for diets of natural foods to supply more than 2000 µg iodine/day, and most diets supply less than 1000 µg iodine/day. People living in the northern coastal regions of Japan, whose diets contain large amounts of seaweed, have been found to have iodine intakes ranging from 50 000 µg to 80 000 µg (50–80 mg) iodine/day.[1]

Iodine deficiency. Iodine supplementation programs in iodine-deficient populations have been associated with an increased incidence of iodine-induced hyperthyroidism (IHH), mainly in older people and those with multinodular goiter. Iodine intakes of 150–200 µg/day have been found to increase the incidence of IHH in iodine-deficient populations. Iodine deficiency increases the risk of developing autonomous thyroid nodules that are unresponsive to the normal thyroid regulation system, resulting in hyperthyroidism after iodine supplementation. IHH is considered by some experts to be an iodine deficiency disorder. In general, the large benefit of iodization programs outweighs the small risk of IHH in iodine-deficient populations.[1,31]

Iodine sufficiency. In iodine-sufficient populations (e.g., the United States), excess iodine intake is most commonly associated with elevated blood levels of TSH, hypothyroidism, and goiter. Although a slightly elevated TSH level does not necessarily indicate inadequate thyroid hormone production, it is the earliest sign of abnormal thyroid function when iodine intake is excessive. In iodine-sufficient adults, elevated TSH levels have been found at iodine intakes between 1700 and 1800 µg/day. In order to minimize the risk of developing hypothyroidism, the FNB set a UL for iodine at 1100 µg/day for adults. Very high (pharmacological) doses of iodine may also produce thyroid enlargement (goiter) due to increased TSH stimulation of the thyroid gland. Prolonged intakes of more than 18 000 µg/day (18 mg/day) have been found to increase the incidence of goiter. The UL values for iodine are listed by life stage in **Table 18.3**. The UL is not meant to apply to individuals who are being treated with iodine under medical supervision.[6]

Table 18.3 Tolerable upper intake level (UL) for iodine

Life stage	Age	UL (µg/day)
Infants	0–12 months	Not possible to establish[a]
Children	1–3 years	200
Children	4–8 years	300
Children	9–13 years	600
Adolescents	14–18 years	900
Adults	≥19 years	1100

[a]Source of intake should be from food and formula only.

Individuals with increased sensitivity to excess iodine intake. Individuals with iodine deficiency, nodular goiter, or autoimmune thyroid disease may be sensitive to intake levels considered safe for the general population and may not be protected by the UL for iodine intake.[6] Children with cystic fibrosis may also be more sensitive to the adverse effects of excess iodine.[32]

Excess iodine and thyroid cancer. Observational studies have found increased iodine intake to be associated with an increased incidence of thyroid papillary cancer. The reasons for this association are not clear. In populations that were previously iodine deficient, salt iodization programs have resulted in relative increases in thyroid papillary cancers and relative decreases in thyroid follicular cancers. In general, thyroid papillary cancers are less aggressive and have a better prognosis than thyroid follicular cancers.[33]

Drug Interactions

Amiodarone, a medication used to prevent abnormal heart rhythms, contains high levels of iodine and may affect thyroid function. Medications used to treat hyperthyroidism, such as propylthiouracil and methimazole, may increase the risk of hypothyroidism. In addition, the use of lithium in combination with pharmacological doses of potassium iodide may result in hypothyroidism. Further, the use of pharmacological doses of potassium iodide may decrease the anticoagulant effect of warfarin.[6,32]

LPI Recommendation

The RDA for iodine is sufficient to ensure normal thyroid function. There is currently no evidence that iodine intakes higher than the RDA are beneficial. Most people in the United States consume more than sufficient iodine in their diets, making supplementation unnecessary. Given the importance of sufficient iodine during fetal development and infancy, pregnant and breastfeeding women should consider taking a supplement that provides 150 μg/day of iodine.

Older Adults

As aging has not been associated with significant changes in the requirement for iodine, our recommendation for iodine intake is no different for older adults.

References

1. Hetzel BS, Clugston GA. Iodine. In: Shils M, Olson JA, Shike M, Ross AC, eds. Modern Nutrition in Health and Disease. 9th ed. Baltimore, MD: Lippincott Williams & Wilkins; 1999:253–264
2. Dunn JT. What's happening to our iodine? J Clin Endocrinol Metab 1998;83(10):3398–3400
3. Larsen PR, Davies TF, Hay ID. The thyroid gland. In: Wilson JD, Foster DW, Kronenberg HM, Larsen PR, eds. Williams Textbook of Endocrinology. 9th ed. Philadelphia, PA: WB Saunders Co.; 1998:389–515
4. World Health Organization, Unicef, ICCIDD. Assessment of iodine deficiency disorders and monitoring their elimination: a guide for programme managers. 3rd ed: World Health Organization; 2007. Available at: http://whqlibdoc.who.int/publications/2007/9789241595827-eng.pdf
5. de Benoist B, McLean E, Andersson M, Rogers L. Iodine deficiency in 2007: global progress since 2003. Food Nutr Bull 2008;29(3):195–202
6. Food and Nutrition Board, Institute of Medicine. Iodine. In: Dietary Reference Intakes for Vitamin A, Vitamin K, Boron, Chromium, Copper, Iodine, Iron, Manganese, Molybdenum, Nickel, Silicon, Vanadium, and Zinc. Washington, DC: National Academy Press; 2001:258–289
7. United Nations Children's Fund. The State of the World's Children 2007. New York: Unicef; 2006: 109
8. Levander OA, Whanger PD. Deliberations and evaluations of the approaches, endpoints and paradigms for selenium and iodine dietary recommendations. J Nutr 1996; 126(9, Suppl):2427S–2434S
9. DeLong GR, Leslie PW, Wang SH, et al. Effect on infant mortality of iodination of irrigation water in a severely iodine-deficient area of China. Lancet 1997;350(9080):771–773
10. Hetzel BS. Iodine and neuropsychological development. J Nutr 2000; 130(2S, Suppl):493S–495S
11. Tiwari BD, Godbole MM, Chattopadhyay N, Mandal A, Mithal A. Learning disabilities and poor motivation to achieve due to prolonged iodine deficiency. Am J Clin Nutr 1996;63(5):782–786
12. Bleichrodt N, Shrestha RM, West CE, Hautvast JG, van de Vijver FJ, Born MP. The benefits of adequate iodine intake. Nutr Rev 1996;54(4 Pt 2):S 72–S 78
13. Becker DV, Braverman LE, Delange F, et al; Public Health Committee of the American Thyroid Association. Iodine supplementation for pregnancy and lactation-United States and Canada: recommendations of the American Thyroid Association. Thyroid 2006;16(10):949–951
14. Zimmermann MB, Jooste PL, Pandav CS. Iodine-deficiency disorders. Lancet 2008;372(9645):1251–1262
15. Hendler SS, Rorvik DM, eds. PDR for Nutritional Supplements, 2nd ed. Montvale, NJ: Thomson Reuters; 2008
16. Knudsen N, Bülow I, Laurberg P, Ovesen L, Perrild H, Jørgensen T. Association of tobacco smoking with goiter in a low-iodine-intake area. Arch Intern Med 2002;162(4):439–443
17. Remer T, Neubert A, Manz F. Increased risk of iodine deficiency with vegetarian nutrition. Br J Nutr 1999;81(1):45–49
18. Davidsson L. Are vegetarians an 'at risk group' for iodine deficiency? Br J Nutr 1999;81(1):3–4
19. Zimmermann MB, Aeberli I, Torresani T, Bürgi H. Increasing the iodine concentration in the Swiss iodized salt program markedly improved iodine status in pregnant women and children: a 5-y prospective national study. Am J Clin Nutr 2005;82(2):388–392
20. Thomson CD, Woodruffe S, Colls A, Doyle TD. Urinary iodine and thyroid status of New Zealand residents. In: Roussel AM, Anderson RA, Favier A, eds. Trace Elements in Man and Animals. Vol 10. New York: Kluwer Academic Press; 2000:343–344
21. Hollowell JG, Staehling NW, Hannon WH, et al. Iodine nutrition in the United States. Trends and public health implications: iodine excretion data from National Health and Nutrition Examination Surveys I and III (1971–1974 and 1988–1994). J Clin Endocrinol Metab 1998;83(10):3401–3408
22. Caldwell KL, Miller GA, Wang RY, Jain RB, Jones RL. Iodine status of the U.S. population, National Health and Nutrition Examination Survey 2003–2004. Thyroid 2008;18(11):1207–1214
23. Iodine level, United States, 2000, CDC. National Center for Health Statistics. Available at: http://www.cdc.gov/nchs/data/hestat/iodine.htm Accessed 4 Jan 2011
24. Zanzonico PB, Becker DV. Effects of time of administration and dietary iodine levels on potassium iodide (KI) blockade of thyroid irradiation by 131I from radioactive fallout. Health Phys 2000;78(6):660–667
25. Nauman J, Wolff J. Iodide prophylaxis in Poland after the Chernobyl reactor accident: benefits and risks. Am J Med 1993;94(5):524–532
26. Nuclear Regulatory Commission. Consideration of potassium iodide in emergency plans. Nuclear Regulatory Commission. Final rule. Fed Regist 2001; 66(13):5427–5440
27. Eskin BA, Grotkowski CE, Connolly CP, Ghent WR. Different tissue responses for iodine and iodide in rat thyroid and mammary glands. Biol Trace Elem Res 1995;49(1):9–19
28. Ghent WR, Eskin BA, Low DA, Hill LP. Iodine replacement in fibrocystic disease of the breast. Can J Surg 1993;36(5):453–460
29. Kessler JH. The effect of supraphysiologic levels of iodine on patients with cyclic mastalgia. Breast J 2004;10(4):328–336
30. Pennington JAT, Schoen SA, Salmon GD, Young B, Johnson RD, Marts RW. Composition of core foods of the U.S. food supply, 1982–1991. III. Copper, manga-

nese, selenium and iodine. J Food Compost Anal 1995;8:171–217

31. Delange F. Risks and benefits of iodine supplementation. Lancet 1998;351(9107):923–924

32. Hendler SS, Rorvik DR, eds. PDR for Nutritional Supplements. Montvale, NJ: Medical Economics Co., Inc.; 2001

33. Feldt-Rasmussen U. Iodine and cancer. Thyroid 2001;11(5):483–486

19 Iron

Iron has the longest and best described history of all the micronutrients. It is a key element in the metabolism of almost all living organisms. In humans, iron is an essential component of hundreds of proteins and enzymes.[1,2]

Function

Oxygen Transport and Storage

Heme is an iron-containing compound found in a number of biologically important molecules. Hemoglobin and myoglobin are heme-containing proteins involved in the transport and storage of oxygen. Hemoglobin is the primary protein found in red blood cells and represents about two-thirds of the body's iron. The vital role of hemoglobin in transporting oxygen from the lungs to the rest of the body is derived from its unique ability to acquire oxygen rapidly during the short time that it spends in contact with the lungs and to release oxygen as needed during its circulation through the tissues. Myoglobin functions in the transport and short-term storage of oxygen in muscle cells, helping to match the supply of oxygen to the demand of working muscles.[3,4]

Electron Transport and Energy Metabolism

Cytochromes are heme-containing compounds that have important roles in mitochondrial electron transport, so cytochromes are critical to cellular energy production and thus life. They serve as electron carriers during the synthesis of ATP, the primary energy storage compound in cells. Cytochrome P450 is a family of enzymes that functions in the metabolism of a number of important biological molecules, as well as the detoxification and metabolism of drugs and pollutants. Nonheme iron-containing enzymes, such as NADH dehydrogenase and succinate dehydrogenase, are also critical to energy metabolism.[3]

Antioxidant and Beneficial Prooxidant Functions

Catalase and peroxidases are heme-containing enzymes that protect cells against the accumulation of hydrogen peroxide, a potentially damaging reactive oxygen species (ROS), by catalyzing a reaction that converts hydrogen peroxide to water and oxygen. As part of the immune response, some white blood cells engulf bacteria and expose them to ROS in order to kill them. The synthesis of one such ROS, hypochlorous acid, by neutrophils is catalyzed by the heme-containing enzyme myeloperoxidase.[3,4]

Oxygen Sensing

Inadequate oxygen (hypoxia), such as that experienced by those who live at high altitudes or have chronic lung disease, induces compensatory physiological responses, including increased red blood cell formation, increased blood vessel growth (angiogenesis), and increased production of enzymes utilized in anaerobic metabolism. Under hypoxic conditions, transcription factors known as *hypoxia inducible factors* (HIFs) bind to response elements in genes that encode various proteins involved in compensatory responses to hypoxia and increase their synthesis. Recent research indicates that an iron-dependent enzyme, prolyl hydroxylase, plays a critical role in regulating HIFs and, consequently, physiological responses to hypoxia. When cellular oxygen tension is adequate, newly synthesized HIF-1α subunits are modified by prolyl hydroxylase in an iron-dependent process that targets HIF-1α for rapid degradation. When cellular oxygen tension drops below a critical threshold, prolyl hydroxylase can no longer target HIF-1α for degradation, allowing HIF-1α to bind to HIF-1β and form an active transcription factor that is able to enter the nucleus and bind to specific response elements on genes.[5,6]

DNA Synthesis

Ribonucleotide reductase is an iron-dependent enzyme that is required for DNA synthesis.[2,7] Thus, iron is required for a number of vital functions, including growth, reproduction, healing, and immune function.

Regulation of Intracellular Iron

Iron response elements are short sequences of nucleotides found in the messenger RNA (mRNA) that code for key proteins in the regulation of iron storage and metabolism. Iron regulatory proteins (IRPs) can bind to iron response elements and affect mRNA translation and stability, thereby regulating the synthesis of specific proteins, such as the iron storage protein ferritin and the transferrin receptor, which is important in maintaining iron homeostasis inside the cell. It has been proposed that, when the iron supply is high, more iron binds to IRPs, thereby preventing them from binding to iron response elements on mRNA. For the ferritin mRNA, this allows for increased translation, thereby promoting iron storage. In the case of the transferrin receptor mRNA, the message is destabilized and becomes degraded to reduce the amount of iron uptake. When the iron supply is low, less iron binds to IRPs, allowing increased binding of IRPs to iron response elements. Thus, when less iron is available, translation of mRNA that codes for ferritin is reduced because iron is not available for storage. Translation of the mRNA that codes for the key regulatory enzyme of heme synthesis in immature red blood cells is also reduced to conserve iron. In contrast, IRP binding to iron response elements in the mRNA that codes for transferrin receptors inhibits mRNA degradation, resulting in increased synthesis of transferrin receptors and increased iron transport to cells.[4,8]

Systemic Regulation of Iron Homeostasis

Although iron is an essential mineral, it is potentially toxic because free iron inside the cell can lead to the generation of free radicals that cause oxidative stress and cellular damage. Thus, it is important for the body to systemically regulate iron homeostasis. The body tightly regulates the transport of iron throughout various body compartments, such as developing red blood cells, circulating macrophages, liver cells that store iron, and other tissues.[9] As mentioned above, intracellular iron levels are regulated according to the body's iron needs, but systemic signals also regulate iron homeostasis in the body. Hepcidin, a peptide hormone synthesized by liver cells, is a key regulator of systemic iron homeostasis. Hepcidin functions to inhibit the release of iron from certain cells, such as enterocytes and macrophages, into plasma.[10] Thus, hepcidin expression is increased when iron requirements are high and decreased when they are low (i.e., when there are sufficient iron stores). Studies in mice have shown that a lack of hepcidin expression is associated with conditions of iron overload,[11] whereas an overexpression of hepcidin is associated with iron-deficiency anemia.[12] Hepcidin expression is in turn regulated by a number of proteins, such as the negative regulator, TMPRSS 6 (transmembrane protease serine 6), and various positive regulators, including transferrin receptor 2, hemojuvelin, and bone morphogenetic proteins.[13]

Nutrient Interactions

Vitamin A. Vitamin A deficiency may exacerbate iron-deficiency anemia. Vitamin A supplementation has been shown to have beneficial effects on iron-deficiency anemia and improve iron status among children and pregnant women. The combination of vitamin A and iron seems to ameliorate anemia more effectively than either iron or vitamin A alone.[14]

Copper. Adequate copper nutritional status appears to be necessary for normal iron metabolism and red blood cell formation. Anemia is a clinical sign of copper deficiency. Animal studies demonstrate a role for copper in iron absorption,[15] and iron has been found to accumulate in the livers of copper-deficient animals, indicating that copper is required for iron transport to the bone marrow for red blood cell formation.[16]

Zinc. High doses of iron supplements taken together with zinc supplements on an empty stomach can inhibit the absorption of zinc. When taken with food, supplemental iron does not appear to inhibit zinc absorption. Iron-fortified foods have no effect on zinc absorption.[17,18]

Calcium. When consumed together in a single meal, calcium has been found to decrease the absorption of heme and nonheme iron.[17] Thus, calcium and iron supplements should not be taken together.

Deficiency

Iron deficiency is the most common nutrient deficiency in the United States and the world. Three levels of iron deficiency are generally identified and are listed below from least to most severe:[3]

1. *Storage iron depletion.* Iron stores are depleted, but the functional iron supply is not limited.
2. *Early functional iron deficiency.* The supply of functional iron is low enough to impair red blood cell formation but not low enough to cause measurable anemia.
3. *Iron-deficiency anemia.* Iron-deficiency anemia results when there is inadequate iron to support normal red blood cell formation. The anemia of iron deficiency is characterized as microcytic and hypochromic, meaning that red blood cells are measurably smaller than normal and their hemoglobin content is decreased. At this stage of iron deficiency, symptoms may be a result of inadequate oxygen delivery due to anemia and/or suboptimal function of iron-dependent enzymes. Low red cell count, low hematocrit, and low hemoglobin concentrations are all used in the clinical diagnosis of iron-deficiency anemia. It is important to remember that iron deficiency is not the only cause of anemia, and that the diagnosis or treatment of iron deficiency solely on the basis of anemia may lead to misdiagnosis or inappropriate treatment of the underlying cause.[19]

Symptoms of Iron Deficiency

Most of the symptoms of iron deficiency are a result of the associated anemia and may include fatigue, rapid heart rate, palpitations, and rapid breathing on exertion. Iron deficiency impairs athletic performance and physical work capacity in several ways. In iron-deficiency anemia, the reduced hemoglobin content of red blood cells results in decreased oxygen delivery to active tissues. Decreased myoglobin levels in muscle cells limit the amount of oxygen that can be delivered to mitochondria for oxidative metabolism. Iron depletion also decreases the oxidative capacity of muscle by diminishing the mitochondrial content of cytochromes and other iron-dependent enzymes required for electron transport and ATP synthesis. Lactic acid production is also increased in iron deficiency.[20] The ability to maintain a normal body temperature on exposure to cold is also impaired in iron-deficient individuals. Severe iron-deficiency anemia may result in brittle and spoon-shaped nails, sores at the corners of the mouth, taste bud atrophy, and a sore tongue. In some cases, advanced iron-deficiency anemia may cause difficulty in swallowing due to the formation of webs of tissue in the throat and esophagus. The development of esophageal webs, also known as Plummer–Vinson syndrome, may require a genetic predisposition in addition to iron deficiency. Further, pica, a behavioral disturbance characterized by the consumption of nonfood items, may be a symptom and a cause of iron deficiency.[19]

Individuals at Increased Risk of Iron Deficiency

Infants and children between the ages of 6 months and 4 years. A full-term infant's iron stores are usually sufficient to last for 6 months. High iron requirements are due to the rapid growth rates sustained during this period.[4]

Adolescents. Early adolescence is another period of rapid growth. In girls, the blood loss that occurs with menstruation adds to the increased iron requirement of adolescence.[4]

Pregnant women. The iron requirement is significantly increased during pregnancy due to increased iron utilization by the developing fetus and placenta, as well as blood volume expansion.[4]

Individuals with chronic blood loss. Chronic bleeding or acute blood loss may result in iron deficiency. One milliliter of blood with a hemoglobin concentration of 150 g/L contains 0.5 mg iron. Thus, chronic loss of very small amounts of blood may result in iron deficiency. A common cause of chronic blood loss and iron deficiency in developing countries is intestinal parasitic infection. Individuals who donate blood frequently, especially menstruating women, may need to increase their iron intake to prevent deficiency because each 500 mL blood donated contains between 200 and 250 mg iron.[7]

Individuals with celiac disease. Celiac disease (celiac sprue) is an autoimmune disorder estimated to occur in 1% of the population. When people with celiac disease consume food or products that contain gluten, the immune system response damages the intestinal villi, which may result in nutrient malabsorption and iron-deficiency anemia.[21]

Individuals with *Helicobacter pylori* infection. *H. pylori* infection is associated with iron-deficiency anemia, especially in children, even in the absence of gastrointestinal bleeding.[22]

Individuals who have had gastric bypass surgery. Some types of gastric bypass (bariatric) surgery increase the risk of iron deficiency by causing malabsorption of iron, among other nutrients.[23]

Vegetarians. As iron from plants is less efficiently absorbed than that from animal sources, the US Food and Nutrition Board (FNB) of the Institute of Medicine has estimated that the bioavailability of iron from a vegetarian diet is only 10%, whereas it is 18% from a mixed diet. Therefore, the recommended dietary allowance (RDA) for iron from a completely vegetarian diet should be adjusted as follows: 14 mg/day for men and postmenopausal women, 33 mg/day for premenopausal women, and 26 mg/day for adolescent girls.[17]

Individuals who engage in regular, intense exercise. Daily iron losses have been found to be greater in athletes involved in intense endurance training. This may be due to increased microscopic bleeding from the gastrointestinal tract or increased fragility and hemolysis of red blood cells. The FNB estimates that the average requirement for iron may be 30% higher for those who engage in regular intense exercise.[17]

Recommended Dietary Allowance

The RDA for iron was revised in 2001 and is based on the prevention of iron deficiency and maintenance of adequate iron stores in individuals eating a mixed diet (**Table 19.1**).[17]

Table 19.1 Recommended dietary allowance for iron

Life stage	Age	Males (mg/day)	Females (mg/day)
Infants	0–6 months	0.27 (AI)	0.27 (AI)
Infants	7–12 months	11	11
Children	1–3 years	7	7
Children	4–8 years	10	10
Children	9–13 years	8	8
Adolescents	14–18 years	11	15
Adults	19–50 years	8	18
Adults	≥51 years	8	8
Pregnancy	All ages	–	27
Breast-feeding	≤18 years	–	10
Breast-feeding	≥19 years	–	9

AI, adequate intake.

Disease Prevention

The following health problems and diseases may be prevented through the treatment or prevention of iron deficiency.

Impaired Intellectual Development in Children

Most observational studies have found relationships between iron-deficiency anemia in children and poor cognitive development, poor school achievement, and behavioral problems. However, it is difficult to separate the effects of iron-deficiency anemia from those of other types of deprivation in such studies, and confounding factors may contribute to the association between iron deficiency and cognitive deficits.[24] In anemic children under the age of 2 years, only one randomized, double-blind trial found a significant benefit of iron supplementation on indices of cognitive development. However, four randomized controlled trials found a significant benefit of iron supplementation on cognition and school achievement in children aged over 2 years, while two studies found no effect. Thus, studies to date indicate improvements in cognitive performance in children aged over 2 years, but children younger than 2 years appear more resistant to such improvements.[25]

A recent systematic review of 17 randomized controlled trials concluded that iron supplementation modestly improves scores of mental development in children aged over 7 years but has no effect on mental development of children under the age of 27 months.[26] Several possible mechanisms link iron-deficiency anemia to altered cognition. Anemic children tend to move around and explore their environment less than children without anemia, which may lead to developmental delays.[27] Conduction of auditory and optic nerve impulses to the brain has been found to be slower in children with iron-deficiency anemia. This effect could be associated with changes in nerve myelination, which have been observed in iron-deficient animals.[28] Neurotransmitter synthesis may also be sensitive to iron deficiency.[20]

Lead Toxicity

Iron deficiency may increase the risk of lead poisoning in children. A number of epidemiological studies have found iron deficiency to be associated with increased blood lead levels in young children. Iron deficiency and lead poisoning share a number of the same risk factors, but iron deficiency has been found to increase the intestinal absorption of lead in humans and animals. However, the use of iron supplementation in lead poisoning should be reserved for those individuals who are truly iron deficient or for those with continuing lead exposure, such as continued residence in lead-exposed housing.[3,29]

Pregnancy Complications

Epidemiological studies provide strong evidence of an association between severe anemia in pregnant women and adverse pregnancy outcomes, such as low birth weight, premature birth, and maternal mortality. Iron deficiency can be a major contributory factor to severe anemia, but evidence that iron-deficiency anemia is a causal factor in poor pregnancy outcomes is still lacking.[30,31] Nevertheless, most experts consider the control of maternal anemia to be an important part of prenatal health care. Elevated hemoglobin, especially in later pregnancy, is also associated with poor pregnancy outcomes, but there is no evidence that this association is related to high iron intakes or iron supplementation. Rather, elevated hemoglobin in pregnancy is more likely to be explained by underlying conditions such as pregnancy-induced hypertension or pre-eclampsia, which are well known to contribute to poor pregnancy outcomes.[31]

Impaired Immune Function

Iron is required by most infectious agents, as well as by the infected host in order to mount an effective immune response. Sufficient iron is critical to several immune functions, including the differentiation and proliferation of T lymphocytes and the generation of ROS by iron-dependent enzymes, which are used for killing pathogens. During an acute inflammatory response, serum iron levels decrease whereas levels of ferritin (the iron storage protein) increase, suggesting that sequestering iron from pathogens is an important host response to infection.[20,32] Despite the critical functions of iron in the immune response, the nature of the relationship between iron deficiency and susceptibility to infection, especially with respect to malaria, remains controversial. High-dose iron supplementation of children living in the tropics has been associated with increased risk of clinical malaria and other infections, such as pneumonia. Studies in cell culture and laboratory animals suggest that the survival of infectious agents that spend part of their life cycle within host cells, such as plasmodia (malaria) and mycobacteria (tuberculosis), may be enhanced by iron therapy. Controlled clinical studies are needed to determine the appropriate use of iron supplementation in regions where malaria is common, as well as in the presence of infectious diseases, such as HIV, tuberculosis, and typhoid.[33]

Disease Treatment

Restless Legs Syndrome

Restless legs syndrome (RLS) is a neurological movement disorder that is often associated with sleep problems. People with RLS experience unpleasant sensations resulting in an irresistible urge to move their legs. These sensations are more common at rest and often interfere with sleep.[34] RLS occurs in some people with iron deficiency, and some RLS patients benefit from iron supplementation. One study found that ferritin levels were lower and transferrin levels higher in the cerebrospinal fluid of individuals with RLS compared with control individuals, suggesting that low iron concentrations in the brain may play a role in RLS.[35] Magnetic resonance imaging (MRI) measurements of brain iron concentrations also indicate that iron insufficiency in certain regions of the brain may occur in patients with RLS.[36] The mechanism by which low iron concentration in the brain contributes to RLS is not known, but may be related to the fact that the activity of an iron-dependent enzyme (tyrosine hydroxylase) is a limiting factor in the synthesis of the neurotransmitter, dopamine.

Sources

Food Sources

The amount of iron in food (or supplements) that is absorbed and used by the body is influenced by the iron nutritional status of the individual and whether or not the iron is in the form of heme. Because heme iron is absorbed by a different mechanism from nonheme iron, it is more readily absorbed and its absorption is less affected by other dietary factors. Individuals who are anemic or iron deficient absorb a larger percentage of the iron that they consume (especially nonheme iron) than individuals who are not anemic and have sufficient iron stores.[3,18]

Heme iron. Heme iron comes mainly from hemoglobin and myoglobin in meat, poultry, and fish. Although heme iron accounts for only 10%–15% of the iron found in the diet, it may provide up to one-third of total absorbed dietary iron. The absorption of heme iron is less influenced by other dietary factors than that of nonheme iron.[2,18]

Nonheme iron. Plants, dairy products, meat, and iron salts added to foods and supplements are all sources of nonheme iron. The absorption of nonheme iron is strongly influenced by enhancers and inhibitors present in the same meal (see below).[3,18]

Enhancers of Nonheme Iron Absorption

Vitamin C (ascorbic acid). Vitamin C strongly enhances the absorption of nonheme iron by reducing dietary ferric iron (Fe^{3+}) to ferrous iron (Fe^{2+}) and forming an absorbable, iron–ascorbic acid complex.

Other organic acids. Citric, malic, tartaric, and lactic acids have some enhancing effects on nonheme iron absorption.

Meat, fish, and poultry. Aside from providing highly absorbable heme iron, meat, fish, and poultry also enhance nonheme iron absorption. The mechanism for this enhancement of nonheme iron absorption is not clear.[17,18]

Table 19.2 Food sources of iron

Food	Serving	Iron (mg)
Raisin bran cereal	1 cup, dry	5.79–18.00
Oysters	6 medium	5.04
Black-strap molasses	1 tablespoon	3.50
Lentils	½ cup, cooked	3.30
Beef	3 ounces,[a] cooked	2.32
Prune juice	6 fluid ounces	2.28
Tofu, firm	¼ block (~⅓ cup)	2.15
Kidney beans	½ cup, cooked	1.97
Cashew nuts	1 ounce	1.89
Potato, with skin	1 medium potato, baked	1.87
Shrimp	8 large, cooked	1.36
Tuna, light	3 ounces,[a] canned	1.30
Chicken, dark meat	3 ounces,[a] cooked	1.13
Raisins, seedless	1 small box (1.5 ounces)	0.81
Prunes	~5 prunes (1.7 ounces)	0.45

[a]A three-ounce serving of meat or seafood is about the size of a deck of cards.

Inhibitors of Nonheme Iron Absorption

Phytic acid (phytate). Phytic acid is present in legumes, grains, and rice and inhibits nonheme iron absorption, probably by binding to it. Small amounts of phytic acid (5–10 mg) can reduce nonheme iron absorption by 50%. The absorption of iron from legumes, such as soybeans, black beans, lentils, mung beans, and split peas, has been shown to be as low as 2%.[7,17]

Polyphenols. Polyphenols, found in some fruit, vegetables, coffee, tea, wines, and spices, can markedly inhibit the absorption of nonheme iron. This effect is reduced by the presence of vitamin C.[7,17]

Soy protein. Soy protein, such as that found in tofu, has an inhibitory effect on iron absorption that is independent of its phytic acid content.[17]

Typical Dietary Intake

National surveys in the United States indicate that the average dietary iron intake is 16–18 mg/day in men, 12 mg/day in pre- and postmenopausal women, and about 15 mg/day in pregnant women.[17] Thus, most premenopausal and pregnant women in the United States consume less than the RDA for iron and many men consume more than the RDA. In the United States, most grain products are fortified with iron. The iron content of some relatively iron-rich foods is listed in **Table 19.2**.

Supplements

Iron supplements are indicated for the prevention and treatment of iron deficiency. Individuals who are not at risk of iron deficiency (e.g., men and postmenopausal women) should not take iron supplements without an appropriate medical evaluation. A number of iron supplements are available, and different forms provide different proportions of elemental iron. Ferrous sulfate (heptahydrate) is 22% elemental iron, ferrous sulfate (monohydrate) is 33% elemental iron, ferrous gluconate is 12% elemental iron, and ferrous fumarate is 33% elemental iron.[37] If not stated otherwise, all the iron doses discussed in this chapter represent elemental iron.

Iron Overload

Several genetic disorders may lead to pathological accumulation of iron in the body. Hereditary hemochromatosis results in iron overload despite normal iron intake. Iron overload due to prolonged iron supplementation is very rare in healthy individuals with no genetic predisposition. This fact emphasizes the degree to which the body's tight control of intestinal iron absorption protects it from the adverse effects of iron overload.[7] However, supplementation of individuals who are not iron deficient should be avoided due to the frequency of undetected hereditary hemochromatosis and recent concerns about the more subtle effects of chronic excess iron intake (see "Safety," p. 164).

Hereditary Hemochromatosis

Hereditary hemochromatosis (HH) refers to genetic disorders of iron metabolism that result in tissue iron overload. If untreated, iron accumulation in the liver and other tissues may lead to cirrhosis of the liver, diabetes, heart muscle damage (cardiomyopathy), or joint problems.[38] There are four main types of HH, which are classified according to the specific gene that is mutated. The most common type of HH, called type 1 or *HFE*-related HH, results from mutations in the *HFE* gene; this mutation was identified in 1996.[39,40] At present, the exact role of the protein encoded by the *HFE* gene is not well understood, but the protein is thought to play a role in regulating intestinal absorption of dietary iron and with sensing the body's iron stores.[41] HH type 2, also referred to as juvenile hemochromatosis (disease onset typically occurs before age 30), results from mutations in genes that encode one of two proteins, hemojuvelin or hepcidin.[42] HH type 3 results from mutations in the transferrin receptor 2 gene, and HH type 4 results from mutations in the gene encoding ferroportin, a protein important in the export of iron from cells.[40]

Iron overload in HH is treated by phlebotomy, the removal of 500 mL blood at a time, at intervals determined by the severity of the iron overload. Individuals with HH are advised to avoid supplemental iron, but are not generally advised to avoid iron-rich foods. Alcohol consumption is strongly discouraged due to the increased risk of cirrhosis of the liver.[7] Genetic testing, which requires a blood sample, is available for those who may be at risk for HH, for example, individuals with a family history of hemochromatosis.

Hereditary Anemias

Iron overload may occur in individuals with severe hereditary anemias that are not caused by iron deficiency. Excessive dietary absorption of iron may occur in response to the body's continued efforts to form red blood cells. Anemic patients at risk of iron overload include those with sideroblastic anemia, pyruvate kinase deficiency, and thalassemia major, especially when they are treated with numerous transfusions. Patients with hereditary spherocytosis and thalassemia minor do not usually develop iron overload unless they are misdiagnosed as having iron deficiency and treated with large doses of iron over many years.[7] The thalassemias (major and minor) are common in individuals of Mediterranean descent. It has been hypothesized that a Mediterranean form of iron overload, distinct from HH, also exists.[43]

Safety

Toxicity

Overdose. Accidental overdose of iron-containing products is the single largest cause of poisoning fatalities in children aged under 6 years. Although the oral lethal dose of elemental iron is approximately 200–250 mg/kg body weight, considerably less has been fatal. Symptoms of acute toxicity may occur with iron doses of 20–60 mg/kg body weight. Iron overdose is an emergency situation because the severity of iron toxicity is related to the amount of elemental iron absorbed. Acute iron poisoning produces symptoms in four stages:

1. Within 1–6 hours of ingestion, symptoms may include nausea, vomiting, abdominal pain, tarry stools, lethargy, weak and rapid pulse, low blood pressure, fever, difficulty breathing, and coma.
2. If not immediately fatal, symptoms may subside for about 24 hours.
3. Symptoms may return 12–48 hours after iron ingestion and include serious signs of failure in the following organ systems: cardiovascu-

lar, kidney, liver, and hematological (blood) systems, and central nervous system (CNS).

4. Long-term damage to the CNS, liver (cirrhosis), and stomach may develop 2–6 weeks after ingestion.[17,37]

Adverse effects. At therapeutic levels for iron deficiency, iron supplements may cause gastrointestinal irritation, nausea, vomiting, diarrhea, or constipation. Stools will often appear darker in color. Iron-containing liquids can temporarily stain teeth, but diluting the liquid helps to prevent this effect. Taking iron supplements with food instead of on an empty stomach may relieve gastrointestinal effects.[37] The FNB based the tolerable upper intake level (UL) for iron on the prevention of gastrointestinal distress (**Table 19.3**). The UL for adolescents and adults over the age of 14 years, including pregnant and breast-feeding women, is 45 mg/day. It should be noted that the UL is not meant to apply to individuals being treated with iron under close medical supervision. Individuals with HH or other conditions of iron overload, as well as individuals with alcoholic cirrhosis and other liver diseases, may experience adverse effects at iron intake levels below the UL.[17]

Diseases Associated with Iron Excess

Cardiovascular diseases. Animal studies suggest a role for iron-induced oxidative stress in the pathology of atherosclerosis and myocardial infarction (heart attack).[44] However, epidemiological studies of iron nutritional status and cardiovascular diseases in humans have yielded conflicting results. A systematic review of 12 prospective cohort studies, including 7800 cases of coronary heart disease (CHD), did not find good evidence to support the existence of strong associations between a number of different measures of iron status and CHD.[45] Serum ferritin concentration is the measure of iron status thought to best reflect

iron stores. However, the same review found no difference in the risk of CHD between individuals with serum ferritin concentrations of 200 µg/L or higher and those with ferritin concentrations of less than 200 µg/L in the five prospective studies that measured serum ferritin. Three large prospective studies found increased dietary heme iron, but not total dietary iron, to be associated with increased risk of either myocardial infarction[46,47] or CHD.[48] When iron stores are high, nonheme iron absorption is inhibited more effectively than heme iron absorption, suggesting that iron from animal sources may play a more important role than total iron intake in CHD risk.[44] Although the relationship between iron stores and CHD requires further clarification, it would be prudent for those who are not at risk of iron deficiency (e.g., men and postmenopausal women) to avoid excess iron intake.

Cancer. A dramatically increased risk of liver cancer (hepatocellular carcinoma) in individuals with cirrhosis due to iron overload in HH has been well documented. However, the relationship between dietary iron and cancer risk in individuals without hemochromatosis is less clear.[17] Several epidemiological studies have reported associations between measures of increased iron status and the incidence of colorectal cancer or the occurrence of precancerous polyps (adenomas), but the associations were not consistent. Dietary iron intake appears to be more consistently related to the risk of colorectal cancer than measures of iron status or iron stores.[49,50]

Increased red meat consumption has been associated with an increased risk of colorectal cancer,[51] but there are a number of potential mechanisms by which increased meat consumption could affect cancer risk other than increasing iron intake. For example, increased red meat consumption increases the secretion of bile acids, which can be toxic to colonic cells, and also increases exposure to carcinogenic compounds generated when meat is cooked.[52] Increased iron in the contents of the colon, rather than increased body iron stores, could increase the risk of colon cancer by exposing colonic cells to potentially damaging ROS derived from iron-catalyzed reactions, especially in the presence of a high-fat diet. Although this possibility is currently under investigation, the interrelationship of dietary iron

Table 19.3 Tolerable upper intake level (UL) for iron

Life stage	Age	UL (mg/day)
Infants	0–12 months	40
Children	1–13 years	40
Adolescents	14–18 years	45
Adults	≥19 years	45

intake, iron stores, and the risk of colorectal cancer remains unclear.

Type 2 diabetes and the metabolic syndrome. Iron has been implicated in the pathogenesis of type 2 diabetes mellitus. Some epidemiological studies have associated high serum or plasma levels of ferritin with an increased risk of type 2 diabetes[53-58] as well as metabolic syndrome.[59,60] Ferritin levels reflect the amount of iron stored in the body. A few studies have reported that people with diabetes have higher ferritin levels than those who are not diabetic.[53,61,62] Other indices of iron excess, such as elevated transferrin saturation, may also be more prevalent in diabetes.[55] Moreover, individuals with the iron overload disease, HH, are known to be at a heightened risk of developing type 2 diabetes.[58] Randomized controlled trials are needed to determine whether lowering body stores of iron will help in the prevention of type 2 diabetes and the metabolic syndrome.

Neurodegenerative disease. Iron is required for normal brain and nerve function through its involvement in cellular metabolism, as well as in the synthesis of neurotransmitters and myelin. However, accumulation of excess iron can result in increased oxidative stress, and the brain is particularly susceptible to oxidative damage. Iron accumulation and oxidative injury are currently under consideration as potential contributors to a number of neurodegenerative diseases, such as Alzheimer disease and Parkinson disease.[63,64] The abnormal accumulation of iron in the brain does not appear to be a result of increased dietary iron, but, rather, a disruption in the complex process of cellular iron regulation. Although the mechanisms for this disruption in iron regulation are not yet known, it is currently an active area of biomedical research.[65,66]

Drug Interactions

Medications that decrease stomach acidity, such as antacids, histamine (H_2)-receptor antagonists (e.g., cimetidine, ranitidine), and proton pump inhibitors (e.g., omeprazole, lansoprazole), may impair iron absorption. Taking iron supplements at the same time as the following medications may result in decreased absorption and efficacy of the medication: levodopa, levothyroxine, methyldopa, penicillamine, quinolones, tetracyclines, and bisphosphonates. Therefore, it is best to take these medications 2 hours before or after iron supplements. Cholestyramine resin, used to lower blood cholesterol levels, should also be taken 2 hours before or after iron supplements because it interferes with iron absorption. Allopurinol, a medication used to treat gout, may increase iron storage in the liver and should not be used in combination with iron supplements.[37,67]

References

1. Wood RJ, Ronnenberg AG. Iron. In: Shils ME, Shike M, Ross AC, Caballero B, Cousins RJ, eds. Modern Nutrition in Health and Disease. 10th ed. Philadelphia, PA: Lippincott Williams & Wilkins; 2006:248–270

2. Beard JL, Dawson HD. Iron. In: O'Dell BL, Sunde RA, eds. Handbook of Nutritionally Essential Minerals. New York: Marcel Dekker, Inc.; 1997:275–334

3. Yip R, Dallman PR. Iron. In: Ziegler EE, Filer LJ, eds. Present Knowledge in Nutrition. 7th ed. Washington, DC: ILSI Press; 1996:277–292

4. Brody T. Nutritional Biochemistry. 2nd ed. San Diego, CA: Academic Press; 1999

5. Ivan M, Kondo K, Yang H, et al. HIFalpha targeted for VHL-mediated destruction by proline hydroxylation: implications for O2 sensing. Science 2001; 292(5516):464–468

6. Jaakkola P, Mole DR, Tian YM, et al. Targeting of HIF-alpha to the von Hippel-Lindau ubiquitylation complex by O2-regulated prolyl hydroxylation. Science 2001;292(5516):468–472

7. Fairbanks VF. Iron in Medicine and Nutrition. In: Shils ME, Olson JA, Shike M, Ross AC, eds. Modern Nutrition in Health and Disease. 9th ed. Philadelphia, PA: Lippincott Williams & Wilkins; 1999:193–221

8. Wallander ML, Leibold EA, Eisenstein RS. Molecular control of vertebrate iron homeostasis by iron regulatory proteins. Biochim Biophys Acta 2006;1763(7): 668–689

9. Anderson GJ, Darshan D, Wilkins SJ, Frazer DM. Regulation of systemic iron homeostasis: how the body responds to changes in iron demand. Biometals 2007; 20(3-4):665–674

10. Fleming MD. The regulation of hepcidin and its effects on systemic and cellular iron metabolism. Hematology (Am Soc Hematol Educ Program) 2008:151–158

11. Nicolas G, Bennoun M, Devaux I, et al. Lack of hepcidin gene expression and severe tissue iron overload in upstream stimulatory factor 2 (USF2) knockout mice. Proc Natl Acad Sci USA 2001;98(15):8780–8785

12. Nicolas G, Bennoun M, Porteu A, et al. Severe iron deficiency anemia in transgenic mice expressing liver hepcidin. Proc Natl Acad Sci USA 2002;99(7):4596–4601

13. Muckenthaler MU. Fine tuning of hepcidin expression by positive and negative regulators. Cell Metab 2008;8(1):1–3

14. Suharno D, West CE, Muhilal, Karyadi D, Hautvast JG. Supplementation with vitamin A and iron for nutritional anaemia in pregnant women in West Java, Indonesia. Lancet 1993;342(8883):1325–1328

15. Vulpe CD, Kuo YM, Murphy TL, et al. Hephaestin, a ceruloplasmin homologue implicated in intestinal iron transport, is defective in the sla mouse. Nat Genet 1999;21(2):195–199

16. Turnlund JR. Copper. In: Shils ME, Shike M, Ross AC, Caballero B, Cousins RJ, eds. Modern Nutrition in Health and Disease. 10th ed. Philadelphia, PA: Lippincott Williams & Wilkins; 2006:286–299

17. Food and Nutrition Board, Institute of Medicine. Iron. In: Dietary Reference Intakes for Vitamin A, Vitamin K, Boron, Chromium, Copper, Iodine, Iron, Manganese, Molybdenum, Nickel, Silicon, Vanadium, and Zinc. Washington, DC: National Academy Press; 2001: 290–393

18. Lynch SR. Interaction of iron with other nutrients. Nutr Rev 1997;55(4):102–110

19. Lee GR. Disorders of iron metabolism and heme synthesis. In: Lee GR, Foerster J, Paraskevas F, Greer JP, Rogers GM, eds. Wintrobe's Clinical Hematology. 10th ed. Baltimore, MD: Lippincott Williams & Wilkins; 1999:979–1070

20. Beard JL. Iron biology in immune function, muscle metabolism and neuronal functioning. J Nutr 2001;131(2S-2):568S–579S, discussion 580S

21. Dewar DH, Ciclitira PJ. Clinical features and diagnosis of celiac disease. Gastroenterology 2005; 128(4, Suppl 1):S19–S24

22. Sherman PM, Macarthur C. Current controversies associated with Helicobacter pylori infection in the pediatric population. Front Biosci 2001;6:E187–E192

23. Bloomberg RD, Fleishman A, Nalle JE, Herron DM, Kini S. Nutritional deficiencies following bariatric surgery: what have we learned? Obes Surg 2005; 15(2):145–154

24. Thomas DG, Grant SL, Aubuchon-Endsley NL. The role of iron in neurocognitive development. Dev Neuropsychol 2009;34(2):196–222

25. McCann JC, Ames BN. An overview of evidence for a causal relation between iron deficiency during development and deficits in cognitive or behavioral function. Am J Clin Nutr 2007;85(4):931–945

26. Sachdev H, Gera T, Nestel P. Effect of iron supplementation on mental and motor development in children: systematic review of randomised controlled trials. Public Health Nutr 2005;8(2):117–132

27. Grantham-McGregor S, Ani C. A review of studies on the effect of iron deficiency on cognitive development in children. J Nutr 2001;131(2S-2):649S–666S, discussion 666S–668S

28. Lozoff B. Iron deficiency and child development. Food Nutr Bull 2007; 28(4, Suppl):S560–S571

29. Wright RO. The role of iron therapy in childhood plumbism. Curr Opin Pediatr 1999;11(3):255–258

30. Rasmussen K. Is there a causal relationship between iron deficiency or iron-deficiency anemia and weight at birth, length of gestation and perinatal mortality? J Nutr 2001;131(2S-2):590S–601S, discussion 601S–603S

31. Yip R. Significance of an abnormally low or high hemoglobin concentration during pregnancy: special consideration of iron nutrition. Am J Clin Nutr 2000; 72(1, Suppl):272S–279S

32. Beard J. Iron. In: Bowman BA, Russell RM,eds. Present Knowledge in Nutrition. 9th ed. Washington, DC: ILSI Press; 2006:430–444

33. Oppenheimer SJ. Iron and its relation to immunity and infectious disease. J Nutr 2001;131(2S-2):616S–633S, discussion 633S–635S

34. Restless legs syndrome: detection and management in primary care. National Heart, Lung, and Blood Institute Working Group on Restless Legs Syndrome. Am Fam Physician 2000;62(1):108–114

35. Earley CJ, Connor JR, Beard JL, Malecki EA, Epstein DK, Allen RP. Abnormalities in CSF concentrations of ferritin and transferrin in restless legs syndrome. Neurology 2000;54(8):1698–1700

36. Allen RP, Barker PB, Wehrl F, Song HK, Earley CJ. MRI measurement of brain iron in patients with restless legs syndrome. Neurology 2001;56(2):263–265

37. Trace elements. Drug Facts and Comparisons, 54th ed St. Louis: Facts and Comparisons; 2000:32

38. Janssen MC, Swinkels DW. Hereditary haemochromatosis. Best Pract Res Clin Gastroenterol 2009;23(2): 171–183

39. Feder JN, Gnirke A, Thomas W, et al. A novel MHC class I-like gene is mutated in patients with hereditary haemochromatosis. Nat Genet 1996;13(4): 399–408

40. Franchini M, Veneri D. Recent advances in hereditary hemochromatosis. Ann Hematol 2005;84(6): 347–352

41. Ayonrinde OT, Milward EA, Chua AC, Trinder D, Olynyk JK. Clinical perspectives on hereditary hemochromatosis. Crit Rev Clin Lab Sci 2008;45(5):451–484

42. Wallace DF, Subramaniam VN. Non-HFE haemochromatosis. World J Gastroenterol 2007;13(35): 4690–4698

43. Pietrangelo A. Hemochromatosis 1998: is one gene enough? J Hepatol 1998;29(3):502–509

44. de Valk B, Marx JJ. Iron, atherosclerosis, and ischemic heart disease. Arch Intern Med 1999;159(14): 1542–1548

45. Danesh J, Appleby P. Coronary heart disease and iron status: meta-analyses of prospective studies. Circulation 1999;99(7):852–854

46. Ascherio A, Willett WC, Rimm EB, Giovannucci EL, Stampfer MJ. Dietary iron intake and risk of coronary disease among men. Circulation 1994;89(3):969–974

47. Klipstein-Grobusch K, Grobbee DE, den Breeijen JH, Boeing H, Hofman A, Witteman JC. Dietary iron and risk of myocardial infarction in the Rotterdam Study. Am J Epidemiol 1999;149(5):421–428

48. van der A DL, Peeters PH, Grobbee DE, Marx JJ, van der Schouw YT, van der AD. Dietary haem iron and coronary heart disease in women. Eur Heart J 2005;26(3): 257–262

49. Kato I, Dnistrian AM, Schwartz M, et al. Iron intake, body iron stores and colorectal cancer risk in women: a nested case-control study. Int J Cancer 1999;80(5): 693–698

50. Wurzelmann JI, Silver A, Schreinemachers DM, Sandler RS, Everson RB. Iron intake and the risk of colorectal cancer. Cancer Epidemiol Biomarkers Prev 1996;5(7):503–507

51. World Cancer Research Fund / American Institute for Cancer Research. Food, Nutrition, Physical Activity, and the Prevention of Cancer: a Global Perspective. Washington, DC: AICR; 2007

52. Bostick R. Diet and nutrition in the prevention of colon cancer. In: Bendich A, Deckelbaum RJ, eds. Preventive Nutrition: The Comprehensive Guide for Health Professionals. 2nd ed. Totowa, NJ: Humana Press, Inc.; 2001:57–95

53. Ford ES, Cogswell ME. Diabetes and serum ferritin concentration among U.S. adults. Diabetes Care 1999; 22(12):1978–1983

54. Hughes K, Choo M, Kuperan P, Ong CN, Aw TC. Cardiovascular risk factors in non-insulin-dependent diabetics compared to non-diabetic controls: a population-based survey among Asians in Singapore. Atherosclerosis 1998;136(1):25–31

55. Thomas MC, MacIsaac RJ, Tsalamandris C, Jerums G. Elevated iron indices in patients with diabetes. Diabet Med 2004;21(7):798–802

56. Hernández C, Lecube A, Carrera A, Simó R. Soluble transferrin receptors and ferritin in Type 2 diabetic patients. Diabet Med 2005;22(1):97–101

57. Jiang R, Manson JE, Meigs JB, Ma J, Rifai N, Hu FB. Body iron stores in relation to risk of type 2 diabetes in apparently healthy women. JAMA 2004;291(6):711–717

58. Swaminathan S, Fonseca VA, Alam MG, Shah SV. The role of iron in diabetes and its complications. Diabetes Care 2007;30(7):1926–1933

59. Jehn M, Clark JM, Guallar E. Serum ferritin and risk of the metabolic syndrome in U.S. adults. Diabetes Care 2004;27(10):2422–2428

60. Sun L, Franco OH, Hu FB, et al. Ferritin concentrations, metabolic syndrome, and type 2 diabetes in middle-aged and elderly Chinese. J Clin Endocrinol Metab 2008;93(12):4690–4696

61. Lecube A, Hernández C, Pelegrí D, Simó R. Factors accounting for high ferritin levels in obesity. Int J Obes (Lond) 2008;32(11):1665–1669

62. Eshed I, Elis A, Lishner M. Plasma ferritin and type 2 diabetes mellitus: a critical review. Endocr Res 2001;27(1-2):91–97

63. Piñero DJ, Hu J, Connor JR. Alterations in the interaction between iron regulatory proteins and their iron responsive element in normal and Alzheimer's diseased brains. Cell Mol Biol (Noisy-le-grand) 2000; 46(4):761–776

64. Altamura S, Muckenthaler MU. Iron toxicity in diseases of aging: Alzheimer's disease, Parkinson's disease and atherosclerosis. J Alzheimers Dis 2009;16(4): 879–895

65. Sayre LM, Perry G, Atwood CS, Smith MA. The role of metals in neurodegenerative diseases. Cell Mol Biol (Noisy-le-grand) 2000;46(4):731–741

66. Benarroch EE. Brain iron homeostasis and neurodegenerative disease. Neurology 2009;72(16):1436–1440

67. Hendler SS, Rorvik D, eds. PDR for Nutritional Supplements. 2nd ed. Montvale, NJ: Physicians' Desk Reference Inc.; 2008

68. Fleming DJ, Jacques PF, Tucker KL, et al. Iron status of the free-living, elderly Framingham Heart Study cohort: an iron-replete population with a high prevalence of elevated iron stores. Am J Clin Nutr 2001; 73(3):638–646

20 Magnesium

Magnesium plays important roles in the structure and function of the human body. The adult human body contains about 25 g magnesium. Over 60% of all the magnesium in the body is found in the skeleton, about 27% in muscle, 6%–7% in other cells, and less than 1% outside cells.[1]

Function

Magnesium is involved in more than 300 essential metabolic reactions, some of which are discussed below.[2]

Energy Production

The metabolism of carbohydrates and fats to produce energy requires numerous magnesium-dependent chemical reactions. Magnesium is required by the ATP-synthesizing protein in mitochondria. ATP (adenosine triphosphate), the molecule that provides energy for almost all metabolic processes, exists primarily as a complex with magnesium (MgATP).[3]

Synthesis of Essential Biomolecules

Magnesium is required for a number of steps during nucleic acid and protein synthesis. Several enzymes participating in the synthesis of carbohydrates and lipids require magnesium for their activity. Glutathione, an important antioxidant, requires magnesium for its synthesis.[3]

Structural Roles

Magnesium plays a structural role in bone, cell membranes, and chromosomes.[3]

Ion Transport across Cell Membranes

Magnesium is required for the active transport of ions such as potassium and calcium across cell membranes. Through its role in ion transport systems, magnesium affects the conduction of nerve impulses, muscle contraction, and normal heart rhythm.[3]

Cell Signaling

Cell signaling requires MgATP for the phosphorylation of proteins and the formation of the cell-signaling molecule, adenosine cyclic 3':5'-monophosphate (cAMP). Cyclic AMP is involved in many processes, including the secretion of parathyroid hormone (PTH) from the parathyroid glands (see Chapters 11 and 14 for more details on the role of PTH).[3]

Cell Migration

Calcium and magnesium levels in the fluid surrounding cells affect the migration of a number of different cell types. Such effects on cell migration may be important in wound healing.[3]

Nutrient Interactions

Zinc. High doses of zinc in supplemental form apparently interfere with the absorption of magnesium. One study reported that zinc supplements of 142 mg/day in healthy men significantly decreased magnesium absorption and disrupted magnesium balance (the difference between magnesium intake and magnesium loss).[2]

Fiber. Large increases in the intake of dietary fiber have been found to decrease magnesium utilization in experimental studies. However, the extent to which dietary fiber affects magnesium nutritional status in individuals with a varied diet outside the studies is not clear.[3,4]

Protein. Dietary protein may affect magnesium absorption. One study in adolescent boys found that magnesium absorption was lower when protein intake was less than 30 g/day, and higher protein intakes (93 g/day vs. 43 g/day) were associated with improved magnesium absorption in adolescents.[5]

Vitamin D and calcium. The active form of vitamin D (calcitriol) may slightly increase intestinal absorption of magnesium. However, magnesium absorption does not seem to be calcitriol dependent as is the absorption of calcium and phosphate. High calcium intake has not been found to affect magnesium balance in most studies. Inadequate blood magnesium levels are known to result in low blood calcium levels, resistance to PTH action, and resistance to some of the effects of vitamin D.[3,4]

Deficiency

Magnesium deficiency in healthy individuals who are consuming a balanced diet is quite rare because magnesium is abundant in both plant and animal foods and because the kidneys are able to limit urinary excretion of magnesium when intake is low. The following conditions increase the risk of magnesium deficiency:[1]

- *Gastrointestinal disorders*: prolonged diarrhea, Crohn disease, malabsorption syndromes, celiac disease, surgical removal of a portion of the intestine, and intestinal inflammation due to radiation may all lead to magnesium depletion.
- *Renal disorders (magnesium wasting)*: diabetes mellitus and long-term use of certain diuretics may result in increased urinary loss of magnesium. Multiple other medications can also result in renal magnesium wasting.[3]
- *Chronic alcoholism*: poor dietary intake, gastrointestinal problems, and increased urinary loss of magnesium may all contribute to magnesium depletion, which is frequently encountered in people who abuse alcohol.
- *Older age*: several studies have found that elderly people have relatively low dietary intakes of magnesium. Intestinal magnesium absorption tends to decrease with age and urinary magnesium excretion tends to increase with age, so suboptimal dietary magnesium intake may increase the risk of magnesium depletion in elderly people.[4]

Although severe magnesium deficiency is uncommon, it has been induced experimentally. When magnesium deficiency was induced in humans, the earliest sign was decreased serum magnesium levels (hypomagnesemia). Over time, serum calcium levels also began to decrease (hy-

pocalcemia) despite adequate dietary calcium and persisted despite increased PTH secretion. Usually, increased PTH secretion quickly results in the mobilization of calcium from bone and normalization of blood calcium levels. As the magnesium depletion progressed, PTH secretion diminished to low levels. Along with hypomagnesemia, signs of severe magnesium deficiency included hypocalcemia, low serum potassium levels (hypokalemia), retention of sodium, low circulating levels of PTH, neurological and muscular symptoms (tremor, muscle spasms, tetany), loss of appetite, nausea, vomiting, and personality changes.[3]

Recommended Dietary Allowance

In 1997, the Food and Nutrition Board (FNB) of the Institute of Medicine increased the recommended dietary allowance (RDA) for magnesium, based on the results of more recent, tightly controlled balance studies that utilized more accurate methods of measuring magnesium (**Table 20.1**).[4] Balance studies are useful for determining the amount of a nutrient that will prevent deficiency; however, such studies provide little information about the amount of a nutrient required for chronic disease prevention or optimum health.

Disease Prevention

Hypertension

Large epidemiological studies suggest a relationship between magnesium and blood pressure. However, the fact that foods high in magnesium (fruit, vegetables, whole grains) are frequently high in potassium and dietary fiber has made it difficult to evaluate independent effects of magnesium on blood pressure. A prospective cohort study of more than 30 000 male health professionals found an inverse association of dietary fiber, potassium, and magnesium, and the development of hypertension over a 4-year period.[6] In a similar study of more than 40 000 female registered nurses, dietary fiber and dietary magnesium were each inversely associated with systolic and diastolic blood pressures in those who did not develop hypertension over the 4-year study period, but neither dietary fiber nor magnesium was related to the risk of developing hyperten-

Table 20.1 Recommended dietary allowance for magnesium

Life stage	Age	Males (mg/day)	Females (mg/day)
Infants	0–6 months	30 (AI)	30 (AI)
Infants	7–12 months	75 (AI)	75 (AI)
Children	1–3 years	80	80
Children	4–8 years	130	130
Children	9–13 years	240	240
Adolescents	14–18 years	410	360
Adults	19–30 years	400	310
Adults	≥31 years	420	320
Pregnancy	≤18 years	–	400
Pregnancy	19–30 years	–	350
Pregnancy	≥31 years	–	360
Breast-feeding	≤18 years	–	360
Breast-feeding	19–30 years	–	310
Breast-feeding	≥31 years	–	320

AI, adequate intake.

sion.[7] The Atherosclerosis Risk in Communities study examined dietary magnesium intake, magnesium blood levels, and risk of developing hypertension in 7731 men and women over a 6-year period.[8] The risk of developing hypertension in both men and women decreased as serum magnesium levels increased, but the trend was statistically significant only in women. Although the investigators found no association between dietary magnesium and the incidence of hypertension, they suggested that low serum magnesium levels may play a modest role in the development of hypertension.

Cardiovascular Diseases

A number of studies have found decreased mortality from cardiovascular diseases in populations who routinely consume "hard" water. Hard (alkaline) water is generally high in magnesium but may also contain more calcium and fluoride than "soft" water, making the cardioprotective effects of hard water difficult to attribute to magnesium alone.[9] One large prospective study (almost 14000 men and women) found a significant trend for increasing serum magnesium levels to be associated with decreased risk of coronary heart disease (CHD) in women but not in men.[10] However, the risk of CHD in the lowest quartile (one-fourth) of dietary magnesium intake was

not significantly higher than the risk in the highest quartile in men or women. In addition, a large prospective study in over 35000 women reported that dietary magnesium, assessed by food frequency questionnaire, was not associated with the risk for various cardiovascular diseases, including stroke, nonfatal myocardial infarction, and CHD.[11] Currently, the relationship between dietary magnesium intake and the risk of cardiovascular disease remains unclear.

Osteoporosis

Although decreased bone mineral density (BMD) is the primary feature of osteoporosis, other osteoporotic changes in the collagenous matrix and mineral components of bone may result in bones that are brittle and more susceptible to fracture. Magnesium comprises about 1% of bone mineral and is known to influence both bone matrix and bone mineral metabolism. As the magnesium content of bone mineral decreases, bone crystals become larger and more brittle. Some studies have found lower magnesium content and larger bone crystals in bones of osteoporotic women compared with nonosteoporotic controls.[12]

Inadequate serum magnesium levels are known to result in low serum calcium levels, resistance to PTH action, and resistance to some of the effects of vitamin D, all of which can lead to increased bone loss. A study of over 900 elderly men and women found that higher dietary magnesium intakes were associated with increased BMD at the hip in both men and women. However, because magnesium and potassium are present in many of the same foods, the effect of dietary magnesium could not be isolated.[13] More recently, a study in over 2000 elderly people reported that magnesium intake was positively associated with total-body BMD in white men and women but not in black men and women.[14] Few studies have addressed the effect of magnesium supplementation on BMD or osteoporosis in humans. In a small group of postmenopausal women with osteoporosis, magnesium supplementation of 750 mg/day for the first 6 months, followed by 250 mg/day for 18 more months, resulted in increased BMD at the wrist after 1 year, with no further increase after 2 years of supplementation.[15] A study in postmenopausal women who were taking estrogen replacement therapy plus a multivitamin found that supplementation with an additional 500 mg/day of magnesium and 600 mg/day of calcium resulted in increased BMD at the heel compared with postmenopausal women receiving only estrogen replacement therapy.[16] Currently, the potential for increased magnesium intake to influence calcium and bone metabolism warrants more research with particular attention to its role in the prevention and treatment of osteoporosis.

Disease Treatment

The use of pharmacological doses of magnesium to treat specific diseases is discussed below. Although many of the cited studies utilized supplemental magnesium in doses considerably higher than the tolerable upper intake level (UL) of 350 mg/day recommended by the FNB for healthy individuals, it is important to note that these studies were all conducted under medical supervision. As a result of the potential risks of high doses of supplemental magnesium, especially in the presence of impaired kidney function, any disease treatment trial using magnesium doses higher than the UL should be conducted under medical supervision.

Hypertension

The results from intervention studies using magnesium supplements to treat hypertension have been conflicting.[4] In uncontrolled trials, hypertensive patients on thiazide diuretics experienced decreases in blood pressure when given magnesium supplements. In general, placebo-controlled trials have not been supportive of a blood pressure-lowering effect for magnesium supplementation.[3] Modest but significant blood pressure-lowering effects have been reported in two placebo-controlled studies using 485 mg/day of supplemental magnesium in individuals with mild-to-moderate hypertension for at least 2 months.[17,18] However, a number of other studies have failed to find any blood pressure-lowering effects with magnesium supplementation.[19] One double-blind, placebo-controlled study found magnesium supplementation to be beneficial in lowering blood pressure in individuals with low magnesium status, suggesting that oral magnesium supplementation may be helpful in hypertensive individuals who are depleted of magnesium due to chronic diuretic use, inadequate dietary intake, or both.[20] However, clinical studies to date are largely conflicting, and two recent reviews concluded that well-controlled, long-term clinical trials are needed to determine whether oral magnesium has any therapeutic benefit in hypertensive individuals.[21,22]

Pre-eclampsia–Eclampsia

Pre-eclampsia–eclampsia is a disease that is unique to pregnancy and may occur any time after 20 weeks of pregnancy through to 6 weeks after birth. Approximately 7% of pregnant women in the United States develop pre-eclampsia–eclampsia. Pre-eclampsia is defined as the presence of elevated blood pressure, protein in the urine, and severe swelling (edema) during pregnancy. Eclampsia occurs with the addition of seizures to the triad of symptoms. Approximately 5% of women with pre-eclampsia go on to develop eclampsia, which is a significant cause of maternal death.[23] For many years, high-dose intravenous magnesium sulfate has been the treatment of choice for preventing eclamptic seizures that may occur in association with pre-eclampsia–eclampsia late in pregnancy or during labor.[24,25] Magnesium is believed to relieve cerebral blood vessel spasm, increasing blood flow to the brain.[26,27]

Cardiovascular Diseases

Myocardial infarction. Results of a meta-analysis of randomized placebo-controlled trials indicated that an intravenous (IV) magnesium infusion given early after suspected myocardial infarction (MI) could decrease the risk of death. The most influential study included in the meta-analysis was a randomized placebo-controlled trial in 2316 patients that found a significant reduction in mortality (7.8% all-cause mortality rate in the experimental group vs. 10.3% all-cause mortality rate in the placebo group) in the group of patients given IV magnesium sulfate within 24 hours of a suspected MI.[28] Follow-up from 1 year to 5 years after treatment revealed that the mortality rate from cardiovascular disease was 21% lower in the magnesium-treated group.[29] However, a larger placebo-controlled trial that included more than 58 000 patients found no significant reduction in 5-week mortality in patients treated with IV magnesium sulfate within 24 hours of a suspected MI, resulting in controversy about the efficacy of the treatment.[30] A US survey of the treatment of more than 173 000 patients with acute MI found that only 5% were given IV magnesium in the first 24 hours after the MI, and that mortality was higher in patients treated with IV magnesium than in those not treated with magnesium.[31] More recently, a systematic review of 26 clinical trials, including 73 363 patients, concluded that IV magnesium likely does not reduce mortality after an MI and thus should not be used as a treatment.[32] Thus, the use of IV magnesium sulfate in the therapy of acute MI remains controversial.

Endothelial dysfunction. Vascular endothelial cells line arterial walls where they are in contact with the blood that flows through the circulatory system. Normally functioning vascular endothelium promotes vasodilation when needed, for example, during exercise, and inhibits the formation of blood clots. In cardiovascular disease, arteries develop atherosclerotic plaque. Atherosclerosis impairs normal endothelial function, increasing the risk of vasoconstriction and clot formation, which may lead to heart attack or stroke. Research indicates that pharmacological doses of oral magnesium may improve endothelial function in individuals with cardiovascular disease. A randomized, double-blind, placebo-controlled trial in 50 men and women with stable coronary artery disease found that 6 months of oral magnesium supplementation (730 mg/day) resulted in a 12% improvement in flow-mediated vasodilation compared with placebo.[33] In other words, the normal dilation response of the brachial (arm) artery to increased blood flow was improved. Magnesium supplementation also resulted in increased exercise tolerance during an exercise stress test compared with placebo.[39]

In another study of 42 patients with coronary artery disease who were already taking low-dose aspirin (an inhibitor of platelet aggregation), 3 months of oral magnesium supplementation (800–1200 mg/day) resulted in an average 35% reduction in platelet-dependent thrombosis, a measure of the propensity of blood to clot.[34] In addition, a recent study in 657 women participating in the Nurses' Health Study reported that dietary magnesium intake was inversely associated with E-selectin, a marker of endothelial dysfunction.[35] Cell culture studies have associated low magnesium concentrations with endothelial dysfunction, namely inhibition of endothelial proliferation.[36] Although preliminary, these studies suggest that magnesium may be of benefit in improving endothelial function in individuals with cardiovascular diseases.

Diabetes Mellitus

Magnesium depletion is commonly associated with both type 1 and type 2 diabetes mellitus. Between 25% and 38% of people with diabetes have been found to have decreased serum levels of magnesium (hypomagnesemia).[37] One cause of the depletion may be increased urinary loss of magnesium, which results from the increased urinary excretion of glucose accompanying poorly controlled diabetes. Magnesium depletion has been shown to increase insulin resistance in a few studies and may adversely affect blood glucose control in diabetes. One study reported that dietary magnesium supplements (400 mg/day) improved glucose tolerance in elderly individuals.[38] More recently, a randomized, double-blind, placebo-controlled study in 63 individuals with type 2 diabetes and hypomagnesemia found that those taking an oral magnesium chloride solution (2.5 g/day) for 16 weeks had improved measures of insulin sensitivity and glycemic control compared with those taking a placebo.[39]

A small study in nine patients with type 2 diabetes reported that supplemental magnesium (300 mg/day for 30 days), in the form of a liquid, magnesium-containing salt solution, improved fasting insulin levels but did not affect fasting glucose levels.[40] Yet, a recent meta-analysis of nine randomized, double-blind, controlled trials concluded that oral supplemental magnesium may lower fasting plasma glucose levels in individuals who have diabetes.[41] Due to conflicting reports, it is currently unclear whether magnesium supplementation has any therapeutic benefit in patients with type 2 diabetes. However, correcting existing magnesium deficiencies may improve glucose metabolism and insulin sensitivity in individuals with diabetes. Large-scale, well-controlled studies are needed to determine whether supplemental magnesium is useful in diabetes.

Migraine Headaches

Individuals who have recurrent migraine headaches have lower intracellular magnesium levels (demonstrated in both red blood cells and white blood cells) than those who do not experience migraines.[42] Oral magnesium supplementation has been shown to increase intracellular magnesium levels in individuals with migraines, leading to the hypothesis that magnesium supplementation might be helpful in decreasing the frequency and severity of migraine headaches. Two placebo-controlled trials have demonstrated modest decreases in the frequency of migraine headaches after supplementation with 600 mg/day of magnesium.[42,43] However, another placebo-controlled study found that 485 mg/day of magnesium did not reduce the frequency of migraine headaches.[44]

More recently, a placebo-controlled trial in 86 children with frequent migraine headaches found that oral magnesium oxide (9 mg/kg body weight per day) reduced headache frequency over the 16-week intervention.[45] Although no serious adverse effects were noted during these migraine headache trials, the investigators did note adverse effects such as diarrhea and gastric (stomach) irritation in about 19%–40% of the individuals taking the magnesium supplements.

Asthma

Serum or red blood cell levels of magnesium have not been found to be lower in patients with asthma compared with those who do not have asthma, even during acute asthmatic attacks. Yet, several clinical trials have examined the effect of IV magnesium infusions on acute asthmatic attacks. One double-blind, placebo-controlled trial in 38 adults, who did not respond to initial treatment in the emergency room, found improved lung function and decreased likelihood of hospitalization when IV magnesium sulfate was infused compared with a placebo.[46] However, another placebo-controlled, double-blind study in 48 adults reported that IV infusion of magnesium sulfate did not improve lung function in patients experiencing an acute asthma attack.[47] A systematic review of seven randomized controlled trials (five adult and two pediatric) concluded that IV magnesium sulfate is beneficial in patients with severe, acute asthma.[48] In addition, a meta-analysis of five randomized placebo-controlled trials, involving 182 children with severe asthma, found that IV infusion of magnesium sulfate was associated with a 71% reduction in the need for hospitalization.[49]

At present, the available evidence indicates that IV magnesium infusion is an efficacious treatment for severe, acute asthma; however, oral magnesium supplementation is of no known value in the management of chronic asthma.[50–52] Nebulized, inhaled magnesium for treating asthma requires further investigation, although a recent systematic review of six randomized controlled trials, including 296 patients, concluded that inhaled magnesium sulfate, along with a β_2 agonist, may improve pulmonary function in patients with acute asthma.[53]

Sources

Food Sources

A large US national survey indicated that the average magnesium intake for men (about 320 mg/day) and the average intake for women (about 230 mg/day) were significantly below the current RDA. Magnesium intakes were even lower in men and women aged over 70 years.[4] Such findings suggest that marginal magnesium deficiency may be relatively common in the United States.

Table 20.2 Food sources of magnesium

Food	Serving	Magnesium (mg)
Oat bran	½ cup dry	96.0
100% bran cereal (e.g., All Bran)	½ cup	93.1
Brown rice	1 cup cooked	86.0
Spinach, frozen, chopped	½ cup cooked	78.0
Almonds	1 ounce (23 almonds)	78.0
Swiss chard, chopped	½ cup cooked	75.0
Lima beans	½ cup cooked	63.0
Shredded wheat	2 biscuits	61.0
Molasses, blackstrap	1 tablespoon	48.0
Peanuts	1 ounce	48.0
Okra, frozen	½ cup cooked	47.0
Hazelnuts	1 ounce (21 hazelnuts)	46.0
Milk 1% fat	8 fluid ounces	34.0
Banana	1 medium	32.0

Table 20.3 Tolerable upper intake level (UL) for supplemental magnesium

Life stage	Age	UL (mg/day)
Infants	0–12 months	Not possible to establish[a]
Children	1–3 years	65
Children	4–8 years	110
Children	9–13 years	350
Adolescents	14–18 years	350
Adults	≥19 years	350

[a]Source of intake should be from food and formula only.

As magnesium is part of chlorophyll, the green pigment in plants, green leafy vegetables are rich in magnesium. Unrefined grains and nuts also have high magnesium content. Meats and milk have an intermediate magnesium content, while refined foods generally have the lowest magnesium content. Water is a variable source of intake; harder water usually has a higher concentration of magnesium salts.[4] Some foods that are relatively rich in magnesium are listed in **Table 20.2,** along with their magnesium content.

Supplements

Magnesium supplements are available as magnesium oxide, magnesium gluconate, magnesium chloride, and magnesium citrate salts, as well as a number of amino acid chelates, including magnesium aspartate. Magnesium hydroxide is used as an ingredient in several antacids.[54]

Safety

Toxicity

Adverse effects have not been identified from magnesium occurring naturally in food. However, adverse effects from excess magnesium have been observed with intakes of various magnesium salts (i.e., supplemental magnesium). The initial symptom of excess magnesium supplementation is diarrhea—a well-known side effect of magnesium that is used therapeutically as a laxative. Individuals with impaired kidney function are at higher risk for adverse effects of magnesium supplementation, and symptoms of magnesium toxicity have occurred in people with impaired kidney function taking moderate doses of magnesium-containing laxatives or antacids. Elevated serum levels of magnesium (hypermagnesemia) may result in a fall in blood pressure (hypotension). Some of the later effects of magnesium toxicity, such as lethargy, confusion, disturbances in normal cardiac rhythm, and deterioration of kidney function, are related to severe hypotension. As hypermagnesemia progresses, muscle weakness and difficulty breathing may occur. Severe hypermagnesemia may result in cardiac arrest.[3,4] The FNB set the UL for magnesium at 350 mg/day (**Table 20.3**). This UL represents the highest level of daily supplemental magnesium intake likely to pose no risk of diarrhea or gastrointestinal disturbance in almost all individuals. The FNB caution that individuals with renal impairment are at higher risk for adverse effects from excess supplemental magnesium intake. However, they also note that there are some conditions that may warrant higher doses of magnesium under medical supervision.[4]

Drug Interactions

Magnesium interferes with the absorption of digoxin (a heart medication), nitrofurantoin (an antibiotic), and certain antimalarial drugs, which could potentially reduce drug efficacy. Bisphosphonates (e.g., alendronate and etidronate), which are drugs used to treat osteoporosis, and magnesium should be taken 2 hours apart so that the absorption of the bisphosphonate is not inhibited. Magnesium has also been found to reduce the efficacy of chlorpromazine (a tranquilizer), penicillamine, oral anticoagulants, and the quinolone and tetracycline classes of antibiotics. As IV magnesium has increased the effects of certain muscle-relaxing medications used during anesthesia, it is advisable to let medical staff know if you are taking oral magnesium supplements, laxatives, or antacids before a surgical procedure. High doses of furosemide and some thiazide diuretics (e.g., hydrochlorothiazide), if taken for extended periods, may result in magnesium depletion.[54,55] Many other medications may also result in renal magnesium loss.[3]

LPI Recommendation

The Linus Pauling Institute supports the latest RDA for magnesium intake (420 mg/day for men aged over 30 years and 320 mg/day for women aged over 30 years). Following the Linus Pauling Institute recommendation to take a daily multivitamin/mineral supplement will ensure an intake of at least 100 mg magnesium/day. Few multivitamin/mineral supplements contain more than 100 mg magnesium due to its bulk. As magnesium is plentiful in foods, eating a varied diet that provides green vegetables and whole grains daily should provide the rest of an individual's magnesium requirement.

Older Adults

Older adults (51 years and older) are less likely than younger adults to consume enough magnesium to meet their needs and should therefore take care to eat magnesium-rich foods in addition to taking a multivitamin/mineral supplement daily. As older adults are more likely to have impaired kidney function, they should avoid taking more than 350 mg/day of supplemental magnesium without medical consultation.

References

1. Shils ME. Magnesium. In: O'Dell BL, Sunde RA, eds. Handbook of Nutritionally Essential Minerals. New York: Marcel Dekker, Inc.; 1997: 117–152
2. Spencer H, Norris C, Williams D. Inhibitory effects of zinc on magnesium balance and magnesium absorption in man. J Am Coll Nutr 1994;13(5):479–484
3. Rude RK, Shils ME. Magnesium. In: Shils ME, Shike M, Ross AC, Caballero B, Cousins RJ, eds. Modern Nutrition in Health and Disease. 10th ed. Baltimore, MD: Lippincott Williams & Wilkins; 2006:223–247
4. Food and Nutrition Board, Institute of Medicine. Magnesium. In: Dietary Reference Intakes for Calcium, Phosphorus, Magnesium, Vitamin D, and Fluoride. Washington, DC: National Academy Press; 1997:190–249
5. Schwartz R, Walker G, Linz MD, MacKellar I. Metabolic responses of adolescent boys to two levels of dietary magnesium and protein. I. Magnesium and nitrogen retention. Am J Clin Nutr 1973;26(5):510–518
6. Ascherio A, Rimm EB, Giovannucci EL, et al. A prospective study of nutritional factors and hypertension among US men. Circulation 1992;86(5):1475–1484
7. Ascherio A, Hennekens C, Willett WC, et al. Prospective study of nutritional factors, blood pressure, and hypertension among US women. Hypertension 1996;27(5):1065–1072
8. Peacock JM, Folsom AR, Arnett DK, Eckfeldt JH, Szklo M. Relationship of serum and dietary magnesium to incident hypertension: the Atherosclerosis Risk in Communities (ARIC) Study. Ann Epidemiol 1999;9(3):159–165
9. Marx A, Neutra RR. Magnesium in drinking water and ischemic heart disease. Epidemiol Rev 1997;19(2):258–272
10. Liao F, Folsom AR, Brancati FL. Is low magnesium concentration a risk factor for coronary heart disease? The Atherosclerosis Risk in Communities (ARIC) Study. Am Heart J 1998;136(3):480–490
11. Song Y, Manson JE, Cook NR, Albert CM, Buring JE, Liu S. Dietary magnesium intake and risk of cardiovascular disease among women. Am J Cardiol 2005;96(8):1135–1141
12. Sojka JE, Weaver CM. Magnesium supplementation and osteoporosis. Nutr Rev 1995;53(3):71–74
13. Tucker KL, Hannan MT, Chen H, Cupples LA, Wilson PW, Kiel DP. Potassium, magnesium, and fruit and vegetable intakes are associated with greater bone mineral density in elderly men and women. Am J Clin Nutr 1999;69(4):727–736
14. Ryder KM, Shorr RI, Bush AJ, et al. Magnesium intake from food and supplements is associated with bone mineral density in healthy older white subjects. J Am Geriatr Soc 2005;53(11):1875–1880
15. Stendig-Lindberg G, Tepper R, Leichter I. Trabecular bone density in a two year controlled trial of peroral magnesium in osteoporosis. Magnes Res 1993;6(2):155–163
16. Abraham GE, Grewal H. A total dietary program emphasizing magnesium instead of calcium. Effect on the mineral density of calcaneous bone in postmenopausal women on hormonal therapy. J Reprod Med 1990;35(5):503–507

17. Kawano Y, Matsuoka H, Takishita S, Omae T. Effects of magnesium supplementation in hypertensive patients: assessment by office, home, and ambulatory blood pressures. Hypertension 1998;32(2):260–265

18. Witteman JC, Grobbee DE, Derkx FH, Bouillon R, de Bruijn AM, Hofman A. Reduction of blood pressure with oral magnesium supplementation in women with mild to moderate hypertension. Am J Clin Nutr 1994;60(1):129–135

19. Whelton PK, Klag MJ. Magnesium and blood pressure: review of the epidemiologic and clinical trial experience. Am J Cardiol 1989;63(14):26G–30G

20. Shils ME. Magnesium. In: Ziegler EE, Filer LJ, eds. Present Knowledge in Nutrition. 7th ed. Washington, DC: ILSI Press; 1996:256–264

21. Sontia B, Touyz RM. Role of magnesium in hypertension. Arch Biochem Biophys 2007;458(1):33–39

22. Dickinson HO, Mason JM, Nicolson DJ, et al. Lifestyle interventions to reduce raised blood pressure: a systematic review of randomized controlled trials. J Hypertens 2006;24(2):215–233

23. Crombleholme WR. Obstetrics. In: Tierney LM, McPhee SJ, Papadakis MA, eds. Current Medical Treatment and Diagnosis. 37th ed. Stamford, CA: Appleton & Lange; 1998: 731–734

24. Sibai BM. Diagnosis, prevention, and management of eclampsia. Obstet Gynecol 2005;105(2):402–410

25. Altman D, Carroli G, Duley L, et al. Magpie Trial Collaboration Group. Do women with pre-eclampsia, and their babies, benefit from magnesium sulphate? The Magpie Trial: a randomised placebo-controlled trial. Lancet 2002;359(9321):1877–1890

26. Ema M, Gebrewold A, Altura BT, Altura BM. Magnesium sulfate prevents alcohol-induced spasms of cerebral blood vessels: an in situ study on the brain microcirculation from male versus female rats. Magnes Trace Elem 1991–1992-1992;10(2-4):269–280

27. Belfort MA, Anthony J, Saade GR, Allen JC Jr; Nimodipine Study Group. A comparison of magnesium sulfate and nimodipine for the prevention of eclampsia. N Engl J Med 2003;348(4):304–311

28. Woods KL, Fletcher S, Roffe C, Haider Y. Intravenous magnesium sulphate in suspected acute myocardial infarction: results of the second Leicester Intravenous Magnesium Intervention Trial (LIMIT-2). Lancet 1992;339(8809):1553–1558

29. Woods KL, Fletcher S. Long-term outcome after intravenous magnesium sulphate in suspected acute myocardial infarction: the second Leicester Intravenous Magnesium Intervention Trial (LIMIT-2). Lancet 1994;343(8901):816–819

30. ISIS-4 Collaborative. ISIS-4: a randomised factorial trial assessing early oral captopril, oral mononitrate, and intravenous magnesium sulphate in 58,050 patients with suspected acute myocardial infarction. ISIS-4 (Fourth International Study of Infarct Survival) Collaborative Group. Lancet 1995;345(8951):669–685

31. Ziegelstein RC, Hilbe JM, French WJ, Antman EM, Chandra-Strobos N. Magnesium use in the treatment of acute myocardial infarction in the United States (observations from the Second National Registry of Myocardial Infarction). Am J Cardiol 2001;87(1):7–10

32. Li J, Zhang Q, Zhang M, Egger M. Intravenous magnesium for acute myocardial infarction. Cochrane Database Syst Rev 2007; (2):CD 002755

33. Shechter M, Sharir M, Labrador MJ, Forrester J, Silver B, Bairey Merz CN. Oral magnesium therapy improves endothelial function in patients with coronary artery disease. Circulation 2000;102(19):2353–2358

34. Shechter M, Merz CN, Paul-Labrador M, et al. Oral magnesium supplementation inhibits platelet-dependent thrombosis in patients with coronary artery disease. Am J Cardiol 1999;84(2):152–156

35. Song Y, Li TY, van Dam RM, Manson JE, Hu FB. Magnesium intake and plasma concentrations of markers of systemic inflammation and endothelial dysfunction in women. Am J Clin Nutr 2007;85(4):1068–1074

36. Maier JA, Malpuech-Brugère C, Zimowska W, Rayssiguier Y, Mazur A. Low magnesium promotes endothelial cell dysfunction: implications for atherosclerosis, inflammation and thrombosis. Biochim Biophys Acta 2004;1689(1):13–21

37. Tosiello L. Hypomagnesemia and diabetes mellitus. A review of clinical implications. Arch Intern Med 1996;156(11):1143–1148

38. Paolisso G, Sgambato S, Gambardella A, et al. Daily magnesium supplements improve glucose handling in elderly subjects. Am J Clin Nutr 1992;55(6):1161–1167

39. Rodríguez-Morán M, Guerrero-Romero F. Oral magnesium supplementation improves insulin sensitivity and metabolic control in type 2 diabetic subjects: a randomized double-blind controlled trial. Diabetes Care 2003;26(4):1147–1152

40. Yokota K, Kato M, Lister F, et al. Clinical efficacy of magnesium supplementation in patients with type 2 diabetes. J Am Coll Nutr 2004;23(5):506S–509S

41. Song Y, He K, Levitan EB, Manson JE, Liu S. Effects of oral magnesium supplementation on glycaemic control in Type 2 diabetes: a meta-analysis of randomized double-blind controlled trials. Diabet Med 2006;23(10):1050–1056

42. Mauskop A, Altura BM. Role of magnesium in the pathogenesis and treatment of migraines. Clin Neurosci 1998;5(1):24–27

43. Peikert A, Wilimzig C, Köhne-Volland R. Prophylaxis of migraine with oral magnesium: results from a prospective, multi-center, placebo-controlled and double-blind randomized study. Cephalalgia 1996;16(4):257–263

44. Pfaffenrath V, Wessely P, Meyer C, et al. Magnesium in the prophylaxis of migraine—a double-blind placebo-controlled study. Cephalalgia 1996;16(6):436–440

45. Wang F, Van Den Eeden SK, Ackerson LM, Salk SE, Reince RH, Elin RJ. Oral magnesium oxide prophylaxis of frequent migrainous headache in children: a randomized, double-blind, placebo-controlled trial. Headache 2003;43(6):601–610

46. Skobeloff EM, Spivey WH, McNamara RM, Greenspon L. Intravenous magnesium sulfate for the treatment of acute asthma in the emergency department. JAMA 1989;262(9):1210–1213

47. Tiffany BR, Berk WA, Todd IK, White SR. Magnesium bolus or infusion fails to improve expiratory flow in acute asthma exacerbations. Chest 1993;104(3):831–834

48. Rowe BH, Bretzlaff JA, Bourdon C, Bota GW, Camargo CA Jr. Magnesium sulfate for treating exacerbations of acute asthma in the emergency department. Cochrane Database Syst Rev 2000; (2):CD 001490

49. Cheuk DK, Chau TC, Lee SL. A meta-analysis on intravenous magnesium sulphate for treating acute asthma. Arch Dis Child 2005;90(1):74–77

50. Monteleone CA, Sherman AR. Nutrition and asthma. Arch Intern Med 1997;157(1):23–34
51. Beasley R, Aldington S. Magnesium in the treatment of asthma. Curr Opin Allergy Clin Immunol 2007;7(1):107–110
52. Fogarty A, Lewis SA, Scrivener SL, et al. Oral magnesium and vitamin C supplements in asthma: a parallel group randomized placebo-controlled trial. Clin Exp Allergy 2003;33(10):1355–1359
53. Blitz M, Blitz S, Beasely R, et al. Inhaled magnesium sulfate in the treatment of acute asthma. Cochrane Database Syst Rev 2007;19(4):CD 003898
54. Hendler SS, Rorvik DR, eds. PDR for Nutritional Supplements. Montvale, NJ: Medical Economics Co., Inc.; 2001
55. Minerals. Drug Facts and Comparisons, 54th ed. St. Louis: Facts and Comparisons, 2000: 29–30

21 Manganese

Manganese is a mineral element that is both nutritionally essential and potentially toxic. The derivation of its name from the Greek word for magic remains appropriate, because scientists are still working to understand the diverse effects of manganese deficiency and manganese toxicity in living organisms.[1]

Function

Manganese plays an important role in a number of physiological processes as a constituent of multiple enzymes and an activator of other enzymes.[2]

Antioxidant Function

Manganese superoxide dismutase (MnSOD) is the principal antioxidant enzyme in mitochondria. As mitochondria consume over 90% of the oxygen used by cells, they are especially vulnerable to oxidative stress. The superoxide radical is one of the reactive oxygen species produced in mitochondria during ATP synthesis. MnSOD catalyzes the conversion of superoxide radicals to hydrogen peroxide, which can be reduced to water by other antioxidant enzymes.[3]

Metabolism

A number of manganese-activated enzymes play important roles in the metabolism of carbohydrates, amino acids, and cholesterol.[4] Pyruvate carboxylase, a manganese-containing enzyme, and phosphoenolpyruvate carboxykinase, a manganese-activated enzyme, are critical in gluconeogenesis—the production of glucose from noncarbohydrate precursors. Arginase, another manganese-containing enzyme, is required by the liver for the urea cycle, a process that detoxifies ammonia generated during amino acid metabolism.[3] In the brain, the manganese-activated enzyme glutamine synthetase converts the amino acid glutamate to glutamine. Glutamate is an excitotoxic neurotransmitter and a precursor to an inhibitory neurotransmitter, γ-aminobutyric acid.[5,6]

Bone Development

Manganese deficiency results in abnormal skeletal development in a number of animal species. Manganese is the preferred cofactor of enzymes called *glycosyltransferases*, which are needed for the synthesis of proteoglycans required for the formation of healthy cartilage and bone.[7]

Wound Healing

Wound healing is a complex process that requires increased production of collagen. Manganese is required for the activation of prolidase, an enzyme that functions to provide the amino acid proline for collagen formation in human skin cells.[8] A genetic disorder known as *prolidase deficiency* results in abnormal wound healing among other problems, and is characterized by abnormal manganese metabolism.[7] Glycosaminoglycan synthesis, which requires manganese-activated glycosyltransferases, may also play an important role in wound healing.[9]

Nutrient Interactions

Iron. Although the specific mechanisms for manganese absorption and transport have not been determined, some evidence suggests that iron and manganese can share common absorption and transport pathways.[10] Absorption of manganese from a meal decreases as the meal's iron content increases.[7] Iron supplementation (60 mg/day for 4 months) was associated with decreased blood manganese levels and decreased MnSOD activity in white blood cells, indicating a reduction in manganese nutritional status.[11] In addition, an individual's iron status can affect manganese bioavailability. Intestinal absorption of manganese is increased during iron deficiency, and increased iron stores (ferritin levels) are associated with decreased manganese absorption.[12] Men generally absorb less manganese

Table 21.1 Adequate intake for manganese

Life stage	Age	Males (mg/day)	Females (mg/day)
Infants	0–6 months	0.003	0.003
Infants	7–12 months	0.6	0.6
Children	1–3 years	1.2	1.2
Children	4–8 years	1.5	1.5
Children	9–13 years	1.9	1.6
Adolescents	14–18 years	2.2	1.6
Adults	≥19 years	2.3	1.8
Pregnancy	All ages	–	2.0
Breast-feeding	All ages	–	2.6

than women; this may be related to the fact that men usually have larger iron stores than women.[13] Further, iron deficiency has been shown to increase the risk of manganese accumulation in the brain.[14]

Magnesium. Supplemental magnesium (200 mg/day) has been shown to slightly decrease manganese bioavailability in healthy adults, either by decreasing manganese absorption or by increasing its excretion.[15]

Calcium. In one set of studies, supplemental calcium (500 mg/day) slightly decreased manganese bioavailability in healthy adults. As a source of calcium, milk had the least effect, while calcium carbonate and calcium phosphate had the greatest effect.[15] Several other studies have found minimal effects of supplemental calcium on manganese metabolism.[16]

Deficiency

Manganese deficiency has been observed in a number of animal species. Signs of manganese deficiency include impaired growth, impaired reproductive function, skeletal abnormalities, impaired glucose tolerance, and altered carbohydrate and lipid metabolism. In humans, demonstration of a manganese deficiency syndrome has been less clear.[2,7] A child on long-term total parenteral nutrition (TPN) lacking manganese developed bone demineralization and impaired growth that were corrected by manganese supplementation.[17] Young men who were fed a low-manganese diet developed decreased serum cho-

lesterol levels and a transient skin rash.[18] Blood calcium, phosphorus, and alkaline phosphatase levels were also elevated, which may indicate increased bone remodeling as a consequence of insufficient dietary manganese. Young women fed a manganese-poor diet developed mildly abnormal glucose tolerance in response to an intravenous infusion of glucose.[16] Overall, manganese deficiency is not common, and there is more concern for toxicity related to manganese overexposure (see "Safety," p. 182).

Adequate Intake

As there was insufficient information on manganese requirements to set a recommended dietary allowance (RDA), the Food and Nutrition Board (FNB) of the Institute of Medicine set an adequate intake (AI). As overt manganese deficiency has not been documented in humans eating natural diets, the FNB based the AI on average dietary intakes of manganese determined by the Total Diet Study—an annual survey of the mineral content of representative American diets.[4] AI values for manganese are listed in **Table 21.1** by age and gender. Manganese requirements are increased in pregnancy and lactation.[4]

Disease Prevention

Low dietary manganese or low levels of manganese in blood or tissue have been associated with several chronic diseases. Although manganese insufficiency is not currently thought to cause the diseases discussed below, more research may be warranted to determine whether suboptimal manganese nutritional status contributes to certain disease processes.

Osteoporosis

Women with osteoporosis have been found to have decreased plasma or serum levels of manganese and also an enhanced plasma response to an oral dose of manganese,[19,20] suggesting that they may have lower manganese status than women without osteoporosis. Yet, a more recent study in postmenopausal women with and without osteoporosis did not find any differences in plasma levels of manganese.[21] A study in healthy postmenopausal women found that a supplement containing manganese (5 mg/day), copper (2.5 mg/day), and zinc (15 mg/day) in combination with a calcium supplement (1000 mg/day) was more effective than the calcium supplement alone in preventing spinal bone loss over a 2-year period.[22] However, the presence of other minerals in the supplement makes it impossible to determine whether manganese supplementation was the beneficial agent for maintaining bone mineral density.

Diabetes Mellitus

Manganese deficiency results in glucose intolerance similar to diabetes mellitus in some animal species, but human studies examining the manganese status of diabetics have generated mixed results. In one study, whole blood manganese levels did not differ significantly between 57 people with diabetes and 28 non-diabetic controls.[23] However, another study found that urinary manganese excretion tended to be slightly higher in 185 people with diabetes compared with 185 non-diabetic controls.[24] A case–control study of 250 diabetic and non-diabetic individuals found that type 2 diabetic individuals had higher serum manganese levels than individuals who did not have diabetes.[25] However, a more recent study in 257 individuals with type 2 diabetes and 166 non-diabetic controls found lower blood levels of manganese in the diabetic patients.[26] In addition, a study of functional manganese status found that the activity of the antioxidant enzyme MnSOD was lower in the white blood cells of people with diabetes than in non-diabetics.[27] Neither 15 mg nor 30 mg oral manganese improved glucose tolerance in diabetics or non-dia-

betic controls when given at the same time as an oral glucose challenge.[28] Although manganese appears to play a role in glucose metabolism, there is little evidence that manganese supplementation improves glucose tolerance in diabetic or non-diabetic individuals.

Seizure Disorders

Manganese-deficient rats are more susceptible to seizures than manganese-sufficient rats, and rats that are genetically prone to epilepsy have lower than normal brain and blood manganese levels. Certain subgroups of humans with epilepsy reportedly have lower whole blood manganese levels than nonepileptic controls. One study found that blood manganese levels of individuals with epilepsy of unknown origin were lower than those of individuals whose epilepsy was induced by trauma (e.g., head injury) or disease, suggesting a possible genetic relationship between epilepsy and abnormal manganese metabolism. Although manganese deficiency does not appear to be a cause of epilepsy in humans, the relationship between manganese metabolism and epilepsy deserves further research.[7,29]

Sources

Food Sources

In the United States, estimated average dietary manganese intakes range from 2.1 mg/day to 2.3 mg/day for men and from 1.6 mg/day to 1.8 mg/day for women. People eating vegetarian diets and Western-type diets may have manganese intakes as high as 10.9 mg/day.[4] Rich sources of manganese include whole grains, nuts, leafy vegetables, and teas. Foods high in phytic acid, such as beans, seeds, nuts, whole grains, and soy products, or foods high in oxalic acid, such as cabbage, spinach, and sweet potatoes, may slightly inhibit manganese absorption. Although teas are rich sources of manganese, the tannins present in tea may moderately reduce its absorption.[15] Intake of other minerals, including iron, calcium, and phosphorus, have been found to limit retention of manganese.[4] The manganese content of some manganese-rich foods is listed in **Table 21.2**.[30]

Table 21.2 Food sources of manganese

Food	Serving	Manganese (mg)
Raisin bran cereal	1 cup	0.78–3.02
Pecans	1 ounce (19 halves)	1.28
Brown rice, cooked	½ cup	1.07
Instant oatmeal (prepared with water)	1 packet	0.99
Spinach, cooked	½ cup	0.84
Pineapple, raw	½ cup, chunks	0.77
Almonds	1 ounce (23 whole kernels)	0.65
Pineapple juice	½ cup (4 fluid ounces)	0.63
Whole-wheat bread	1 slice	0.60
Peanuts	1 ounce	0.55
Lima beans, cooked	½ cup	0.49
Pinto beans, cooked	½ cup	0.39
Navy beans, cooked	½ cup	0.48
Sweet potato, cooked	½ cup, mashed	0.44
Tea (green)	1 cup (8 ounces)	0.41–1.58
Tea (black)	1 cup (8 ounces)	0.18–0.77

Breast Milk and Infant Formulas

Infants are exposed to varying amounts of manganese depending on their source of nutrition. Manganese concentrations in breast milk, cow-based formula, and soy-based formula are in the range 3–10 µg/L, 30–50 µg/L, and 200–300 µg/L, respectively. However, bioavailability of manganese from breast milk is higher than from infant formulas, and manganese deficiencies in breast-fed infants or toxicities in formula-fed infants have not been reported.[31]

Water

Manganese concentrations in drinking water range from 1 µg/L to 100 µg/L, but most sources contain less than 10 µg/L.[32] The US Environmental Protection Agency (EPA) recommends 0.05 mg (50 µg)/L as the maximum allowable manganese concentration in drinking water.[33]

Supplements

Several forms of manganese are found in supplements, including manganese gluconate, manganese sulfate, manganese ascorbate, and amino acid chelates of manganese. Manganese is available as a stand-alone supplement or in combination products.[34] Relatively high levels of manganese ascorbate may be found in a bone/joint health product containing chondroitin sulfate and glucosamine hydrochloride.

Safety

Toxicity

Inhaled manganese. Manganese toxicity may result in multiple neurological problems and is a well-recognized health hazard for people who inhale manganese dust, such as welders and smelters.[1,4] Unlike ingested manganese, inhaled manganese is transported directly to the brain before it can be metabolized in the liver.[35] The symptoms of manganese toxicity generally appear slowly over a period of months to years. In its worst form, manganese toxicity can result in a permanent neurological disorder with symptoms similar to those of Parkinson disease, including tremors, difficulty walking, and facial muscle spasms. This syndrome, often called *manganism*, is sometimes preceded by psychiatric symptoms, such as irritability, aggressiveness, and even hallucinations.[36,37] In addition, environmental or occupational inhalation of manganese can cause an inflammatory response in the lungs.[38] Clinical symptoms of effects to the lung include cough, acute bronchitis, and decreased lung function.[39]

Methylcyclopentadienyl manganese tricarbonyl. Methylcyclopentadienyl manganese tricarbonyl (MMT) is a manganese-containing compound used in gasoline as an anti-knock additive. Although it has been used for this purpose in Canada for more than 20 years, uncertainty about adverse health effects from inhaled exhaust emissions kept the US EPA from approving its use in unleaded gasoline. In 1995, a US court decision made MMT available for widespread use in unleaded gasoline.[35] A study in Montreal, where MMT had been used for more than 10 years, found airborne manganese levels to be similar to those in areas where MMT was not used.[40] A more recent Canadian study found higher concentrations of respirable manganese in an urban versus a rural area, but average concentrations in both areas were below the safe level set by the US EPA.[41] The impact of long-term exposure to low levels of MMT combustion products has not, however, been thoroughly evaluated and will require additional study.[42]

Ingested manganese. Limited evidence suggests that high manganese intakes from drinking water may be associated with neurological symptoms similar to those of Parkinson disease. Severe neurological symptoms were reported in 25 people who drank water contaminated with manganese, and probably other contaminants, from dry cell batteries for 2–3 months.[43] Water manganese levels were found to be 14 mg/L almost 2 months after symptoms began and may have already been declining.[1] A study of older adults in Greece found a high prevalence of neurological symptoms in those exposed to water manganese levels of 1.8–2.3 mg/L,[44] while a study in Germany found no evidence of increased neurological symptoms in people drinking water with manganese levels ranging from 0.3 mg/L to 2.2 mg/L compared with those drinking water containing less than 0.05 mg/L.[45] Manganese in drinking water may be more bioavailable than manganese in food. However, none of the studies measured dietary manganese, so total manganese intake in these cases is unknown. In the United States, the EPA recommends 0.05 mg/L as the maximum allowable manganese concentration in drinking water.[33]

In addition, more recent studies have shown that children exposed to high levels of manganese through drinking water experience cognitive and behavioral deficits.[46] For instance, a cross-sectional study in 142 10-year-old children, who were exposed to a mean manganese water concentration of 0.8 mg/L, found that children exposed to higher manganese levels had significantly lower scores on three tests of intellectual function.[47] Another study associated high levels of manganese in tap water with hyperactive behavioral disorders in children.[48] These and other recent reports have raised concern over the neurobehavioral effects of manganese exposure in children.[46]

A single case of manganese toxicity was reported in a person who took large amounts of mineral supplements for years,[49] while another case was reported as a result of a person taking a Chinese herbal supplement.[36] Manganese toxicity resulting from foods alone has not been reported in humans, even though certain vegetarian diets could provide up to 20 mg/day of manganese.[4,32]

Intravenous manganese. Manganese neurotoxicity has been observed in individuals receiving TPN, both as a result of excessive manganese in the solution and as an incidental contaminant.[50] Neonates are especially vulnerable to manganese-related neurotoxicity.[51] Infants receiving manganese-containing TPN can be exposed to manganese concentrations about 100-fold higher than breast-fed infants.[31] As a result of potential toxicities, some argue against including manganese in parenteral nutrition.[52]

Individuals with Increased Susceptibility to Manganese Toxicity

Chronic liver disease. Manganese is eliminated from the body mainly in bile, so impaired liver function may lead to decreased manganese excretion. Manganese accumulation in individuals with cirrhosis or liver failure may contribute to neurological problems and Parkinson disease–like symptoms.[1,34]

Newborn. The newborn brain may be more susceptible to manganese toxicity due to a greater expression of receptors for the manganese transport protein (transferrin) in developing nerve

Table 21.3 Tolerable upper intake level (UL) for manganese

Life stage	Age	UL (mg/day)
Infants	0–12 months	Not possible to establish[a]
Children	1–3 years	2
Children	4–8 years	3
Children	9–13 years	6
Adolescents	14–18 years	9
Adults	≥19 years	11

[a]Source of intake should be from food and formula only.

cells and the immaturity of the liver's bile elimination system.[4]

Children. Compared with adults, infants and children have higher intestinal absorption, as well as lower biliary excretion, of manganese.[46] Thus, children are especially susceptible to any negative, neurotoxic effects of manganese. Indeed, several recent studies in school-aged children have reported deleterious cognitive and behavioral effects after excessive manganese exposure.[47,48,53]

Iron-deficient populations. Iron deficiency has been shown to increase the risk of manganese accumulation in the brain.[14]

Due to the severe implications of manganese neurotoxicity, the FNB set very conservative upper intake levels (UL) for manganese; these are listed in **Table 21.3** by age group.[4]

Drug Interactions

Magnesium-containing antacids and laxatives and the antibiotic medication tetracycline may decrease the absorption of manganese if taken together with manganese-containing foods or supplements.[34]

High Levels of Manganese in Supplements Marketed for Bone/Joint Health

Two studies have found that supplements containing a combination of glucosamine hydrochloride, chondroitin sulfate, and manganese ascorbate are beneficial in relieving pain due to mild or moderate osteoarthritis of the knee when compared with a placebo.[54,55] The dose of elemental manganese supplied by the supplements was 30 mg/day for 8 weeks in one study[55] and 40 mg/day for 6 months in the other.[54] No adverse effects were reported during either study, and blood manganese levels were not measured. Neither study compared the treatment containing manganese ascorbate with a treatment containing glucosamine hydrochloride and chondroitin sulfate without manganese ascorbate, so it is impossible to determine whether the supplement would have resulted in the same benefit without high doses of manganese.

LPI Recommendation

The AI for manganese (2.3 mg/day for men and 1.8 mg/day for women) appears sufficient to prevent deficiency in most individuals. The daily intake of manganese most likely to promote optimum health is not known. Following the Linus Pauling Institute recommendation to take a multivitamin/mineral supplement containing 100% of the daily values (DVs) of most nutrients will generally provide 2 mg/day of manganese in addition to that in food. As a result of the potential for toxicity and the lack of information about benefit, manganese supplementation beyond 100% of the DV (2 mg/day) is not recommended. There is currently no evidence that the consumption of a manganese-rich plant-based diet results in manganese toxicity.

Older Adults

The requirement for manganese is not known to be higher for older adults. However, liver disease is more common in older adults and may increase the risk of manganese toxicity by decreasing the elimination of manganese from the body. Manganese supplementation beyond 100% of the DV (2 mg/day) is not recommended.

References

1. Keen CL, Ensunsa JL, Watson MH, et al. Nutritional aspects of manganese from experimental studies. Neurotoxicology 1999;20(2-3):213–223
2. Nielsen FH. Ultratrace minerals. In: Shils M, Olson JA, Shike M, Ross AC, eds. Modern Nutrition in Health and Disease. 9th ed. Baltimore, MD: Lippincott Williams & Wilkins; 1999:283–303
3. Leach RM, Harris ED. Manganese. In: O'Dell BL, Sunde RA, eds. Handbook of Nutritionally Essential Minerals. New York: Marcel Dekker, Inc.; 1997:335–355
4. Food and Nutrition Board, Institute of Medicine. Manganese. In: Dietary Reference Intakes for Vitamin A, Vitamin K, Boron, Chromium, Copper, Iodine, Iron, Manganese, Molybdenum, Nickel, Silicon, Vanadium,

and Zinc. Washington, DC: National Academy Press; 2001:394–419

5. Wedler FC. Biochemical and nutritional role of manganese: an overview. In: Klimis-Tavantzis DJ, ed. Manganese in Health and Disease. Boca Raton, FL: CRC Press, Inc.; 1994:1–37

6. Albrecht J, Sonnewald U, Waagepetersen HS, Schousboe A. Glutamine in the central nervous system: function and dysfunction. Front Biosci 2007;12: 332–343

7. Keen CL, Zidenberg-Cherr S. Manganese. In: Ziegler EE, Filer LJ, eds. Present Knowledge in Nutrition. 7th ed. Washington, DC: ILSI Press; 1996:334–343

8. Muszyńska A, Pałka J, Gorodkiewicz E. The mechanism of daunorubicin-induced inhibition of prolidase activity in human skin fibroblasts and its implication to impaired collagen biosynthesis. Exp Toxicol Pathol 2000;52(2):149–155

9. Shetlar MR, Shetlar CL. The role of manganese in wound healing. In: Klimis-Tavantzis DL, ed. Manganese in Health and Disease. Boca Raton, FL: CRC Press, Inc.; 1994:145–157

10. Fitsanakis VA, Zhang N, Garcia S, Aschner M. Manganese (Mn) and iron (Fe): interdependency of transport and regulation. Neurotox Res 2010;18(2): 124–131

11. Davis CD, Greger JL. Longitudinal changes of manganese-dependent superoxide dismutase and other indexes of manganese and iron status in women. Am J Clin Nutr 1992;55(3):747–752

12. Finley JW. Manganese absorption and retention by young women is associated with serum ferritin concentration. Am J Clin Nutr 1999;70(1):37–43

13. Finley JW, Johnson PE, Johnson LK. Sex affects manganese absorption and retention by humans from a diet adequate in manganese. Am J Clin Nutr 1994;60(6): 949–955

14. Aschner M, Dorman DC. Manganese: pharmacokinetics and molecular mechanisms of brain uptake. Toxicol Rev 2006;25(3):147–154

15. Kies C. Bioavailability of manganese. In: Klimis-Tavantzis DL, ed. Manganese in Health and Disease. Boca Raton, FL: CRC Press, Inc.; 1994:39–58

16. Johnson PE, Lykken GI. Manganese and calcium absorption and balance in young women fed diets with varying amounts of manganese and calcium. J Trace Elem Exp Med 1991;4:19–35

17. Norose N, Terai M, Norose K. Manganese deficiency in a child with very short bowel syndrome receiving long-term parenteral nutrition. J Trace Elem Exp Med 1992;5:100–101 (abstract)

18. Friedman BJ, Freeland-Graves JH, Bales CW, et al. Manganese balance and clinical observations in young men fed a manganese-deficient diet. J Nutr 1987;117(1):133–143

19. Freeland-Graves J, Llanes C. Models to study manganese deficiency. In: Klimis-Tavantzis DL, ed. Manganese in Health and Disease. Boca Raton, FL: CRC Press, Inc.; 1994:59–86

20. Reginster JY, Strause LG, Saltman P, Franchimont P. Trace elements and postmenopausal osteoporosis: a preliminary study of decreased serum manganese. Med Sci Res 1988;16:337–338

21. Odabasi E, Turan M, Aydin A, Akay C, Kutlu M. Magnesium, zinc, copper, manganese, and selenium levels in postmenopausal women with osteoporosis. Can magnesium play a key role in osteoporosis? Ann Acad Med Singapore 2008;37(7):564–567

22. Strause L, Saltman P, Smith KT, Bracker M, Andon MB. Spinal bone loss in postmenopausal women supplemented with calcium and trace minerals. J Nutr 1994;124(7):1060–1064

23. Walter RM Jr, Uriu-Hare JY, Olin KL, et al. Copper, zinc, manganese, and magnesium status and complications of diabetes mellitus. Diabetes Care 1991; 14(11):1050–1056

24. el-Yazigi A, Hannan N, Raines DA. Urinary excretion of chromium, copper, and manganese in diabetes mellitus and associated disorders. Diabetes Res 1991;18(3): 129–134

25. Ekin S, Mert N, Gunduz H, Meral I. Serum sialic acid levels and selected mineral status in patients with type 2 diabetes mellitus. Biol Trace Elem Res 2003; 94(3):193–201

26. Kazi TG, Afridi HI, Kazi N, et al. Copper, chromium, manganese, iron, nickel, and zinc levels in biological samples of diabetes mellitus patients. Biol Trace Elem Res 2008;122(1):1–18

27. Nath N, Chari SN, Rathi AB. Superoxide dismutase in diabetic polymorphonuclear leukocytes. Diabetes 1984;33(6):586–589

28. Walter RM, Aoki TT, Keen CL. Acute oral manganese does not consistently affect glucose tolerance in nondiabetic and type II diabetic humans. J Trace Elem Exp Med 1991;4:(2)73–79

29. Carl GF, Gallagher BB. Manganese and epilepsy. In: Klimis-Tavantzis DL, ed. Manganese in Health and Disease. Boca Raton, FL: CRC Press, Inc.; 1994: 133–157

30. U.S. Department of Agriculture, Agricultural Research Service. USDA National Nutrient Database for Standard Reference, Release 22. 2009. Available at: www.nal.usda.gov/fnic/foodcomp/search (accessed 3 March, 2010)

31. Aschner JL, Aschner M. Nutritional aspects of manganese homeostasis. Mol Aspects Med 2005;26 (4-5):353–362

32. Keen CL, Zidenberg-Cherr S. Manganese toxicity in humans and experimental animals. In: Klimis-Tavantzis DL, ed. Manganese in Health and Disease. Boca Raton, FL: CRC Press, Inc.; 1994: 193–205

33. EPA Office of Water. Current Drinking Water Standards. Environmental Protection Agency [Web page]. Available at: http://www.epa.gov/safewater/mcl. html (accessed 4 Jan 2011)

34. Hendler SS, Rorvik DR, eds. PDR for Nutritional Supplements. Montvale, NJ: Medical Economics Co., Inc.; 2001

35. Davis JM. Methylcyclopentadienyl manganese tricarbonyl: health risk uncertainties and research directions. Environ Health Perspect 1998;106(Suppl 1):191–201

36. Pal PK, Samii A, Calne DB. Manganese neurotoxicity: a review of clinical features, imaging and pathology. Neurotoxicology 1999;20(2-3):227–238

37. Aschner M, Aschner JL. Manganese neurotoxicity: cellular effects and blood-brain barrier transport. Neurosci Biobehav Rev 1991;15(3):333–340

38. Han J, Lee JS, Choi D, et al. Manganese (II) induces chemical hypoxia by inhibiting HIF-prolyl hydroxylase: implication in manganese-induced pulmonary inflammation. Toxicol Appl Pharmacol 2009;235(3): 261–267

39. Roels H, Lauwerys R, Buchet JP, et al. Epidemiological survey among workers exposed to manganese: ef-

fects on lung, central nervous system, and some biological indices. Am J Ind Med 1987;11(3):307–327

40. Zayed J, Thibault C, Gareau L, Kennedy G. Airborne manganese particulates and methylcyclopentadienyl manganese tricarbonyl (MMT) at selected outdoor sites in Montreal. Neurotoxicology 1999;20(2–3): 151–157

41. Bolté S, Normandin L, Kennedy G, Zayed J. Human exposure to respirable manganese in outdoor and indoor air in urban and rural areas. J Toxicol Environ Health A 2004;67(6):459–467

42. Aschner M. Manganese: brain transport and emerging research needs. Environ Health Perspect 2000; 108(Suppl 3):429–432

43. Kawamura R. Intoxication by manganese in well water. Kitasato Arch Exp Med 1941;18:145–169

44. Kondakis XG, Makris N, Leotsinidis M, Prinou M, Papapetropoulos T. Possible health effects of high manganese concentration in drinking water. Arch Environ Health 1989;44(3):175–178

45. Vieregge P, Heinzow B, Korf G, Teichert HM, Schleifenbaum P, Mösinger HU. Long term exposure to manganese in rural well water has no neurological effects. Can J Neurol Sci 1995;22(4):286–289

46. Ljung K, Vahter M. Time to re-evaluate the guideline value for manganese in drinking water? Environ Health Perspect 2007;115(11):1533–1538

47. Wasserman GA, Liu X, Parvez F, et al. Water manganese exposure and children's intellectual function in Araihazar, Bangladesh. Environ Health Perspect 2006;114(1):124–129

48. Bouchard M, Laforest F, Vandelac L, Bellinger D, Mergler D. Hair manganese and hyperactive behaviors: pilot study of school-age children exposed through tap water. Environ Health Perspect 2007;115(1): 122–127

49. Keen C, Zidenberg-Cherr S. Manganese toxicity in humans and experimental animals. In: Klimis-Tavantzis D, ed. Manganese in Health and Disease. Boca Raton, FL: CRC Press, Inc.; 1994

50. Dobson AW, Erikson KM, Aschner M. Manganese neurotoxicity. Ann N Y Acad Sci 2004;1012:115–128

51. Erikson KM, Thompson K, Aschner J, Aschner M. Manganese neurotoxicity: a focus on the neonate. Pharmacol Ther 2007;113(2):369–377

52. Hardy IJ, Gillanders L, Hardy G. Is manganese an essential supplement for parenteral nutrition? Curr Opin Clin Nutr Metab Care 2008;11(3):289–296

53. Wright RO, Amarasiriwardena C, Woolf AD, Jim R, Bellinger DC. Neuropsychological correlates of hair arsenic, manganese, and cadmium levels in school-age children residing near a hazardous waste site. Neurotoxicology 2006;27(2):210–216

54. Das A Jr, Hammad TA. Efficacy of a combination of FCHG49 glucosamine hydrochloride, TRH122 low molecular weight sodium chondroitin sulfate and manganese ascorbate in the management of knee osteoarthritis. Osteoarthritis Cartilage 2000;8(5):343–350

55. Leffler CT, Philippi AF, Leffler SG, Mosure JC, Kim PD. Glucosamine, chondroitin, and manganese ascorbate for degenerative joint disease of the knee or low back: a randomized, double-blind, placebo-controlled pilot study. Mil Med 1999;164(2):85–91

22 Molybdenum

Molybdenum is an essential trace element for virtually all life forms. It functions as a cofactor for a number of enzymes that catalyze important chemical transformations in the global carbon, nitrogen, and sulfur cycles.[1] Thus, molybdenum-dependent enzymes are required not only for human health, but also for the health of our ecosystem.

Function

The biological form of molybdenum, present in almost all molybdenum-containing enzymes (molybdoenzymes), is an organic molecule known as the *molybdenum cofactor*.[2] In humans, molybdenum is known to function as a cofactor for three enzymes.

1. *Sulfite oxidase* catalyzes the transformation of sulfite to sulfate, a reaction that is necessary for the metabolism of sulfur-containing amino acids (methionine and cysteine).
2. *Xanthine oxidase* catalyzes the breakdown of nucleotides (precursors to DNA and RNA) to form uric acid, which contributes to the plasma antioxidant capacity of the blood.
3. *Aldehyde oxidase* and xanthine oxidase catalyze hydroxylation reactions that involve a number of different molecules with similar chemical structures.

Xanthine oxidase and aldehyde oxidase also play a role in the metabolism of drugs and toxins.[3] Of these three enzymes, only sulfite oxidase is known to be crucial for human health.[4]

Nutrient Interactions

Copper. Excess dietary molybdenum has been found to result in copper deficiency in grazing animals (ruminants). In ruminants, the formation of compounds containing sulfur and molybdenum, known as *thiomolybdates*, appears to prevent the absorption of copper. This interaction between thiomolybdates and copper does not occur to a significant degree in humans. One early study reported that molybdenum intakes of 500 µg/day and 1500 µg/day from sorghum increased urinary copper excretion.[2] However, the results of a more recent, well-controlled study indicated that very high dietary molybdenum intakes (up to 1500 µg/day) did not adversely affect copper nutritional status in eight healthy young men.[5]

Deficiency

Dietary molybdenum deficiency has never been observed in healthy people.[2] The only documented case of acquired molybdenum deficiency occurred in a patient with Crohn disease on long-term total parenteral nutrition (TPN) without molybdenum added to the TPN solution.[6] The patient developed rapid heart and respiratory rates, headache, and night blindness, and ultimately became comatose. He also demonstrated biochemical signs of molybdenum deficiency, including low plasma uric acid levels, decreased urinary excretion of uric acid and sulfate, and increased urinary excretion of sulfite. Thus, the patient was diagnosed with defects in uric acid production and sulfur amino acid metabolism. The patient's clinical condition improved and the amino acid intolerance disappeared when the TPN solution was discontinued and instead supplemented with molybdenum (160 µg/day).[6]

Current understanding of the essential nature of molybdenum in humans is based largely on the study of individuals with very rare inborn errors of metabolism that result in a deficiency of the molybdoenzyme, sulfite oxidase. Two forms of sulfite oxidase deficiency have been identified:

1. Isolated sulfite oxidase deficiency, in which only sulfite oxidase activity is affected.
2. Molybdenum cofactor deficiency, in which the activities of all three molybdoenzymes are affected.

As molybdenum functions only in the form of the molybdenum cofactor in humans, any disturbance of molybdenum cofactor metabolism can

Table 22.1 Recommended dietary allowance for molybdenum

Life stage	Age	Males (µg/day)	Females (µg/day)
Infants	0–6 months	2 (AI)	2 (AI)
Infants	7–12 months	3 (AI)	3 (AI)
Children	1–3 years	17	17
Children	4–8 years	22	22
Children	9–13 years	34	34
Adolescents	14–18 years	43	43
Adults	≥19 years	45	45
Pregnancy	All ages	–	50
Breast-feeding	All ages	–	50

AI, adequate intake.

disrupt the function of all molybdoenzymes. Together, molybdenum cofactor deficiency and isolated sulfite oxidase deficiency have been diagnosed in more than 100 individuals worldwide. Both disorders result from recessive traits, meaning that only individuals who inherit two copies of the abnormal gene (one from each parent) develop the disease. Individuals who inherit only one copy of the abnormal gene are known as carriers of the trait but do not exhibit any symptoms. The symptoms of isolated sulfite oxidase deficiency and molybdenum cofactor deficiency are identical and usually include severe brain damage, which appears to be due to the loss of sulfite oxidase activity. At present, it is not clear whether the neurological effects are a result of the accumulation of a toxic metabolite, such as sulfite, or inadequate sulfate production. Isolated sulfite oxidase deficiency and molybdenum cofactor deficiency can be diagnosed relatively early in pregnancy (10–14 weeks' gestation) through chorionic villous sampling and, in some cases, carriers of molybdenum cofactor deficiency can be identified through genetic testing. No cure is currently available for either disorder, although anti-seizure medications and dietary restriction of sulfur-containing amino acids may be beneficial in some cases.[7]

Recommended Dietary Allowance

The recommended dietary allowance (RDA) for molybdenum was most recently revised in January 2001.[2] It was based on the results of nutritional balance studies conducted in eight healthy young men under controlled laboratory conditions.[8,9] The RDA values for molybdenum are listed in **Table 22.1** by age and gender. Adequate intake (AI) was set for infants based on mean molybdenum intake from human milk, exclusively.

Disease Prevention

Gastroesophageal Cancer

Linxian is a small region in northern China where the incidence of cancer of the esophagus and stomach is very high (10 times higher than the average in China and 100 times higher than the average in the United States). The soil in this region is low in molybdenum and other mineral elements, so dietary molybdenum intake is also low. Increased intake of nitrosamines, which are known carcinogens, may be one of a number of dietary and environmental factors that contributes to the development of gastroesophageal cancer in this population. Plants require molybdenum to synthesize nitrate reductase, a molybdoenzyme necessary for converting nitrates from the soil to amino acids. Thus, when molybdenum content in the soil is low, plants preferentially convert nitrates to nitrosamines instead of using nitrate to synthesize amino acids. This results in increased nitrosamine exposure for those who consume the plants. Adding molybdenum to the soil in the form of ammonium molybdenate may help decrease the risk of gastroesophageal cancer by limiting nitrosamine exposure. It is not clear whether dietary molybdenum supplementation is beneficial in decreasing the risk of gastroesophageal cancer. In a large intervention trial, dietary supplementation of molybdenum (30 µg/

day) and vitamin C (120 mg/day) did not decrease the incidence of gastroesophageal cancer or other cancers in residents of Linxian over a 5-year period.[10]

Sources

Food Sources

The Total Diet Study, an annual survey of the mineral content in the typical American diet, indicates that the dietary intake of molybdenum averages 76 µg/day for women and 109 µg/day for men. Thus, usual molybdenum intakes are well above the RDA for molybdenum. Legumes, such as beans, lentils, and peas, are the richest sources of molybdenum. Grain products and nuts are considered good sources, while animal products, fruit, and many vegetables are generally low in molybdenum.[2] As the molybdenum content of plants depends on the soil molybdenum content and other environmental conditions, the molybdenum content of foods can vary considerably.[11]

Supplements

Molybdenum in nutritional supplements is generally in the form of sodium molybdate or ammonium molybdate.[12]

Safety

Toxicity

The toxicity of molybdenum compounds appears to be relatively low in humans. Increased serum levels of uric acid and ceruloplasmin (an iron-oxidizing enzyme) have been reported in occupationally exposed workers in a molybdenite roasting plant.[13] Goutlike symptoms have also been reported in an Armenian population consuming 10–15 mg molybdenum from food daily.[14] In other studies, blood and urinary uric acid levels were not elevated by molybdenum intakes up to 1.5 mg/day.[2] There has been only one report of acute toxicity related to molybdenum from a dietary supplement: a man reportedly consumed a total of 13.5 mg molybdenum over a period of 18 days (300–800 µg/day) and developed acute psychosis with hallucinations, seizures, and other neurological symptoms.[12] However, a controlled study in four healthy young men found that mo-

Table 22.2 Tolerable upper intake level (UL) for molybdenum

Life stage	Age	UL (µg/day)
Infants	0–12 months	Not possible to establish[a]
Children	1–3 years	300
Children	4–8 years	600
Children	9–13 years	1100
Adolescents	14–18 years	1700
Adults	≥19 years	2000

[a]Source of intake should be from food and formula only.

lybdenum intakes ranging from 22 µg/day to 1490 µg/day (almost 1.5 mg/day) elicited no serious adverse effects when molybdenum was given for 24 days.[9]

The Food and Nutrition Board (FNB) of the Institute of Medicine found little evidence that molybdenum excess was associated with adverse health outcomes in generally healthy people. To determine the tolerable upper intake level (UL), the FNB selected adverse reproductive effects in rats as the most sensitive index of toxicity and applied a large uncertainty factor because animal data were used.[2] The ULs for molybdenum are listed by life stage in **Table 22.2**.

Drug Interactions

High doses of molybdenum have been found to inhibit the metabolism of acetaminophen in rats;[15] however, it is not known whether this occurs at clinically relevant doses in humans.

LPI Recommendation

The RDA for molybdenum (45 µg/day for adults) is sufficient to prevent deficiency. Although the intake of molybdenum most likely to promote optimum health is not known, there is currently no evidence that intakes higher than the RDA are beneficial. Most people in the United States consume more than sufficient molybdenum in their diets, making supplementation unnecessary. Following the Linus Pauling Institute's general recommendation to take a multivitamin/mineral supplement that contains 100% of the daily values (DVs) for most nutrients is likely to provide 75 µg/day of molybdenum because the DV for molybdenum has not been revised to reflect the most recent RDA. Although the amount of molybdenum currently found in most multivitamin/mineral supplements is higher than the RDA, it is well below the UL of 2000 µg/day and should be safe for adults.

Older Adults

Because aging has not been associated with significant changes in the requirement for molybdenum,[2] our recommendation for older adults is the same as that for adults aged 50 and younger.

References

1. Wuebbens MM, Liu MT, Rajagopalan K, Schindelin H. Insights into molybdenum cofactor deficiency provided by the crystal structure of the molybdenum cofactor biosynthesis protein MoaC. Structure 2000; 8(7):709–718
2. Food and Nutrition Board, Institute of Medicine. Molybdenum. In: Dietary Reference Intakes for Vitamin A, Vitamin K, Boron, Chromium, Copper, Iodine, Iron, Manganese, Molybdenum, Nickel, Silicon, Vanadium, and Zinc. Washington, DC: National Academy Press; 2001:420–441
3. Eckhert C. Other trace elements In: Shils ME, Shike M, Ross AC, Caballero B, Cousins RJ, eds. Modern Nutrition in Health and Disease. 10th ed. Philadelphia, PA: Lippincott Williams & Wilkins; 2006:338–350
4. Beedham C. Molybdenum hydroxylases as drug-metabolizing enzymes. Drug Metab Rev 1985;16(1-2): 119–156
5. Turnlund JR, Keyes WR. Dietary molybdenum: Effect on copper absorption, excretion, and status in young men. In: Roussel AM, ed. Trace Elements in Man and Animals. Vol 10. New York: Kluwer Academic Press; 2000:951–953
6. Abumrad NN, Schneider AJ, Steel D, Rogers LS. Amino acid intolerance during prolonged total parenteral nutrition reversed by molybdate therapy. Am J Clin Nutr 1981;34(11):2551–2559
7. Johnson JL, Duran M. Molybdenum cofactor deficiency and isolated sulfite deficiency. In: Scriver RC, ed. Metabolic and Molecular Bases of Inherited Disease. New York: McGraw-Hill; 2001:3163–3177
8. Turnlund JR, Keyes WR, Peiffer GL, Chiang G. Molybdenum absorption, excretion, and retention studied with stable isotopes in young men during depletion and repletion. Am J Clin Nutr 1995;61(5):1102–1109
9. Turnlund JR, Keyes WR, Peiffer GL. Molybdenum absorption, excretion, and retention studied with stable isotopes in young men at five intakes of dietary molybdenum. Am J Clin Nutr 1995;62(4):790–796
10. Blot WJ, Li JY, Taylor PR, et al. Nutrition intervention trials in Linxian, China: supplementation with specific vitamin/mineral combinations, cancer incidence, and disease-specific mortality in the general population. J Natl Cancer Inst 1993;85(18):1483–1492
11. Mills CF, Davis GK. Molybdenum. In: Mertz W, ed. Trace Elements in Human and Animal Nutrition. 5th ed. San Diego, CA: Academic Press; 1987:429–463
12. Hendler SS, Rorvik DR, eds. PDR for Nutritional Supplements. Montvale, NJ: Medical Economics Co., Inc.; 2001:308–311
13. Walravens PA, Moure-Eraso R, Solomons CC, Chappell WR, Bentley G. Biochemical abnormalities in workers exposed to molybdenum dust. Arch Environ Health 1979;34(5):302–308
14. Vyskocil A, Viau C. Assessment of molybdenum toxicity in humans. J Appl Toxicol 1999;19(3):185–192
15. Boles JW, Klaassen CD. Effects of molybdate and pentachlorophenol on the sulfation of acetaminophen. Toxicology 2000;146(1):23–35

23 Phosphorus

Phosphorus is an essential mineral that is required by every cell in the body for normal function.[1] Most of the phosphorus in the body is found as phosphate (PO_4^{3-}). Approximately 85% of the body's phosphorus is found in bone.[2]

Function

Phosphorus is a major structural component of bone in the form of a calcium phosphate salt called *hydroxyapatite*. Phospholipids (e.g., phosphatidylcholine) are major structural components of cell membranes. All energy production and storage are dependent on phosphorylated compounds, such as adenosine triphosphate (ATP) and creatine phosphate. Nucleic acids, which are responsible for the storage and transmission of genetic information, are long chains of phosphate-containing molecules. A number of enzymes, hormones, and cell-signaling molecules depend on phosphorylation for their activation. Phosphorus also helps to maintain normal acid–base balance (pH) by acting as one of the body's most important buffers. In addition, the phosphorus-containing molecule 2,3-diphosphoglycerate (2,3-DPG) binds to hemoglobin in red blood cells and affects oxygen delivery to the tissues of the body.[1]

Nutrient Interactions

Fructose. A study of 11 men found that a diet high in fructose (20% of total calories) resulted in increased urinary loss of phosphorus and a negative phosphorus balance (i.e., daily loss of phosphorus higher than daily intake). This effect was more pronounced when the diet was also low in magnesium.[3] A potential mechanism for this effect is the lack of feedback inhibition of the conversion of fructose to fructose 1-phosphate in the liver. In other words, fructose 1-phosphate accumulates in the cell but does not inhibit the enzyme that phosphorylates fructose, which consumes large amounts of phosphate. This phenomenon is known as *phosphate trapping*.[1] This

study's finding is relevant because fructose consumption in the United States has been increasing rapidly since the introduction of high fructose corn syrup in 1970, while magnesium intake has decreased over the past century.[3]

Calcium and vitamin D. Dietary phosphorus is readily absorbed in the small intestine, and any excess phosphorus absorbed is excreted by the kidneys. The regulation of blood calcium and phosphorus levels is interrelated through the actions of parathyroid hormone (PTH) and vitamin D (**Fig. 23.1**). A slight drop in blood calcium levels (e.g., in the case of inadequate calcium intake) is sensed by the parathyroid glands, resulting in their increased secretion of PTH. PTH stimulates conversion of vitamin D to its active form (calcitriol) in the kidneys. Increased calcitriol levels in turn result in increased intestinal absorption of both calcium and phosphorus. Both PTH and vitamin D stimulate bone resorption, resulting in the release of bone mineral (calcium and phosphate) into the blood. Although PTH stimulation causes decreased urinary excretion of calcium, it results in increased urinary excretion of phosphorus, which is advantageous in bringing blood calcium levels up to normal because high blood levels of phosphate suppress the conversion of vitamin D to its active form in the kidneys.[4]

Is high phosphorus intake detrimental to bone health? Some investigators are concerned about the increasing amounts of phosphates in the diet which can be attributed to phosphoric acid in soft drinks and phosphate additives in a number of commercially prepared foods.[5,6] As phosphorus is not as tightly regulated by the body as calcium, serum phosphate levels can rise slightly with a high phosphorus diet, especially after meals. High phosphate levels in the blood reduce the formation of the active form of vitamin D (calcitriol) in the kidneys, reduce blood calcium, and lead to increased PTH release by the parathyroid glands. However, high serum phosphorus levels also lead to decreased urinary calcium excretion.[2] If sustained, elevated PTH levels could

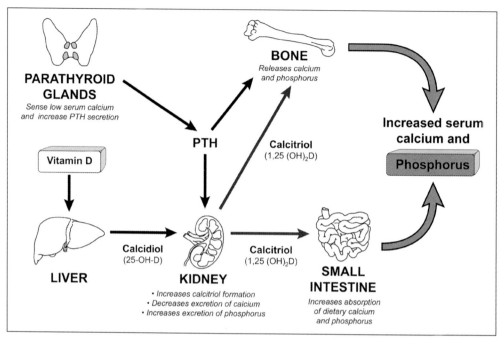

Fig. 23.1 Calcium and phosphorus homeostasis. Calcium-sensing proteins in the parathyroid glands sense serum calcium levels. In response to slight declines in serum calcium, the parathyroid glands secrete parathyroid hormone (PTH). PTH stimulates the activity of the 1-hydroxylase enzyme in the kidney, resulting in increased production of calcitriol, the biologically active form of vitamin D. Calcitriol activates the vitamin D-dependent transport system in the small intestine, increasing the absorption of dietary calcium and phosphorus. Calcitriol and PTH act on the skeleton to increase the mobilization of calcium and phosphorus into the circulation. In the kidneys, calcitriol and PTH increase calcium reabsorption and increase phosphorus excretion.

have an adverse effect on bone mineral content, but this effect has been observed only in humans on diets that were high in phosphorus and low in calcium. Moreover, similarly elevated PTH levels have been reported in diets that were low in calcium without being high in phosphorus.[7]

More recently, a controlled trial in young women found no adverse effects of a phosphorus-rich diet (3000 mg/day) on bone-related hormones and biochemical markers of bone resorption when dietary calcium intakes were maintained at almost 2000 mg/day.[8] At present, there is no convincing evidence that the dietary phosphorus levels experienced in the United States adversely affect bone mineral density. However, the substitution of phosphate-containing soft drinks and snack foods for milk and other calcium-rich foods does represent a serious risk to bone health.

Deficiency

Inadequate phosphorus intake results in abnormally low serum phosphate levels (hypophosphatemia). The effects of hypophosphatemia may include loss of appetite, anemia, muscle weakness, bone pain, rickets (in children), osteomalacia (in adults), increased susceptibility to infection, numbness and tingling of the extremities, and difficulty walking. Severe hypophosphatemia may result in death. Because phosphorus is so widespread in food, dietary phosphorus deficiency is usually seen only in cases of near-total starvation. Other individuals at risk of hypophosphatemia include people who abuse alcohol, those with diabetes recovering from an episode of diabetic ketoacidosis, and starving or anorexic patients on re-feeding regimens that are high in calories but too low in phosphorus.[1,2]

The Recommended Dietary Allowance

The recommended dietary allowance (RDA) for phosphorus was based on the maintenance of normal serum phosphate levels in adults, which was believed to represent adequate phosphorus intake to meet cellular and bone formation needs (**Table 23.1**).[2]

Sources

Food Sources

Phosphorus is found in most foods because it is a critical component of all living organisms. Dairy products, meat, and fish are particularly rich sources of phosphorus. Phosphorus is also a component of many polyphosphate food additives and is present in most soft drinks as phosphoric acid. Dietary phosphorus derived from food additives is not calculated in most food databases, so the total amount of phosphorus consumed by the average person in the United States is not entirely clear. A large survey of nutrient consumption in the United States found that the average phosphorus intake was 1495 mg/day in men and 1024 mg/day in women. The Food and Nutrition Board (FNB) of the Institute of Medicine estimates that phosphorus consumption in the United States has increased 10%–15% over the past 20 years.[2]

The phosphorus in all plant seeds (beans, peas, cereals, and nuts) is present in a storage form of phosphate called *phytic acid* or *phytate*. Only about 50% of the phosphorus from phytate is available to humans because we lack enzymes (phytases) that liberate phosphorus from phytate.[9] Yeasts possess phytases, so whole grains incorporated into leavened breads have more bioavailable phosphorus than whole grains incorporated into breakfast cereals or flat breads.[2] **Table 23.2** lists a number of phosphorus-rich foods along with their phosphorus content.

Supplements

Sodium phosphate and potassium phosphate salts are used for the treatment of hypophosphatemia, and their use requires medical supervision. Calcium phosphate salts are sometimes used as calcium supplements.[10]

Safety

Toxicity

The most serious adverse effect of abnormally elevated blood levels of phosphate (hyperphosphatemia) is the calcification of nonskeletal tissues, most commonly the kidneys. Such calcium phosphate deposition can lead to organ damage, especially kidney damage. Because the kidneys are very efficient at eliminating excess phosphate

Table 23.1 Recommended dietary allowance for phosphorus

Life stage	Age	Males (mg/day)	Females (mg/day)
Infants	0–6 months	100 (AI)	100 (AI)
Infants	7–12 months	275 (AI)	275 (AI)
Children	1–3 years	460	460
Children	4–8 years	500	500
Children	9–13 years	1250	1250
Adolescents	14–18 years	1250	1250
Adults	≥19 years	700	700
Pregnancy	≤18 years	–	1250
Pregnancy	≥19 years	–	700
Breast-feeding	≤18 years	–	1250
Breast-feeding	≥19 years	–	700

AI, adequate intake.

Table 23.2 Food sources of phosphorus

Food	Serving	Phosphorus (mg)
Yogurt, plain nonfat	8 ounces	385
Fish, salmon	3 ounces, cooked[a]	252
Milk, skimmed	8 ounces	247
Fish, halibut	3 ounces, cooked[a]	242
Lentils[b]	½ cup, cooked	178
Beef	3 ounces, cooked[a]	173
Turkey	3 ounces, cooked[a]	173
Chicken	3 ounces, cooked[a]	155
Almonds[b]	1 ounce (23 nuts)	134
Cheese, mozzarella; part skimmed	1 ounce	131
Peanuts[b]	1 ounce	107
Egg	1 large, cooked	104
Bread, whole-wheat	1 slice	57
Carbonated cola drink	12 ounces	40
Bread, enriched white	1 slice	25

[a]A 3-ounce serving of meat or fish is about the size of a deck of cards.
[b]Phosphorus from nuts, seeds, and grains is about 50% less bioavailable than phosphorus from other sources.[9]

from the circulation, hyperphosphatemia from dietary causes is usually a problem only in people with kidney failure (end-stage renal disease) or hypoparathyroidism. When kidney function is only 20% of normal, even typical levels of dietary phosphorus may lead to hyperphosphatemia. Pronounced hyperphosphatemia has also occurred due to increased intestinal absorption of phosphate salts taken by mouth as well as to colonic absorption of the phosphate salts in enemas.[1] To avoid the adverse effects of hyperphosphatemia, the FNB set a tolerable upper intake level (UL) for oral phosphorus intake (**Table 23.3**).[2] The lower UL for individuals aged over 70 years reflects the increased likelihood of impaired kidney function in elderly individuals. The UL does not apply to individuals with significantly impaired kidney function or other health conditions known to increase the risk of hyperphosphatemia.

Drug Interactions

Aluminum-containing antacids reduce the absorption of dietary phosphorus by forming aluminum phosphate, which is nonabsorbable. When consumed in high doses, aluminum-containing antacids can produce abnormally low blood phosphate levels (hypophosphatemia) as

well as aggravate phosphate deficiency due to other causes.[11] As little as 1 ounce (28 g) of aluminum hydroxide gel three times a day for several weeks can diminish serum phosphate levels and lead to increased urinary calcium loss.[12] Excessively high doses of calcitriol, the active form of vitamin D, or its analogs may result in hyperphosphatemia.[2]

Potassium supplements or potassium-sparing diuretics taken together with a phosphate may result in high blood levels of potassium (hyperkalemia). Hyperkalemia can be a serious problem, resulting in life-threatening heart rhythm abnor-

Table 23.3 Tolerable upper intake level (UL) for phosphorus

Life stage	Age	UL (g/day)
Infants	0–12 months	Not possible to establish[a]
Children	1–8 years	3
Children	9–13 years	4
Adolescents	14–18 years	4
Adults	19–70 years	4
Adults	>70 years	3
Pregnancy	–	3.5
Breast-feeding	–	4

[a]Source of intake should be from food and formula only.

malities (arrhythmias). People taking such a combination must inform their health-care provider and have their serum potassium levels checked regularly.[11]

LPI Recommendation

The Linus Pauling Institute supports the RDA for phosphorus (700 mg/day for adults). Although few multivitamin/mineral supplements contain more than 15% of the current RDA for phosphorus, a varied diet should easily provide adequate phosphorus for most people.

Older Adults

At present, there is no evidence that the phosphorus requirements of older adults differ from those of younger adults (700 mg/day). Although few multivitamin/mineral supplements contain more than 15% of the current RDA for phosphorus, a varied diet should easily provide adequate phosphorus for most people.

References

1. Knochel JP. Phosphorus. In: Shils ME, Shike M, Ross AC, Caballero B, Cousins RJ, eds. Modern Nutrition in Health and Disease. 10th ed. Baltimore, MD: Lippincott Williams & Wilkins; 2006:211–222
2. Food and Nutrition Board, Institute of Medicine. Phosphorus. In: Dietary Reference Intakes for Calcium, Phosphorus, Magnesium, Vitamin D, and Fluoride. Washington, DC: National Academy Press; 1997: 146–189
3. Milne DB, Nielsen FH. The interaction between dietary fructose and magnesium adversely affects macromineral homeostasis in men. J Am Coll Nutr 2000;19(1):31–37
4. Bringhurst FR, Demay MB, Kronenberg HM. Hormones and disorders of mineral metabolism. In: Wilson JD, Foster DW, Kronenberg HM, Larsen PR, eds. Williams Textbook of Endocrinology. 9th ed. Philadelphia, PA: WB Saunders Co.; 1998:1155–1210
5. Calvo MS, Park YK. Changing phosphorus content of the U.S. diet: potential for adverse effects on bone. J Nutr 1996;126(4, Suppl):1168S–1180S
6. Calvo MS. Dietary considerations to prevent loss of bone and renal function. Nutrition 2000;16(7-8): 564–566
7. Weaver CM, Heaney RP. Calcium. In: Shils M, Olson JA, Shike M, Ross AC, eds. Modern Nutrition in Health and Disease. 9th ed. Baltimore, MD: Lippincott Williams & Wilkins; 1999:141–155
8. Grimm M, Müller A, Hein G, Fünfstück R, Jahreis G. High phosphorus intake only slightly affects serum minerals, urinary pyridinium crosslinks and renal function in young women. Eur J Clin Nutr 2001;55(3): 153–161
9. National Research Council, Food and Nutrition Board. Recommended Dietary Allowances. 10th ed. Washington, DC: National Academy Press; 1989:184–187
10. Hendler SS, Rorvik DR, eds. PDR for Nutritional Supplements. Montvale, NJ: Medical Economics Co., Inc.; 2001
11. Minerals. Drug Facts and Comparisons, 54th ed. St. Louis: Facts and Comparisons; 2000:29
12. Knochel JP. Phosphorus. In: Shils M, Olson JA, Shike M, Ross AC, eds. Modern Nutrition in Health and Disease. 9th ed. Baltimore, MD: Lippincott Williams & Wilkins; 1999:157–167

24 Potassium

Potassium is an essential dietary mineral and electrolyte. The term *electrolyte* refers to a substance that dissociates into ions (charged particles) in solution, making it capable of conducting electricity. Normal body function depends on tight regulation of potassium concentrations both inside and outside cells.[1]

Function

Maintenance of Membrane Potential

Potassium is the principal positively charged ion (cation) in the fluid inside cells, whereas sodium is the principal cation in the fluid outside cells. Potassium concentrations are about 30 times higher inside than outside cells, whereas sodium concentrations are more than 10 times lower inside than outside cells. The concentration differences between potassium and sodium across cell membranes create an electrochemical gradient known as the *membrane potential*. A cell's membrane potential is maintained by ion pumps in the cell membrane, especially the Na$^+$/K$^+$ ATPase pumps. These pumps use ATP (energy) to pump sodium out of the cell in exchange for potassium (**Fig. 24.1**). Their activity has been estimated to account for 20%–40% of the resting energy expenditure in a typical adult. The large proportion of energy dedicated to maintaining sodium/potassium concentration gradients emphasizes the importance of this function in sustaining life. Tight control of cell membrane potential is critical for nerve impulse transmission, muscle contraction, and heart function.[2,3]

Cofactor for Enzymes

A limited number of enzymes require the presence of potassium for their activity. The activation of Na$^+$/K$^+$ ATPase requires the presence of sodium and potassium. The presence of potassium is also required for the activity of pyruvate kinase, an important enzyme in carbohydrate metabolism.[2]

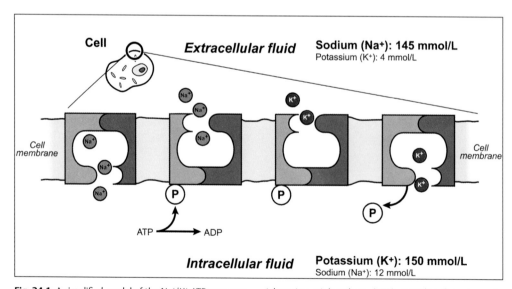

Fig. 24.1 A simplified model of the Na$^+$/K$^+$ ATPase pump. The concentration differences between potassium (K$^+$) and sodium (Na$^+$) across cell membranes create an electrochemical gradient known as the membrane potential. Adenosine triphosphate (ATP) provides the energy to pump three Na$^+$ ions out of the cell in exchange for two K$^+$ ions, thus maintaining the membrane potential.

Table 24.1 Adequate intake for potassium

Life stage	Age	Males (mg/day)	Females (mg/day)
Infants	0–6 months	400	400
Infants	7–12 months	700	700
Children	1–3 years	3000	3000
Children	4–8 years	3800	3800
Children	9–13 years	4500	4500
Adolescents	14–18 years	4700	4700
Adults	≥19 years	4700	4700
Pregnancy	All ages	–	4700
Breast-feeding	All ages	–	5100

Deficiency

An abnormally low plasma potassium concentration is referred to as *hypokalemia*. Hypokalemia is most commonly a result of excessive loss of potassium, e.g., from prolonged vomiting, the use of some diuretics, some forms of kidney disease, or metabolic disturbances. The symptoms of hypokalemia are related to alterations in membrane potential and cellular metabolism. They include fatigue, muscle weakness and cramps, and intestinal paralysis, which may lead to bloating, constipation, and abdominal pain. Severe hypokalemia may result in muscular paralysis or abnormal heart rhythms (cardiac arrhythmias) that can be fatal.[2,4]

Conditions that Increase the Risk of Hypokalemia

Conditions that increase the risk of hypokalemia include the following: the use of potassium-wasting diuretics (e.g., thiazide diuretics or furosemide), alcoholism, severe vomiting or diarrhea, overuse or abuse of laxatives, anorexia or bulimia nervosa, magnesium depletion, and congestive heart failure.[5]

In rare cases, habitual consumption of large amounts of black licorice has resulted in hypokalemia.[6,7] Licorice contains a compound (i.e., glycyrrhizic acid) with similar physiological effects to those of aldosterone, a hormone that increases urinary excretion of potassium. Low dietary intakes of potassium do not generally result in hypokalemia,[5] but research indicates that insufficient dietary potassium increases the risk of a number of chronic diseases.

Adequate Intake

In 2004, the Food and Nutrition Board (FNB) of the Institute of Medicine established an adequate intake (AI) for potassium based on intake levels that have been found to lower blood pressure, reduce salt sensitivity, and minimize the risk of kidney stones (**Table 24.1**).[4]

Disease Prevention

The diets of Western industrialized cultures are quite different from those of prehistoric cultures and the few remaining isolated primitive cultures. Among other differences, the daily intake of sodium chloride (salt) in Western industrialized cultures is about three times higher than the daily intake of potassium on a molar basis, whereas salt intake in primitive cultures is about seven times lower than potassium intake.[8] The relative deficiency of dietary potassium in the modern diet may play a role in the pathology of some chronic diseases.

Stroke

Several large epidemiological studies have suggested that increased potassium intake is associated with decreased risk of stroke. A prospective study of more than 43 000 men followed for 8 years found that men in the top quintile (one-fifth) of dietary potassium intake (median intake 4300 mg/day) were only 62% as likely to have a stroke as those in the lowest quintile of potassium intake (median intake 2400 mg/day).[9] The inverse association was especially high in men with hypertension. However, a similar prospective study of more than 85 000 women followed for 14 years found a much more modest association between potassium intake and the risk of stroke.[10] Another large study that followed more than 9000 people for an average of 16 years found that potassium intake was inversely related to stroke only in black men and men with hypertension.[11] However, black men and women reported significantly lower potassium intakes than white men and women (1606 mg/day vs. 2178 mg/day).

More recent data from the same population indicate that those with potassium intakes higher than 1352 mg/day were only 72% as likely to have a stroke as those with potassium intakes lower than 1352 mg/day.[12] A prospective study in 5600 men and women older than 65 years found that low potassium intake was associated with a significantly increased incidence of stroke in individuals not taking diuretics.[13] More recently, a prospective study in a cohort of 26 556 men who smoked reported that higher intake of potassium was associated with a nonsignificant reduction in risk of cerebral infarction.[14] Taken together, the epidemiological data suggest that a modest increase in fruit and vegetable intake (rich sources of dietary potassium), especially in those with hypertension and/or relatively low potassium intakes, could significantly reduce the risk of stroke.

Osteoporosis

At least four cross-sectional studies have reported significant positive associations between dietary potassium intake and bone mineral density (BMD) in populations of premenopausal, perimenopausal, and postmenopausal women as well as elderly men.[15–17] The average dietary potassium intakes of the study participants ranged from about 3000 mg/day to 3400 mg/day, whereas the highest potassium intakes exceeded 6000 mg/day and the lowest intakes ranged from 1400 mg/day to 1600 mg/day. In all of these studies, BMD was also positively and significantly associated with fruit and vegetable intake. One study that examined changes in BMD over time found that higher dietary potassium intakes (and fruit and vegetable intakes) were associated with significantly less decline in BMD at the hip in men, but not in women, over a 4-year period.[17] However, a prospective study that followed 266

elderly women found that women in the highest quartile (one-fourth) of potassium excretion had higher BMD measures after 5 years compared with women in the lowest quartile of potassium excretion,[18] suggesting that eating potassium-rich foods may help to prevent osteoporosis.

Potassium-rich foods, such as fruit and vegetables, are also rich in precursors to bicarbonate ions, which buffer acids in the body. The modern Western diet tends to be relatively low in sources of alkali (fruit and vegetables) and high in sources of acid (fish, meats, and cheeses). When the quantity of bicarbonate ions is insufficient to maintain normal pH, the body is capable of mobilizing alkaline calcium salts from bone in order to neutralize acids consumed in the diet and generated by metabolism.[19] Increased consumption of fruit and vegetables reduces the net acid content of the diet and may preserve calcium in bones, which might otherwise be mobilized to maintain normal pH. Support for this theory was provided by a study of 18 postmenopausal women, which found that potassium bicarbonate supplementation decreased urinary acid and calcium excretion, resulting in increased biomarkers of bone formation and decreased biomarkers of bone resorption.[20] Other studies have reported that short-term (3 months or less) supplementation with potassium citrate decreased urinary acid excretion and biomarkers of bone resorption in postmenopausal women[21] and also ameliorated the negative effects of a high-salt diet on bone metabolism.[22] However, a recent 2-year randomized controlled trial found that potassium citrate supplementation did not reduce bone turnover or increase BMD in postmenopausal women.[23] Overall, consumption of potassium-rich fruits and vegetables may improve BMD and help lower the risk of osteoporosis.

Kidney Stones

Abnormally high urinary calcium (hypercalciuria) increases the risk of developing kidney stones. In individuals with a history of developing calcium-containing kidney stones, increased dietary acid load was significantly associated with increased urinary calcium excretion.[24] Increasing dietary potassium (and alkali) intake, by increasing fruit and vegetable intake or by taking potassium bicarbonate supplements, has been found to decrease urinary calcium excretion. In addition, potassium deprivation has been found to increase urinary calcium excretion.[25,26] A large prospective study of more than 45 000 men followed for 4 years found that men whose potassium intake averaged more than 4042 mg/day were only half as likely to develop symptomatic kidney stones as men whose intake averaged less than 2895 mg/day.[27] A similar study that followed more than 90 000 women over a period of 12 years found that women in the highest quintile of potassium intake (averaging 3458 mg/day) were only 65% as likely to develop symptomatic kidney stones as women in the lowest quintile of potassium intake (averaging 2703 mg/day).[28] In both of these prospective studies, dietary potassium intake was derived almost entirely from potassium-rich food, such as fruit and vegetables.

Disease Treatment

Hypertension

A number of studies indicate that groups with relatively high dietary potassium intakes have lower blood pressures than comparable groups with relatively low potassium intakes.[29] Data on more than 17 000 adults who participated in the third National Health and Nutrition Examination Survey (NHANES III) indicated that higher dietary potassium intakes were associated with significantly lower blood pressures.[30] The results of the Dietary Approaches to Stop Hypertension (DASH) trial provided further support for the beneficial effects of a potassium-rich diet on blood pressure.[31] Compared with a control diet providing only 3.5 servings per day of fruit and vegetables and 1700 mg/day of potassium, consumption of a diet including 8.5 servings per day of fruit and vegetables and 4100 mg/day of potassium lowered blood pressure by an average of 2.8/1.1 mmHg (systolic BP/diastolic BP) in all subjects and by an average of 7.2/2.8 mm Hg in those with hypertension.

In 1997, a meta-analysis of 33 randomized controlled trials, including 2609 individuals, assessed the effects of increased potassium intake, mostly in the form of potassium chloride (KCl) supplements, on blood pressure.[32] Increased potassium intake (2300–3900 mg/day) resulted in slight but significant blood pressure reductions that averaged 1.8/1.0 mmHg in people with normal blood pressure and 4.4/2.5 mmHg in people

with hypertension. Subgroup analysis indicated that the blood pressure-lowering effect of potassium was more pronounced in individuals with higher salt intakes and in trials where black individuals made up a majority of the participants. A clinical trial in 150 Chinese men and women with borderline-to-mild hypertension found that moderate supplementation with 500 mg/day of potassium chloride for 12 weeks resulted in a significant 5 mmHg reduction in systolic BP compared with placebo; no changes in diastolic BP were observed in this study.[32] Similar to many Western diets, the customary diet of this population was high in sodium and low in potassium. A crossover trial in 14 hypertensive individuals reported that supplementation with potassium citrate was equally as effective in lowering blood pressure as potassium chloride.[33] A more recent crossover trial in 42 adults with mild, untreated high blood pressure compared the effects of supplemental potassium chloride or potassium bicarbonate with a placebo.[34] Supplementation with potassium chloride slightly decreased ambulatory systolic BP but had no effect on office systolic BP, whereas supplementation with potassium bicarbonate did not affect blood pressure measurements. Both supplements resulted in improved endothelial function and other cardiovascular benefits.[34] However, a crossover trial in 48 adults with early hypertension (defined as a diastolic BP of greater than 80 mmHg but less than 100 mmHg), who were not taking antihypertensive medication, reported that increased potassium intake through dietary or supplemental (potassium citrate) means did not improve blood pressure or vascular function.[35]

Thus, increasing potassium intake by consuming a diet rich in fruits and vegetables may help lower blood pressure and may have other health benefits. Supplemental potassium might help lower blood pressure in some individuals, but potassium supplements should only be used in consultation with a medical provider.

Sources

Food Sources

The richest sources of potassium are fruits and vegetables. A dietary survey in the United States indicated that the average dietary potassium intake is about 2300 mg/day for women and

Table 24.2 Food sources of potassium

Food	Serving	Potassium (mg)
Potato, baked with skin	1 medium	926
Plums, dried (prunes)	½ cup	637
Raisins	½ cup	598
Prune juice	6 fluid ounces	528
Lima beans, cooked	½ cup	485
Acorn squash, cooked	½ cup (cubed)	448
Banana	1 medium	422
Spinach, cooked	½ cup	420
Tomato juice	6 fluid ounces	417
Orange juice	6 fluid ounces	372
Artichoke, cooked	1 medium	343
Raisin bran cereal	1 cup	335–362
Molasses	1 tablespoon	293
Tomato	1 medium	292
Orange	1 medium	237
Sunflower seeds	1 ounce	241
Almonds	1 ounce	200

3100 mg/day for men.[30] The potassium content of some relatively potassium-rich foods is listed in **Table 24.2**.[36]

Supplements

Multivitamin/mineral supplements in the United States do not contain more than 99 mg potassium per serving. Higher doses of supplemental potassium are generally prescribed to prevent and treat potassium depletion and hypokalemia. The use of more potent potassium supplements in potassium deficiency requires close monitoring of serum potassium concentrations. Potassium supplements are available as a number of different salts, including potassium chloride, citrate, gluconate, bicarbonate, aspartate, and orotate.[37] As a result of the potential for serious side effects, the decision to use a potent potassium supplement should be made in collaboration with a health-care provider.

Safety

Toxicity (Excess)

Abnormally elevated serum potassium concentrations are referred to as hyperkalemia. Hyperkalemia occurs when potassium intake exceeds the capacity of the kidneys to eliminate it. Acute or chronic renal (kidney) failure, the use of potassium-sparing diuretics, and insufficient aldosterone secretion (hypoaldosteronism) may result in the accumulation of excess potassium due to decreased urinary potassium excretion. Oral doses greater than 18 g taken at one time in individuals not accustomed to high intakes may lead to severe hyperkalemia, even in those with normal kidney function.[4] Hyperkalemia may also result from a shift of intracellular potassium into the circulation, which may occur with the rupture of red blood cells (hemolysis) or tissue damage (e.g., trauma or severe burns). Symptoms of hyperkalemia may include tingling of the hands and feet, muscular weakness, and temporary paralysis. The most serious complication of hyperkalemia is the development of an abnormal heart rhythm (cardiac arrhythmia), which can lead to cardiac arrest.[38] The FNB did not set a tolerable upper intake level (UL) for potassium because adverse effects from high dietary intakes of potassium have not been reported in healthy individuals.[4]

Adverse Reactions to Potassium Supplements

Gastrointestinal symptoms are the most common side effects of potassium supplements, including nausea, vomiting, abdominal discomfort, and diarrhea. Intestinal ulceration has been reported after the use of enteric-coated potassium chloride tablets. Taking potassium with meals or taking a microencapsulated form of potassium may reduce gastrointestinal side effects. The most serious adverse reaction to potassium supplementation is hyperkalemia. Individuals with abnormal kidney function and those on potassium-sparing medications should be monitored closely to prevent hyperkalemia.[5,37]

Table 24.3 Medications associated with hyperkalemia[27]

Medication family	Specific medications
Potassium-sparing agents	Spironolactone, triamterene, amiloride
Angiotensin-converting enzyme inhibitors	Captopril, enalapril, fosinopril
Nonsteroidal anti-inflammatory agents	Indometacin, ibuprofen, ketorolac
Anti-infective agents	Trimethoprim–sulfamethoxazole, pentamidine
Anticoagulant	Heparin
Cardiac glycoside	Digitalis
Antihypertensive agents	β-Blockers and α-blockers
Angiotensin receptor blockers	Losartan, valsartan, irbesartan, candesartan

Table 24.4 Medications associated with hypokalemia[5]

Medication family	Specific medications
β-Adrenergic agonists	Epinephrine
Decongestants	Pseudoephedrine, phenylpropanolamine
Bronchodilators	Albuterol, terbutaline, pirbuterol, isoetharine, fenoterol, ephedrine, isoproterenol, metaproterenol, theophylline
Tocolytic (labor-suppressing) agents	Ritodrine, buphenin
Diuretics	Acetazolamide, thiazides, chlorthalidone, indapamide, metolazone, quinethazone, bumetanide, ethacrynic acid, furosemide, torsemide
Mineralocorticoids	Fludrocortisone
Substances with mineralocorticoid effects	Licorice, carbenoxolone, gossypol
High-dose glucocorticoids	
High-dose antibiotics	Penicillin, nafcillin, carbenicillin
Other	Caffeine, sodium polystyrene sulfonate

Drug Interactions

The classes of medication listed in **Table 24.3** are known to increase the risk of hyperkalemia (elevated serum potassium);[38] individuals are encouraged to consult their physicians regarding any dietary restriction that may apply when taking such medications. Medications that are known to increase the risk of hypokalemia (low serum potassium) are listed in **Table 24.4**.[5]

LPI Recommendation

There is considerable evidence that a diet supplying at least 4.7 g/day of potassium is associated with a decreased risk of stroke, hypertension, osteoporosis, and kidney stones. Fruit and vegetables are among the richest sources of dietary potassium, and a large body of evidence supports the association of increased fruit and vegetable intakes with reduced risk of cardiovascular disease.[39,40] Consequently, the Linus Pauling Institute recommends increasing potassium intake to at least 4.7 g/day by increasing consumption of potassium-rich foods, especially fruit, vegetables, and nuts.

Older Adults

A diet supplying at least 4.7 g/day of potassium is also appropriate for healthy older adults because such diets are associated with decreased risk of stroke, hypertension, osteoporosis, and kidney stones. This recommendation does not apply to individuals who have been advised to limit potassium consumption by a health-care professional.

References

1. Peterson LN. Potassium in nutrition. In: O'Dell BL, Sunde RA, eds. Handbook of Nutritionally Essential Minerals. New York: Marcel Dekker, Inc.; 1997: 153–183
2. Sheng H-W. Sodium, chloride and potassium. In: Stipanuk M, ed. Biochemical and Physiological Aspects of Human Nutrition. Philadelphia, PA: WB Saunders Co.; 2000:686–710
3. Brody T. Nutritional Biochemistry. 2nd ed. San Diego, CA: Academic Press; 1999
4. Food and Nutrition Board, Institute of Medicine. Potassium. In: Dietary Reference Intakes for Water, Potassium, Sodium, Chloride, and Sulfate. Washington, DC: National Academies Press; 2005:186–268
5. Gennari FJ. Hypokalemia. N Engl J Med 1998;339(7): 451–458
6. Walker BR, Edwards CR. Licorice-induced hypertension and syndromes of apparent mineralcorticoid excess. Endocrin Metab Clin North Am 1994;23(2):359–377
7. Mumoli N, Cei M. Licorice-induced hypokalemia. Int J Cardiol 2008;124(3):e42–44
8. Young DB, Lin H, McCabe RD. Potassium's cardiovascular protective mechanisms. Am J Physiol 1995;268 (4 Pt 2):R825–837
9. Ascherio A, Rimm EB, Hernan MA, et al. Intake of potassium, magnesium, calcium, and fiber and risk of

stroke among US men. Circulation 1998;98(12): 1198–1204

10. Iso H, Stampfer MJ, Manson JE, et al. Prospective study of calcium, potassium, and magnesium intake and risk of stroke in women. Stroke 1999;30(9):1772–1779

11. Fang J, Madhavan S, Alderman MH. Dietary potassium intake and stroke mortality. Stroke 2000;31(7): 1532–1537

12. Bazzano LA, He J, Ogden LG, et al. Dietary potassium intake and risk of stroke in US men and women: National Health and Nutrition Examination Survey I epidemiologic follow-up study. Stroke 2001;32(7): 1473–1480

13. Green DM, Ropper AH, Kronmal RA, Psaty BM, Burke GL; Cardiovascular Health Study. Serum potassium level and dietary potassium intake as risk factors for stroke. Neurology 2002;59(3):314–320

14. Larsson SC, Virtanen MJ, Mars M, et al. Magnesium, calcium, potassium, and sodium intakes and risk of stroke in male smokers. Arch Intern Med 2008;168(5): 459–465

15. New SA, Bolton-Smith C, Grubb DA, Reid DM. Nutritional influences on bone mineral density: a cross-sectional study in premenopausal women. Am J Clin Nutr 1997;65(6):1831–1839

16. New SA, Robins SP, Campbell MK, et al. Dietary influences on bone mass and bone metabolism: further evidence of a positive link between fruit and vegetable consumption and bone health? Am J Clin Nutr 2000;71(1):142–151

17. Tucker KL, Hannan MT, Chen H, Cupples LA, Wilson PW, Kiel DP. Potassium, magnesium, and fruit and vegetable intakes are associated with greater bone mineral density in elderly men and women. Am J Clin Nutr 1999;69(4):727–736

18. Zhu K, Devine A, Prince RL. The effects of high potassium consumption on bone mineral density in a prospective cohort study of elderly postmenopausal women. Osteoporos Int 2009;20(2):335–340

19. Morris RC, Frassetto LA, Schmidlin O, Forman A, Sebastian A. Expression of osteoporosis as determined by diet-disordered electrolyte and acid-base metabolism. In: Burkhardt P, Dawson-Hughes B, Heaney R, eds. Nutritional Aspects of Osteoporosis. San Diego, CA: Academic Press; 2001:357–378

20. Sebastian A, Harris ST, Ottaway JH, Todd KM, Morris RC Jr. Improved mineral balance and skeletal metabolism in postmenopausal women treated with potassium bicarbonate. N Engl J Med 1994;330(25): 1776–1781

21. Marangella M, Di Stefano M, Casalis S, Berutti S, D'Amelio P, Isaia GC. Effects of potassium citrate supplementation on bone metabolism. Calcif Tissue Int 2004;74(4):330–335

22. Sellmeyer DE, Schloetter M, Sebastian A. Potassium citrate prevents increased urine calcium excretion and bone resorption induced by a high sodium chloride diet. J Clin Endocrinol Metab 2002;87(5):2008–2012

23. Macdonald HM, Black AJ, Aucott L, et al. Effect of potassium citrate supplementation or increased fruit and vegetable intake on bone metabolism in healthy postmenopausal women: a randomized controlled trial. Am J Clin Nutr 2008;88(2):465–474

24. Trinchieri A, Zanetti G, Currò A, Lizzano R. Effect of potential renal acid load of foods on calcium metabolism of renal calcium stone formers. Eur Urol 2001; 39(Suppl 2):33–36, discussion 36–37

25. Lemann J Jr, Pleuss JA, Gray RW. Potassium causes calcium retention in healthy adults. J Nutr 1993;123(9): 1623–1626

26. Morris RC Jr, Schmidlin O, Tanaka M, Forman A, Frassetto L, Sebastian A. Differing effects of supplemental KCl and KHCO3: pathophysiological and clinical implications. Semin Nephrol 1999;19(5):487–493

27. Curhan GC, Willett WC, Rimm EB, Stampfer MJ. A prospective study of dietary calcium and other nutrients and the risk of symptomatic kidney stones. N Engl J Med 1993;328(12):833–838

28. Curhan GC, Willett WC, Speizer FE, Spiegelman D, Stampfer MJ. Comparison of dietary calcium with supplemental calcium and other nutrients as factors affecting the risk for kidney stones in women. Ann Intern Med 1997;126(7):497–504

29. Barri YM, Wingo CS. The effects of potassium depletion and supplementation on blood pressure: a clinical review. Am J Med Sci 1997;314(1):37–40

30. Hajjar IM, Grim CE, George V, Kotchen TA. Impact of diet on blood pressure and age-related changes in blood pressure in the US population: analysis of NHANES III. Arch Intern Med 2001;161(4):589–593

31. Appel LJ, Moore TJ, Obarzanek E, et al; DASH Collaborative Research Group. A clinical trial of the effects of dietary patterns on blood pressure. N Engl J Med 1997;336(16):1117–1124

32. Whelton PK, He J, Cutler JA, et al. Effects of oral potassium on blood pressure. Meta-analysis of randomized controlled clinical trials. JAMA 1997;277(20): 1624–1632

33. He FJ, Markandu ND, Coltart R, Barron J, MacGregor GA. Effect of short-term supplementation of potassium chloride and potassium citrate on blood pressure in hypertensives. Hypertension 2005;45(4):571–574

34. He FJ, Marciniak M, Carney C, et al. Effects of potassium chloride and potassium bicarbonate on endothelial function, cardiovascular risk factors, and bone turnover in mild hypertensives. Hypertension 2010;55(3):681–688

35. Berry SE, Mulla UZ, Chowienczyk PJ, Sanders TA. Increased potassium intake from fruit and vegetables or supplements does not lower blood pressure or improve vascular function in UK men and women with early hypertension: a randomised controlled trial. Br J Nutr 2010:1–9

36. U.S. Department of Agriculture, Agricultural Research Service. USDA National Nutrient Database for Standard Reference, Release 22. 2009. Available at: http://www.nal.usda.gov/fnic/foodcomp/search/. Accessed 15 March 2010

37. Hendler SS, Rorvik DR, eds. PDR for Nutritional Supplements. Montvale, NJ: Medical Economics Company, Inc; 2001

38. Mandal AK. Hypokalemia and hyperkalemia. Med Clin North Am 1997;81(3):611–639

39. Liu S, Manson JE, Lee IM, et al. Fruit and vegetable intake and risk of cardiovascular disease: the Women's Health Study. Am J Clin Nutr 2000;72(4):922–928

40. Joshipura KJ, Ascherio A, Manson JE, et al. Fruit and vegetable intake in relation to risk of ischemic stroke. JAMA 1999;282(13):1233–1239

25 Selenium

Selenium is a trace element that is essential in small amounts, but like all essential elements, it is toxic at high levels. Humans and animals require selenium for the function of a number of selenium-dependent enzymes, also known as *selenoproteins*. During selenoprotein synthesis, selenocysteine is incorporated into a very specific location in the amino acid sequence in order to form a functional protein. Unlike animals, plants do not appear to require selenium for survival. However, when selenium is present in the soil, plants incorporate it nonspecifically into compounds that usually contain sulfur.[1]

Function

Selenoproteins

At least 25 selenoproteins have been identified, but the metabolic functions have been identified for only about half of them.[2]

Glutathione peroxidases. Five selenium-containing glutathione peroxidases have been identified: cellular or classic peroxidase (GPx), plasma or extracellular GPx, phospholipid hydroperoxide GPx, gastrointestinal GPx, and olfactory GPx.[2] Although each GPx is a distinct selenoprotein, they are all antioxidant enzymes that reduce potentially damaging reactive oxygen species (ROS), such as hydrogen peroxide and lipid hydroperoxides, to produce harmless products such as water and alcohols by coupling their reduction with the oxidation of glutathione (**Fig. 25.1**). Sperm mitochondrial capsule selenoprotein, an antioxidant enzyme that protects developing sperm from oxidative damage and later forms a structural protein required by mature sperm, was once thought to be a distinct selenoprotein but now appears to be phospholipid hydroperoxide GPx.[3]

Thioredoxin reductase. Together with the compound thioredoxin, thioredoxin reductase participates in the regeneration of several antioxidants, possibly including vitamin C. Maintenance of thioredoxin in a reduced form by thioredoxin reductase is important for regulating cell growth and viability.[2,4]

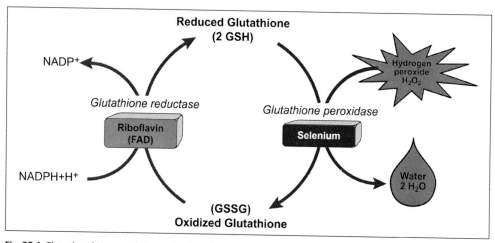

Fig. 25.1 The glutathione oxidation–reduction (redox) cycle. One molecule of hydrogen peroxide is reduced to two molecules of water, while two molecules of glutathione (GSH) are oxidized in a reaction catalyzed by the sele-noenzyme, glutathione peroxidase. Oxidized glutathione may be reduced by the flavin adenine dinucleotide (FAD)-dependent enzyme, glutathione reductase.

Iodothyronine deiodinases (thyroid hormone deiodinases). The thyroid gland releases very small amounts of biologically active thyroid hormone (triiodothyronine or T_3) and larger amounts of an inactive form of thyroid hormone (thyroxine or T_4) into the circulation. Most of the biologically active T_3 in the circulation and inside cells is created by the removal of one iodine atom from T_4 in a reaction catalyzed by selenium-dependent iodothyronine deiodinases. Three different selenium-dependent iodothyronine deiodinases (types I, II, and III) can both activate and inactivate thyroid hormone by acting on T_3, T_4, or other thyroid hormone metabolites. Thus, selenium is an essential element for normal development, growth, and metabolism because of its role in the regulation of thyroid hormones.[2,5]

Selenoprotein P. Selenoprotein P is found in plasma and also associated with vascular endothelial cells (cells that line the inner walls of blood vessels). The primary function of selenoprotein P appears to be a transport protein for selenium.[6] It also functions as an antioxidant that protects endothelial cells from damage induced by such compounds as peroxynitrite, a reactive nitrogen species.[7]

Selenoprotein W. Selenoprotein W is found in muscle. Although its function is currently unknown, it is thought to play a role in muscle metabolism.[8] There is about 80% homology of this selenoprotein from six different species of animals.[9]

Selenophosphate synthetase. Incorporation of selenocysteine into selenoproteins is directed by the genetic code and requires the enzyme selenophosphate synthetase. A selenoprotein itself, selenophosphate synthetase catalyzes the synthesis of monoselenium phosphate, a precursor of selenocysteine that is required for the synthesis of selenoproteins.[2]

Methionine-*R*-sulfoxide reductase. Methionine-*R*-sulfoxide reductase was initially identified as selenoprotein R and selenoprotein X by two different laboratories. However, later studies revealed that the protein catalyzes stereospecific reduction of oxidized methionine residues in reactions that use thioredoxin as a reducing agent.

There are two forms of this specific selenoprotein.[2]

Sep15 (15-kDA selenoprotein). Sep15 is mammalian protein located in the endoplasmic reticulum of the cell. Here, it binds uridyl diphosphate (UDP)-glucose:glycoprotein glucosyltransferase, an enzyme that senses protein folding. Sep15 has a redox function and is also implicated in cancer prevention.[2]

Selenoprotein V. Selenoprotein V is expressed exclusively in testes and is thought to function in spermatogenesis.[2]

Selenoprotein S. Selenoprotein S is involved in retrotranslocation of misfolded proteins from the endoplasmic reticulum to the cytosol. This protein may also be involved in inflammatory and immune responses.[2]

Nutrient Interactions

Antioxidant nutrients. As an integral part of the glutathione GPxs and thioredoxin reductase, selenium interacts with nutrients that affect cellular redox status (i.e., prooxidant/antioxidant balance). Other minerals that are critical components of antioxidant enzymes include copper (as superoxide dismutase), zinc (as superoxide dismutase), and iron (as catalase). Selenium as GPx also appears to support the activity of vitamin E (α-tocopherol) in limiting the oxidation of lipids. Animal studies indicate that selenium and vitamin E tend to spare each other and that selenium can prevent some of the damage resulting from vitamin E deficiency in models of oxidative stress.[10] Further, thioredoxin reductase maintains the antioxidant function of vitamin C by catalyzing its regeneration from its oxidized form, dehydroascorbic acid.[6]

Iodine. Selenium deficiency may exacerbate the effects of iodine deficiency. Iodine is essential for the synthesis of thyroid hormone; however, the *iodothyronine deiodinases* are also required for the conversion of T_4 to the biologically active thyroid hormone T_3. Selenium supplementation in a small group of elderly individuals decreased plasma T_4, indicating increased deiodinase activity and thus increased conversion of T_4 to T_3.[1]

Deficiency

Insufficient selenium intake results in decreased activity of the GPx enzymes, as well as some other thioredoxin reductase and thyroid deiodinases. Even when severe, isolated selenium deficiency does not usually result in obvious clinical illness. However, selenium-deficient individuals appear to be more susceptible to additional physiological stresses.[11]

Individuals at Increased Risk of Selenium Deficiency

Clinical selenium deficiency has been observed in chronically ill patients who were receiving total parenteral nutrition (TPN) without added selenium for prolonged periods of time. Muscular weakness, muscle wasting, and cardiomyopathy (inflammation and damage to the heart muscle) have been observed in these patients. TPN solutions are now supplemented with selenium to prevent such problems. People who have had a large portion of the small intestine surgically removed or those with severe gastrointestinal problems, such as Crohn disease, are also at risk for selenium deficiency due to impaired absorption. Specialized medical diets used to treat metabolic disorders, such as phenylketonuria, are often low in selenium. Specialized diets that are to be used exclusively over long periods of time should have their selenium content assessed to determine the need for selenium supplementation.[11]

Keshan Disease

Keshan disease is a cardiomyopathy that affects young women and children in a selenium-deficient region of China. The acute form of the disease is characterized by the sudden onset of cardiac insufficiency, whereas the chronic form results in moderate-to-severe heart enlargement with varying degrees of cardiac insufficiency. The incidence of Keshan disease is closely associated with very low dietary intakes of selenium and poor selenium nutritional status. Selenium supplementation protects people from developing Keshan disease but cannot reverse heart muscle damage once it occurs.[11,12] Despite the strong evidence that selenium deficiency is a fundamental factor in the etiology of Keshan disease, the seasonal and annual variation in its occurrence suggests that an infectious agent is involved in addition to selenium deficiency. Coxsackievirus is one virus type that has been isolated from Keshan disease patients, and studies in selenium-deficient mice show that this virus is capable of causing an inflammation of the heart called *myocarditis*. Studies in mice also indicate that oxidative stress induced by selenium deficiency results in changes in the viral genome; such genomic changes are capable of converting a relatively harmless viral strain to a myocarditis-causing strain.[13,14] Although not proven in Keshan disease, selenium deficiency may result in a more virulent strain of virus with the potential to invade and damage the heart muscle.

Kashin–Beck Disease

Kashin–Beck disease is characterized by the degeneration of articular cartilage between joints (osteoarthritis) and is associated with poor selenium status in areas of northern China, North Korea, and eastern Siberia. The disease affects children between the ages of 5 and 13 years. Severe forms of the disease may result in joint deformities and dwarfism. Unlike Keshan disease, there is little evidence that improving selenium nutritional status prevents Kashin–Beck disease. Thus, the role of selenium deficiency in the etiology of Kashin–Beck disease is less certain. A number of other causative factors have been suggested for Kashin–Beck disease, including fungal toxins in grain, iodine deficiency, and contaminated drinking water.[11,12]

Recommended Dietary Allowance

The recommended dietary allowance (RDA) was revised in 2000 by the Food and Nutrition Board (FNB) of the Institute of Medicine. The most recent RDA is based on the amount of dietary selenium required to maximize the activity of GPx in plasma (**Table 25.1**).[15]

Table 25.1 Recommended dietary allowance for selenium

Life stage	Age	Males (µg/day)	Females (µg/day)
Infants	0–6 months	15 (AI)	15 (AI)
Infants	7–12 months	20 (AI)	20 (AI)
Children	1–3 years	20	20
Children	4–8 years	30	30
Children	9–13 years	40	40
Adolescents	14–18 years	55	55
Adults	≥19 years	55	55
Pregnancy	All ages	–	60
Breast-feeding	All ages	–	70

AI, adequate intake.

Disease Prevention

Immune Function

Selenium deficiency has been associated with impaired function of the immune system.[16] Moreover, selenium supplementation in individuals who are not overtly selenium deficient appears to stimulate the immune response. In two small studies, healthy[17,18] and immunosuppressed individuals[19] supplemented with 200 µg/day of selenium as sodium selenite for 8 weeks showed an enhanced immune cell response to foreign antigens compared with those taking a placebo. A considerable amount of basic research also indicates that selenium plays a role in regulating the expression of cell-signaling molecules called *cytokines*, which orchestrate the immune response.[20]

Viral Infection

Selenium deficiency appears to enhance the virulence or progression of some viral infections. The increased oxidative stress resulting from selenium deficiency may induce mutations or changes in the expression of some viral genes. When selenium-deficient mice are inoculated with a relatively harmless strain of Coxsackievirus, mutations occur in the viral genome that result in a more virulent form of the virus, which causes an inflammation of the heart muscle known as *myocarditis*. Once mutated, this form of the virus also causes myocarditis in mice that are not selenium deficient, demonstrating that the increased virulence is due to a change in the virus rather than the effects of selenium deficiency on the host immune system. A study in mice that lack cellular (classic) GPx-1 (knockout mice) demonstrated that cellular GPx provides protection against myocarditis resulting from mutations in the genome of a previously benign virus. Selenium deficiency results in decreased activity of GPx, increasing oxidative damage and the likelihood of mutations in the viral genome. Coxsackievirus has been isolated from the blood of some sufferers of Keshan disease, suggesting that it may be a cofactor in the development of the cardiomyopathy associated with selenium deficiency in humans.[21]

Cancer

Animal studies. There is a great deal of evidence indicating that selenium supplementation at high levels reduces the incidence of cancer in animals. More than two-thirds of over 100 published studies in 20 different animal models of spontaneous, viral, and chemically induced cancers found that selenium supplementation significantly reduces tumor incidence.[22] The evidence indicates that the methylated forms of selenium are the active species against tumors, and these methylated selenium compounds are produced at the greatest amounts with excess selenium intakes.[23] The relationships of selenium intake to cancer in humans and selenium status to tumor incidence in animals have been summarized.[24]

Epidemiological studies. Geographic studies have consistently observed higher cancer mortality rates in populations living in areas with low soil selenium and relatively low dietary selenium intakes. Results of epidemiological studies of cancer incidence in groups with less variable selenium intakes have been less consistent, but such studies also show a trend for individuals with lower selenium levels (blood and nails) to have a higher incidence of several different types of cancer. However, this trend is less pronounced in women, and a prospective study of more than 60 000 female nurses in the United States found no association between toenail selenium levels and total cancer risk.[25]

Hepatitis infection and cigarette smoking are known to increase one's risk for various types of cancer, and low dietary selenium intake may heighten cancer risk. Chronic infection with viral hepatitis B or C significantly increases risk of liver cancer. In a study of Taiwanese men with chronic viral hepatitis B or C infection, low plasma selenium concentrations were associated with an even greater risk of liver cancer; the inverse association between selenium levels and liver cancer was stronger in cigarette smokers and in those with lower plasma levels of vitamin A and certain carotenoids.[26] A case–control study within a prospective study of over 9000 Finnish men and women examined serum selenium levels in 95 individuals subsequently diagnosed with lung cancer and 190 matched controls.[27] Lower serum selenium levels were associated with an increased risk of lung cancer, and the association was more pronounced in those who smoked. In this Finnish population, selenium levels were only about 60% of the level commonly observed in other Western countries. Results of a meta-analysis of 16 studies suggest that selenium may protect against lung cancer. In this analysis, a significantly lower risk (54% reduction) of lung cancer was found when studies assessing selenium exposure by toenail selenium content were pooled. A nonsignificant decrease (20% reduction) in lung cancer risk was found when studies assessing selenium status by serum levels were collectively analyzed.[28]

Some studies have reported that low dietary selenium intakes are associated with increased risk of prostate cancer. A case–control study within a prospective study of over 50 000 male health professionals in the United States found a significant inverse relationship between toenail selenium content and the risk of prostate cancer; 181 men diagnosed with advanced prostate cancer and 181 matched controls were included in this study.[29] In this study, individuals whose toenail selenium content was consistent with an average dietary intake of 159 µg/day of selenium had a 65% lower risk of advanced prostate cancer compared with those with toenail selenium content consistent with an average intake of 86 µg/day. Within a prospective study of more than 9000 Japanese–American men, a case–control study that examined 249 confirmed cases of prostate cancer and 249 matched controls found the risk of developing prostate cancer was 50% less in men with serum selenium levels in the highest quartile (one-fourth) compared with those in the lowest quartile.[30] A case–control study found that men with prediagnostic plasma selenium levels in the lowest quartile were four to five times more likely to develop prostate cancer than those in the highest quartile.[31]

A case–control study that compared 724 prostate cancer cases with 879 matched controls reported that serum selenium levels were not associated with prostate cancer.[32] In contrast, one of the largest case–control studies to date found a significant inverse association between toenail selenium and the risk of colon cancer, but no associations between toenail selenium and the risk of breast cancer or prostate cancer were observed.[33] A meta-analysis of 20 epidemiological studies, mainly case–control studies, found that selenium levels in the serum or toenails were significantly lower in those with prostate cancer.[34] However, a recent prospective study in a cohort of over 295 000 men reported that frequent multivitamin use (more than seven times a week) and use of selenium supplements, together, was associated with significant increases in advanced and fatal prostate cancer.[35] Clearly, more prospective studies as well as clinical trials are needed to understand whether selenium status is linked to prostate cancer.

Human intervention trials. An intervention trial of selenium supplementation was undertaken among a general population of 130 471 individuals in five townships of Quidong, China, a high-risk area for viral hepatitis B infection and liver cancer. This trial provided table salt enriched with sodium selenite to the population of one township (20 847 people), using the other four townships as controls. During an 8-year follow-up period, the average incidence of liver cancer was reduced by 35% in the selenium-enriched population, while no reduction was found in the control populations. In a clinical trial in the same region, 226 individuals with evidence of chronic hepatitis B infection were supplemented with either 200 µg selenium in the form of a selenium-enriched yeast tablet or a placebo yeast tablet daily. During the 4-year follow-up period, seven of 113 individuals on the placebo developed primary liver cancer, whereas none of the 113 individuals supplemented with selenium developed liver cancer.[36]

In the United States, a double-blind, placebo-controlled study of more than 1300 older adults with a history of nonmelanoma skin cancer found that supplementation with 200 µg/day of selenium-enriched yeast for an average of 7.4 years was associated with a 49% decrease in prostate cancer incidence in men.[37] The protective effect of selenium supplementation was greatest in men with lower baseline plasma selenium and prostate-specific antigen levels. Surprisingly, the most recent results from this study indicate that selenium supplementation increased the risk of one type of skin cancer (squamous cell carcinoma) by 25%,[38] but did not significantly decrease the risk of lung cancer.[39] Although selenium supplementation shows promise for the prevention of prostate cancer, its effects on the risk for other types of cancer are unclear. In response to the need to confirm these findings, several large placebo-controlled trials designed to further investigate the role of selenium supplementation in prostate cancer prevention are currently under way.[24,40,41] However, a large, randomized, placebo-controlled intervention study using selenium and vitamin E supplementation (i.e., the Selenium and Vitamin E Cancer Prevention Trial or SELECT study) was recently halted because there was no evidence of benefit in preventing prostate cancer.[42] After 5.5 years of follow-up in the SELECT study, selenium supplementation (200 µg/day), alone or when co-supplemented with vitamin E, did not alter the risk for prostate, lung, or colorectal cancer.[67]

Possible mechanisms. Several mechanisms have been proposed for the cancer prevention effects of selenium:

- maximizing the activity of antioxidant selenoenzymes and improving antioxidant status
- improving immune system function
- affecting the metabolism of carcinogens
- increasing the levels of selenium metabolites that inhibit tumor cell growth
- influence of selenium on apoptosis
- influence of selenium on DNA repair
- selenium as an antiangiogenic agent

A two-stage model has been proposed to explain the different anticarcinogenic activities of selenium at different doses. At nutritional or physiological doses (about 40–100 µg/day in adults), selenium maximizes antioxidant selenoenzyme activity, probably enhances immune system function, and may affect carcinogen metabolism. At supranutritional or pharmacological levels (approximately 200–300 µg/day in adults), the formation of selenium metabolites, especially methylated forms of selenium, may also exert anticarcinogenic effects.[22,23]

Cardiovascular Diseases

Theoretically, optimizing selenoenzyme activity could decrease the risk of cardiovascular disease by decreasing lipid peroxidation and influencing the metabolism of cell-signaling molecules known as *prostaglandins*. However, prospective studies in humans have not demonstrated strong support for the cardioprotective effects of selenium. Although one study found a significant increase in illness and death from cardiovascular disease in individuals with serum selenium levels below 45 µg/L compared to matched pairs with levels above 45 µg/L,[43] another study, using the same cutoff points for serum selenium, found a significant difference only in deaths from stroke.[44] One study in middle-aged and elderly Danish men found an increased risk of cardiovascular disease in men with serum selenium levels below 79 µg/L,[45] but several other studies found no clear inverse association between selenium nutritional status and cardiovascular disease risk.[46] In a multicenter study in Europe, toenail selenium levels and risk of myocardial infarction (heart attack) were associated in the center only where selenium levels were the lowest.[47] Although some epidemiological evidence suggests that low levels of selenium (lower than those commonly found in the United States) may increase the risk of cardiovascular diseases, definitive evidence about the role of selenium in preventing cardiovascular diseases will require controlled clinical trials.

Type 2 Diabetes Mellitus

Only a few studies have examined whether selenium status influences risk for type 2 diabetes mellitus and the results are conflicting. One study found lower toenail selenium levels in men with type 2 diabetes than in non-diabetic men;[48] in contrast, another study reported higher serum selenium levels in people with type 2 diabetes.[49] A recent, randomized, double-blind, placebo-controlled study in 1202 men and women participating in the Nutritional Prevention of Cancer trial found that selenium supplementation (200 µg/day, mean follow-up 7.7 years) was linked to an increase in prevalence of type 2 diabetes.[50] In the SELECT study, selenium supplementation (200 µg/day, median follow-up 5.5 years) was associated with a statistically nonsignificant increased risk of type 2 diabetes.[67]

Disease Treatment

HIV/AIDS

There appears to be a unique interaction between selenium and the human immunodeficiency virus (HIV) that causes acquired immune deficiency syndrome (AIDS). Declining selenium levels in HIV-infected individuals are sensitive markers of disease progression and severity, even before malnutrition becomes a factor. Low levels of plasma selenium have also been associated with a significantly increased risk of death from HIV. Adequate selenium nutritional status may increase resistance to HIV infection by enhancing the function of important immune system cells known as *T cells* and modifying their production of intracellular messengers known as *cytokines*.[20,51] In HIV infection, increased oxidative stress appears to favor viral replication, possibly by activating specific transcription pathways. As an integral component of GPx and thioredoxin reductase, selenium plays an important role in decreasing oxidative stress in HIV-infected cells and possibly suppressing the rate of HIV replication.[51] Recent research indicates that HIV may be capable of incorporating host selenium into viral

selenoproteins that have GPx activity. Although the significance of these findings requires further clarification, they suggest that both the human immune system and the activity of the virus are affected by selenium nutritional status.[51-53]

Only a few trials of selenium supplementation in HIV-infected individuals have been published. Two uncontrolled trials of selenium supplementation (one using 400 µg/day of selenium-enriched yeast and the other using 80 µg/day of sodium selenite plus 25 mg/day of vitamin C) reported subjective improvement but did not demonstrate any improvement in biological parameters related to AIDS progression.[54] Another trial followed 15 HIV-infected patients supplemented with 100 µg/day of sodium selenite and 22 unsupplemented patients for 1 year and found that selenium-supplemented patients had evidence of decreased oxidative stress and significant reductions in a biological marker of immunological activation and HIV progression. However, there were no differences in the CD4 T-cell count (an important biological marker of the progress of HIV infection) or mortality between the supplemented and unsupplemented patients.[55,56] A randomized controlled trial in 186 HIV-positive men and women found that selenium supplementation at 200 µg/day for 2 years significantly decreased hospitalization rates.[57] A recent, randomized, double-blind, placebo-controlled trial in 174 HIV-1-positive individuals reported that selenium supplementation (200 µg/day of selenium-enriched yeast) for 9 months was associated with increased serum selenium concentrations, increased CD4 T-cell counts, and no progression of the HIV-1 viral load.[58]

Sources

Food Sources

The richest food sources of selenium are organ meats and seafood, followed by muscle meats. In general, there is wide variation in the selenium content of plants and grains because plants do not appear to require selenium. Thus, the incorporation of selenium into plant proteins is dependent only on soil selenium content. Brazil nuts grown in areas of Brazil with selenium-rich soil may provide more than 100 µg selenium in one nut, whereas those grown in selenium-poor soil may provide 10 times less.[59] In the United

Table 25.2 Food sources of selenium

Food	Serving	Selenium (µg)
Brazil nuts (from selenium-rich soil)	1 ounce (6 kernels)	544[a]
Crab meat	3 ounces[b]	41
Salmon	3 ounces[b]	40
Halibut	3 ounces[b]	40
Noodles, enriched	1 cup, cooked	38
Pork	3 ounces[2]	35
Shrimp	3 ounces[b] (10–12)	34
Whole-wheat bread	2 slices	23
Rice, brown	1 cup, cooked	19
Beef	3 ounces[b]	16
Chicken (light meat)	3 ounces[b]	13
Milk, skimmed	8 ounces (1 cup)	5
Walnuts, black	1 ounce, shelled	5

[a]Above the tolerable upper intake level of 400 µg/day.
[b]A 3-ounce serving of meat or seafood is about the size of a deck of cards.

States, grains are a good source of selenium, but fruit and vegetables tend to be relatively poor sources. In general, drinking water is not a significant source of selenium in North America. The average dietary intake of adults in the United States has been found to range from about 80 µg/day to 110 µg/day. As a result of food distribution patterns in the United States, people living in areas with low soil selenium avoid deficiency because they eat foods produced in areas with higher soil selenium.[11,15] **Table 25.2** lists some good food sources of selenium and their selenium content.

Supplements

Selenium supplements are available in several forms. Sodium selenite and sodium selenate are inorganic forms of selenium. Selenate is almost completely absorbed, but a significant amount is excreted in the urine before it can be incorporated into proteins. Selenite is only about 50% absorbed but is better retained than selenate once it is absorbed. Selenomethionine, an organic form of selenium that occurs naturally in foods, is about 90% absorbed.[15] Selenomethionine and selenium-enriched yeast, which mainly supply selenomethionine, are also available as supplements. The consumer should be aware that some forms of selenium yeast on the market contain yeast plus mainly inorganic forms of selenium. Both inorganic and organic forms of selenium can be metabolized to selenocysteine by the body and incorporated into selenoenzymes.[60]

Selenium-enriched Vegetables

Selenium-enriched garlic, broccoli, onions, and ramps (wild leeks) have been shown to reduce chemically induced tumors in rats.[24,61,62] Selenium-enriched vegetables are of interest to scientists because some of the forms of selenium that they produce (e.g., methylated forms of selenium) may be more potent inhibitors of tumor formation than the forms currently available in supplements.

Safety

Toxicity

Although selenium is required for health, similar to other nutrients, high doses of selenium can be toxic. Acute and fatal toxicities have occurred with accidental or suicidal ingestion of gram quantities of selenium. Clinically significant selenium toxicity was reported in 13 individuals after taking supplements that contained 27.3 mg (27 300 µg) per tablet due to a manufacturing error. Chronic selenium toxicity (selenosis) may occur with smaller doses of selenium over long periods of time. The most frequently reported symptoms of selenosis are hair and nail brittleness and loss. Other symptoms may include gastrointestinal disturbances, skin rashes, a garlic breath odor, fatigue, irritability, and nervous system abnormalities. In an area of China with a high prevalence of selenosis, toxic effects occurred with increasing frequency when blood selenium concentrations reached a level corresponding to an intake of 850 µg/day. The FNB set the tolerable upper intake level (UL) for selenium at 400 µg/day in adults based on the prevention of hair and nail brittleness and loss and early signs of chronic selenium toxicity (**Table 25.3**).[15] The UL of 400 µg/day for adults includes selenium obtained from food, which averages about

Table 25.3 Tolerable upper intake level (UL) for selenium

Life stage	Age	UL (µg/day)
Infants	0–6 months	45
Infants	6–12 months	60
Children	1–3 years	90
Children	4–8 years	150
Children	9–13 years	280
Adolescents	14–18 years	400
Adults	≥19 years	400

100 µg/day for adults in the United States, as well as selenium from supplements.

Drug Interactions

At present, few interactions between selenium and medications are known.[63] The anticonvulsant medication valproic acid has been found to decrease plasma selenium levels. Animal studies have found that supplemental sodium selenite decreases the toxicities of the antibiotic nitrofurantoin and the herbicide paraquat.[64]

Antioxidant supplements and HMG-CoA reductase inhibitors (statins). A 3-year randomized controlled trial in 160 patients with documented coronary heart disease and low high-density lipoprotein (HDL) levels found that a combination of simvastatin and niacin increased HDL2 levels, inhibited the progression of coronary artery stenosis (narrowing), and decreased the frequency of cardiovascular events, including myocardial infarction (heart attack) and stroke.[65] Surprisingly, when an antioxidant combination (1000 mg vitamin C, 800 IU α-tocopherol, 100 µg selenium, and 25 mg β-carotene daily) was taken with the simvastatin–niacin combination, the protective effects were diminished. Although the individual contribution of selenium to this effect cannot be determined, these findings highlight the need for further research on potential interactions between antioxidant supplements and cholesterol-lowering agents such as hydroxymethylglutaryl coenzyme A (HMG-CoA) reductase inhibitors (statins).

LPI Recommendation

The average American diet is estimated to provide about 100 µg/day of selenium, an amount that is well above the current RDA (55 µg/day) and appears sufficient to maximize plasma and cellular glutathione peroxidase activity. Although the amount of selenium in multivitamin/mineral supplements varies considerably, such supplements rarely provide more than the daily value (DV) of 70 µg. Eating a varied diet and taking a daily multivitamin supplement should provide sufficient selenium for most people in the United States.

Men
A controlled trial that examined the effect of selenium supplementation on cancer risk in a well-nourished population found that 200 µg/day of supplemental selenium significantly decreased the risk of prostate cancer in men by 49%.[37] However, the risk of one type of skin cancer was increased by 25%.[38] Although mortality from prostate cancer is considerably higher than mortality from squamous cell cancer of the skin, these findings suggest that the overall effects of selenium supplementation on cancer risk are not yet clear enough to support a general recommendation for an extra selenium supplement. More recently, a much larger, randomized, placebo-controlled intervention study, the SELECT study, found that 200 µg/day of selenium did not alter risk of prostate cancer.[67] Men taking supplemental selenium in order to reduce the risk of prostate cancer should not exceed 200 µg/day and should take precautions to reduce the risk of squamous cell carcinoma, such as using sunscreen and avoiding prolonged sun exposure.

Women
Because there is no evidence that selenium supplementation decreases the risk of cancer in women who are not selenium deficient, there is no reason for women to take an extra selenium supplement. However, animal studies suggest that mammary tumors are significantly reduced by selenium,[66] and the two human trials currently under way should yield more definitive information on this relationship in women.[24]

Older Adults
Because aging has not been associated with significant changes in the requirement for selenium, the Linus Pauling Institute recommendation for selenium is the same for older men and women.

References

1. Rayman MP. The importance of selenium to human health. Lancet 2000;356(9225):233–241
2. Gladyshev VN. Selenoproteins and selenoproteomes. In: Hatfield DL, Berry MJ, Gladyshev VN, eds. Selenium: Its Molecular Biology and Role in Human Health. 2nd ed. New York: Springer; 2006:99–114
3. Ursini F, Heim S, Kiess M, et al. Dual function of the selenoprotein PHGPx during sperm maturation. Science 1999;285(5432):1393–1396
4. Mustacich D, Powis G. Thioredoxin reductase. Biochem J 2000;346(Pt 1):1–8
5. Bianco AC, Larsen PR. Selenium, deiodinases and endocrine function. In: Hatfield DL, Berry MJ, Gladyshev VN, eds. Selenium: Its Molecular Biology and Role in Human Health, 2nd ed. New York: Springer; 2006: 207–219
6. Burk RF, Olson GE, Hill KE. Deletion of selenoprotein P gene in the mouse. In: Hatfield DL, Berry MJ, Gladyshev VN, eds. Selenium: Its Molecular Biology and Role in Human Health. 2nd ed. New York: Springer; 2006:111–122
7. Arteel GE, Briviba K, Sies H. Protection against peroxynitrite. FEBS Lett 1999;445(2-3):226–230
8. Kioussi C, Whanger PD. Selenoprotein W in development and oxidative stress. In: Hatfield DL, Berry MJ, Gladyshev VN, eds. Selenium: Its Molecular Biology and Role in Human Health. 2nd ed. New York: Springer; 2006:135–140
9. Gu QP, Beilstein MA, Vendeland SC, Lugade A, Ream W, Whanger PD. Conserved features of selenocysteine insertion sequence (SECIS) elements in selenoprotein W cDNAs from five species. Gene 1997;193(2):187–196
10. Sword JT, Pope AL, Hoekstra WG. Endotoxin and lipid peroxidation in vitro in selenium- and vitamin E-deficient and -adequate rat tissues. J Nutr 1991;121(2):258–264
11. Burk RF, Levander OA. Selenium. In: Shils M, Olson JA, Shike M, Ross AC, eds. Modern Nutrition in Health and Disease. 9th ed. Baltimore, MD: Lippincott Williams & Wilkins; 1999:265–276
12. Foster LH, Sumar S. Selenium in health and disease: a review. Crit Rev Food Sci Nutr 1997;37(3):211–228
13. Levander OA. Coxsackievirus as a model of viral evolution driven by dietary oxidative stress. Nutr Rev 2000;58(2 Pt 2):S17–S24
14. Beck MA, Esworthy RS, Ho YS, Chu FF. Glutathione peroxidase protects mice from viral-induced myocarditis. FASEB J 1998;12(12):1143–1149
15. Food and Nutrition Board, Institute of Medicine. Selenium. In: Dietary Reference Intakes for Vitamin C, Vitamin E, Selenium, and Carotenoids. Washington, DC: National Academy Press; 2000:284–324
16. McKenzie RC, Beckett GJ, Arthur JR. Effects of selenium on immunity and aging. In: Hatfield DL, Berry MJ, Gladyshev VN, eds. Selenium: Its Molecular Biology and Role in Human Health. 2nd ed. New York: Springer; 2006: 311–323
17. Roy M, Kiremidjian-Schumacher L, Wishe HI, Cohen MW, Stotzky G. Supplementation with selenium and human immune cell functions. I. Effect on lymphocyte proliferation and interleukin 2 receptor expression. Biol Trace Elem Res 1994;41(1-2):103–114
18. Kiremidjian-Schumacher L, Roy M, Wishe HI, Cohen MW, Stotzky G. Supplementation with selenium and human immune cell functions. II. Effect on cytotoxic lymphocytes and natural killer cells. Biol Trace Elem Res 1994;41(1-2):115–127
19. Kiremidjian-Schumacher L, Roy M, Glickman R, et al. Selenium and immunocompetence in patients with head and neck cancer. Biol Trace Elem Res 2000;73(2):97–111
20. Baum MK, Miguez-Burbano MJ, Campa A, Shor-Posner G. Selenium and interleukins in persons infected with human immunodeficiency virus type 1. J Infect Dis 2000;182(Suppl 1):S69–S73
21. Beck MA. Selenium and viral infections. In: Hatfield DL, Berry MJ, Gladyshev VN, eds. Selenium: Its Molecular Biology and Role in Human Health. 2nd ed. New York: Springer; 2006:287–298
22. Combs GF Jr, Gray WP. Chemopreventive agents: selenium. Pharmacol Ther 1998;79(3):179–192
23. Ip C. Lessons from basic research in selenium and cancer prevention. J Nutr 1998;128(11):1845–1854
24. Whanger PD. Selenium and its relationship to cancer: an update. Br J Nutr 2004;91(1):11–28
25. Garland M, Morris JS, Stampfer MJ, et al. Prospective study of toenail selenium levels and cancer among women. J Natl Cancer Inst 1995;87(7):497–505
26. Yu MW, Horng IS, Hsu KH, Chiang YC, Liaw YF, Chen CJ. Plasma selenium levels and risk of hepatocellular carcinoma among men with chronic hepatitis virus infection. Am J Epidemiol 1999;150(4):367–374
27. Knekt P, Marniemi J, Teppo L, Heliövaara M, Aromaa A. Is low selenium status a risk factor for lung cancer? Am J Epidemiol 1998;148(10):975–982
28. Zhuo H, Smith AH, Steinmaus C. Selenium and lung cancer: a quantitative analysis of heterogeneity in the current epidemiological literature. Cancer Epidemiol Biomarkers Prev 2004;13(5):771–778
29. Yoshizawa K, Willett WC, Morris SJ, et al. Study of prediagnostic selenium level in toenails and the risk of advanced prostate cancer. J Natl Cancer Inst 1998;90(16):1219–1224
30. Nomura AM, Lee J, Stemmermann GN, Combs GF Jr. Serum selenium and subsequent risk of prostate cancer. Cancer Epidemiol Biomarkers Prev 2000;9(9):883–887
31. Brooks JD, Metter EJ, Chan DW, et al. Plasma selenium level before diagnosis and the risk of prostate cancer development. J Urol 2001;166(6):2034–2038
32. Peters U, Foster CB, Chatterjee N, et al. Serum selenium and risk of prostate cancer-a nested case-control study. Am J Clin Nutr 2007;85(1):209–217
33. Ghadirian P, Maisonneuve P, Perret C, et al. A case-control study of toenail selenium and cancer of the breast, colon, and prostate. Cancer Detect Prev 2000;24(4):305–313
34. Brinkman M, Reulen RC, Kellen E, Buntinx F, Zeegers MP. Are men with low selenium levels at increased risk of prostate cancer? Eur J Cancer 2006;42(15):2463–2471
35. Lawson KA, Wright ME, Subar A, et al. Multivitamin use and risk of prostate cancer in the National Institutes of Health-AARP Diet and Health Study. J Natl Cancer Inst 2007;99(10):754–764
36. Yu SY, Zhu YJ, Li WG. Protective role of selenium against hepatitis B virus and primary liver cancer in Qidong. Biol Trace Elem Res 1997;56(1):117–124
37. Duffield-Lillico AJ, Dalkin BL, Reid ME, et al; Nutritional Prevention of Cancer Study Group. Selenium supplementation, baseline plasma selenium status and incidence of prostate cancer: an analysis of the

complete treatment period of the Nutritional Prevention of Cancer Trial. BJU Int 2003;91(7):608–612

38. Duffield-Lillico AJ, Slate EH, Reid ME, et al; Nutritional Prevention of Cancer Study Group. Selenium supplementation and secondary prevention of nonmelanoma skin cancer in a randomized trial. J Natl Cancer Inst 2003;95(19):1477–1481

39. Reid ME, Duffield-Lillico AJ, Garland L, Turnbull BW, Clark LC, Marshall JR. Selenium supplementation and lung cancer incidence: an update of the nutritional prevention of cancer trial. Cancer Epidemiol Biomarkers Prev 2002;11(11):1285–1291

40. Klein EA, Thompson IM, Lippman SM, et al. SELECT: the Selenium and Vitamin E Cancer Prevention Trial: rationale and design. Prostate Cancer Prostatic Dis 2000;3(3):145–151

41. Clark LC, Marshall JR. Randomized, controlled chemoprevention trials in populations at very high risk for prostate cancer: Elevated prostate-specific antigen and high-grade prostatic intraepithelial neoplasia. Urology 2001; 57(4, Suppl 1):185–187

42. National Cancer Institute. Review of Prostate Cancer Prevention Study Shows No Benefit for Use of Selenium and Vitamin E Supplements. [Web page]. Available at: http://www.cancer.gov/newscenter/pressreleases/SELECTresults2008 (accessed 4 Jan 2011)

43. Salonen JT, Alfthan G, Huttunen JK, Pikkarainen J, Puska P. Association between cardiovascular death and myocardial infarction and serum selenium in a matched-pair longitudinal study. Lancet 1982; 2(8291):175–179

44. Virtamo J, Valkeila E, Alfthan G, Punsar S, Huttunen JK, Karvonen MJ. Serum selenium and the risk of coronary heart disease and stroke. Am J Epidemiol 1985;122(2):276–282

45. Suadicani P, Hein HO, Gyntelberg F. Serum selenium concentration and risk of ischaemic heart disease in a prospective cohort study of 3000 males. Atherosclerosis 1992;96(1):33–42

46. Salvini S, Hennekens CH, Morris JS, Willett WC, Stampfer MJ. Plasma levels of the antioxidant selenium and risk of myocardial infarction among U.S. physicians. Am J Cardiol 1995;76(17):1218–1221

47. Kardinaal AF, Kok FJ, Kohlmeier L, et al. Association between toenail selenium and risk of acute myocardial infarction in European men. The EURAMIC Study. European Antioxidant Myocardial Infarction and Breast Cancer. Am J Epidemiol 1997;145(4):373–379

48. Rajpathak S, Rimm E, Morris JS, Hu F. Toenail selenium and cardiovascular disease in men with diabetes. J Am Coll Nutr 2005;24(4):250–256

49. Bleys J, Navas-Acien A, Guallar E. Serum selenium and diabetes in U.S. adults. Diabetes Care 2007;30(4):829–834

50. Stranges S, Marshall JR, Natarajan R, et al. Effects of long-term selenium supplementation on the incidence of type 2 diabetes: a randomized trial. Ann Intern Med 2007;147(4):217–223

51. Baum MK, Campa A. Role of selenium in HIV/AIDS. In: Hatfield DL, Berry MJ, Gladyshev VN, eds. Selenium: Its Molecular Biology and Role in Human Health. 2nd ed. New York: Springer; 2006:299–310

52. Zhao L, Cox AG, Ruzicka JA, Bhat AA, Zhang W, Taylor EW. Molecular modeling and in vitro activity of an HIV-1-encoded glutathione peroxidase. Proc Natl Acad Sci U S A 2000;97(12):6356–6361

53. Zhang W, Ramanathan CS, Nadimpalli RG, Bhat AA, Cox AG, Taylor EW. Selenium-dependent glutathione peroxidase modules encoded by RNA viruses. Biol Trace Elem Res 1999;70(2):97–116

54. Constans J, Conri C, Sergeant C. Selenium and HIV infection. Nutrition 1999;15(9):719–720

55. Delmas-Beauvieux MC, Peuchant E, Couchouron A, et al. The enzymatic antioxidant system in blood and glutathione status in human immunodeficiency virus (HIV)-infected patients: effects of supplementation with selenium or beta-carotene. Am J Clin Nutr 1996;64(1):101–107

56. Constans J, Delmas-Beauvieux MC, Sergeant C, et al. One-year antioxidant supplementation with beta-carotene or selenium for patients infected with human immunodeficiency virus: a pilot study. Clin Infect Dis 1996;23(3):654–656

57. Burbano X, Miguez-Burbano MJ, McCollister K, et al. Impact of a selenium chemoprevention clinical trial on hospital admissions of HIV-infected participants. HIV Clin Trials 2002;3(6):483–491

58. Hurwitz BE, Klaus JR, Llabre MM, et al. Suppression of human immunodeficiency virus type 1 viral load with selenium supplementation: a randomized controlled trial. Arch Intern Med 2007;167(2):148–154

59. Chang JC, Gutenmann WH, Reid CM, Lisk DJ. Selenium content of Brazil nuts from two geographic locations in Brazil. Chemosphere 1995;30(4):801–802

60. Schrauzer GN. Selenomethionine: a review of its nutritional significance, metabolism and toxicity. J Nutr 2000;130(7):1653–1656

61. Whanger PD, Ip C, Polan CE, Uden PC, Welbaum G. Tumorigenesis, metabolism, speciation, bioavailability, and tissue deposition of selenium in selenium-enriched ramps (Allium tricoccum). J Agric Food Chem 2000;48(11):5723–5730

62. Ip C, Birringer M, Block E, et al. Chemical speciation influences comparative activity of selenium-enriched garlic and yeast in mammary cancer prevention. J Agric Food Chem 2000;48(6):2062–2070

63. Azrak RG, Cao S, Pendyala L, et al. Efficacy of increasing the therapeutic index of irinotecan, plasma and tissue selenium concentrations is methylselenocysteine dose dependent. Biochem Pharmacol 2007; 73(9):1280–1287

64. Flodin NW. Micronutrient supplements: toxicity and drug interactions. Prog Food Nutr Sci 1990;14(4):277–331

65. Brown BG, Zhao XQ, Chait A, et al. Simvastatin and niacin, antioxidant vitamins, or the combination for the prevention of coronary disease. N Engl J Med 2001;345(22):1583–1592

66. Ip C, Ganther HE. Novel strategies in selenium cancer chemoprevention research. In: Burk RF, ed. Selenium in Biology and Human Health. New York: Springer-Verlag; 1994:169–180

67. Lippman SM, Klein EA, Goodman PJ, et al. Effect of selenium and vitamin E on risk of prostate cancer and other cancers: the Selenium and Vitamin E Cancer Prevention Trial (SELECT). JAMA 2009;301(1):39–51

26 Sodium Chloride

Salt (sodium chloride) is essential for life. The tight regulation of the body's sodium and chloride concentrations is so important that multiple mechanisms work in concert to control them. Although scientists agree that a minimal amount of salt is required for survival, the health implications of excess salt intake represent an area of continued investigation among scientists, clinicians, and public health experts.[1]

Function

Sodium (Na^+) and chloride (Cl^-) are the principal ions in the fluid outside cells (extracellular fluid), which includes blood plasma. As such, they play critical roles in a number of life-sustaining processes.[2]

Maintenance of Membrane Potential

Sodium and chloride are electrolytes that contribute to the maintenance of concentration and charge differences across cell membranes. Potassium is the principal positively charged ion (cation) inside cells, whereas sodium is the principal cation in extracellular fluid. Potassium concentrations are about 30 times higher inside than outside cells, while sodium concentrations are more than 10 times lower inside than outside cells. The concentration differences between potassium and sodium across cell membranes create an electrochemical gradient known as the *membrane potential*. A cell's membrane potential is maintained by ion pumps in the cell membrane, especially the Na^+/K^+ ATPase pumps. These pumps use ATP (energy) to pump sodium out of the cell in exchange for potassium (**Fig. 26.1**). Their activity has been estimated to account for 20%–40% of the resting energy expenditure in a typical adult. The large proportion of energy dedicated to maintaining sodium/potassium concentration gradients emphasizes the importance of this function in sustaining life. Tight control of cell membrane potential is critical for nerve impulse transmission, muscle contraction, and cardiac function.[3,4]

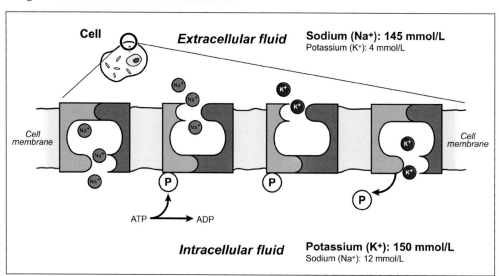

Fig. 26.1 A model of the Na^+/K^+ ATPase pump. The concentration differences between potassium (K^+) and sodium (Na^+) across cell membranes create an electrochemical gradient known as the membrane potential. Adenosine triphosphate (ATP) provides the energy to pump three Na^+ ions out of the cell in exchange for two K+ ions, thus maintaining the membrane potential.

Nutrient Absorption and Transport

Absorption of sodium in the small intestine plays an important role in the absorption of chloride, amino acids, glucose, and water. Similar mechanisms are involved in the reabsorption of these nutrients after they have been filtered from the blood by the kidneys. Chloride, in the form of hydrochloric acid (HCl), is also an important component of gastric juice, which helps the digestion and absorption of many nutrients.[2,5]

Maintenance of Blood Volume and Blood Pressure

As sodium is the primary determinant of extracellular fluid volume, including blood volume, a number of physiological mechanisms that regulate blood volume and blood pressure work by adjusting the body's sodium content. In the circulatory system, pressure receptors (baroreceptors) sense changes in blood pressure and send excitatory or inhibitory signals to the nervous system and/or endocrine glands to affect sodium regulation by the kidneys. In general, sodium retention results in water retention and sodium loss results in water loss.[4,5] Below are descriptions of two of the many systems that affect blood volume and blood pressure through sodium regulation.

Renin–angiotensin–aldosterone system. In response to a significant decrease in blood volume or pressure (e.g., serious blood loss or dehydration), the kidneys release renin into the circulation. Renin is an enzyme that splits a small peptide (angiotensin I) from a larger protein (angiotensinogen) produced by the liver. Angiotensin I is split into a smaller peptide (angiotensin II) by angiotensin-converting enzyme (ACE), an enzyme present on the inner surface of blood vessels and in the lungs, liver, and kidneys. Angiotensin II stimulates the constriction of small arteries, resulting in increased blood pressure. It is also a potent stimulator of aldosterone synthesis by the adrenal glands. Aldosterone is a steroid hormone that acts on the kidneys to increase the reabsorption of sodium and the excretion of potassium. Retention of sodium by the kidneys increases the retention of water, resulting in increased blood volume and blood pressure.[4]

Antidiuretic hormone. Secretion of antidiuretic hormone (ADH) by the posterior pituitary gland is stimulated by a significant decrease in blood volume or pressure. ADH acts on the kidneys to increase the reabsorption of water.[4]

Deficiency

Sodium (and chloride) deficiency does not generally result from inadequate dietary intake, even in those on very low-salt diets.[5]

Hyponatremia

Hyponatremia, defined as a serum sodium concentration of less than 136 mmol/L, may result from increased fluid retention (dilutional hyponatremia) or increased sodium loss. Dilutional hyponatremia may be due to inappropriate ADH secretion, which is associated with disorders affecting the central nervous system and with use of certain drugs. In some cases, excessive water intake may also lead to dilutional hyponatremia. Conditions that increase the loss of sodium and chloride include severe or prolonged vomiting or diarrhea, excessive and persistent sweating, the use of some diuretics, and some forms of kidney disease. Symptoms of hyponatremia include headache, nausea, vomiting, muscle cramps, fatigue, disorientation, and fainting. Complications of severe and rapidly developing hyponatremia may include cerebral edema (swelling of the brain), seizures, coma, and brain damage. Acute or severe hyponatremia may be fatal without prompt and appropriate medical treatment.[6]

Prolonged endurance exercise and hyponatremia. Hyponatremia has recently been recognized as a potential problem in individuals competing in very long endurance exercise events, such as marathons, ultramarathons, and ironman triathlons. In 1997, 25 of 650 participants in an ironman triathlon (almost 4%) received medical attention for hyponatremia.[7] Participants who developed hyponatremia during an ironman triathlon had evidence of fluid overload despite relatively modest fluid intakes, suggesting that fluid excretion was inadequate and/or the fluid needs of these ultradistance athletes may be less than currently recommended.[8] It has been speculated that the use of nonsteroidal anti-inflam-

Table 26.1 Adequate intake (AI) for sodium, with estimated sodium chloride (salt) equivalence

Life stage	Age	Males and females	
		Sodium (g/day)	Salt (g/day)
Infants	0–6 months	0.12	0.30
Infants	7–12 months	0.37	0.93
Children	1–3 years	1.0	2.5
Children	4–8 years	1.2	3.0
Children	9–13 years	1.5	3.8
Adolescents	14–18 years	1.5	3.8
Adults	19–50 years	1.5	3.8
Adults	51–70 years	1.3	3.3
Adults	≥71 years	1.2	3.0
Pregnancy	All ages	1.5	3.8
Breast-feeding	All ages	1.5	3.8

matory drugs (NSAIDs) may increase the risk of exercise-related hyponatremia by impairing water excretion,[9] but firm evidence is currently lacking.

Adequate Intake for Sodium

In 2004, the Food and Nutrition Board (FNB) of the Institute of Medicine established an adequate intake (AI) for sodium based on the amount needed to replace losses through sweat in moderately active people and to achieve a diet that provides sufficient amounts of other essential nutrients (**Table 26.1**).[5] This recommended intake is well below the average dietary intakes of most people in the United States.

Disease Prevention (Dietary Sodium and Disease)

Gastric Cancer

Epidemiological studies, conducted mainly in Asian countries, indicate that high intakes of salted, smoked, and pickled foods increase the risk of gastric cancer.[10,11] Although these foods are high in salt, they may also contain carcinogens, such as nitrosamines. In addition, populations with high intakes of salted foods tend to have low intakes of fruit and vegetables, which protect against gastric cancer.[12] The risk of developing stomach cancer is increased by chronic inflam-

mation of the stomach and infection by the bacterium, *Helicobacter pylori*. High concentrations of salt may damage the cells lining the stomach, potentially increasing the risk of *H. pylori* infection and cancer-promoting genetic damage. Although there is little evidence that salt itself is a carcinogen, high intakes of certain salted foods, such as salted fish, may increase the risk of gastric cancer in susceptible individuals.[11,13,14]

Osteoporosis

Osteoporosis is a multifactorial skeletal disorder in which bone strength is compromised, resulting in an increased risk of fracture. Nutrition is one of many factors contributing to the development and progression of osteoporosis. Increased salt intake has been found to increase urinary excretion of calcium. Each 2.3 g increment of sodium (5.8 g salt) excreted by the kidneys draws about 24–40 mg calcium into the urine.[15] Salt intake has been associated with biochemical markers of bone resorption in some studies but not in others. In general, cross-sectional studies have not found an association between sodium intake and bone mineral density (BMD).[16] However, a 2-year study of postmenopausal women found that increased urinary sodium excretion (an indicator of increased sodium intake) was associated with decreased BMD at the hip.[17] More recently, a longitudinal study in 40 postmenopausal women found that adherence to a low sodium diet (2 g/day) for 6 months was associated with significant reductions in sodium excretion, calcium excretion, and the amino-terminal propeptide of type I collagen, a biomarker of bone resorption. However, these associations were observed only in women with baseline urinary sodium excretions of 3.4 g/day or more (i.e., the mean sodium intake for the US adult population).[18] Long-term prospective studies are needed to determine whether decreasing salt intake has clinically significant effects on BMD and fracture risk in individuals at risk for osteoporosis. For more information on osteoporosis, see Chapter 14.

Kidney Stones

Most kidney stones contain calcium as a main constituent. Although their cause is often unknown, abnormally elevated urinary calcium (hypercalciuria) increases the risk of developing calcium stones.[19] Increased dietary salt has been found to increase urinary calcium excretion, and this effect may be more pronounced in patients with a history of calcium-containing kidney stones.[20] A large prospective study that followed more than 90 000 women over a 12-year period found that women with a sodium intake averaging 4.9 g/day (12.6 g/day of salt) had a 30% higher risk of developing symptomatic kidney stones than women whose sodium intake averaged 1.5 g/day (4.0 g/day of salt).[21] However, a similar study in men did not find an association between sodium intake and symptomatic kidney stones.[22] Clinical studies have shown that salt restriction reduces urinary calcium in individuals with a tendency to form calcium stones,[23] and a 5-year randomized trial of two different diets in men with recurrent calcium oxalate stones found that a diet low in salt and animal protein significantly decreased stone recurrence compared with a low-calcium diet.[24]

Hypertension

Several lines of research, conducted over several decades, have suggested that sodium intake is causally related to blood pressure. Animal studies have provided much information on the physiology of this relationship. Of particular importance, a key animal experiment conducted in 26 adult chimpanzees, a species closely related to humans, showed that blood pressure levels rose and fell as a result of experimentally induced high and low levels of sodium, providing strong evidence that higher sodium intake causes blood pressure to increase and reduced intake causes it to decrease.[25]

In human studies, cross-cultural population studies comparing cultures with very low salt intakes to those with high intakes, and observational studies, most of which were cross-sectional, have suggested that increased salt consumption is associated with higher blood pressure. However, populations in cross-cultural studies may differ in a number of other ways that could affect blood pressure, and observational studies have varied in their ability to control for confounding factors.[26] The largest and most rigorously designed observational study of sodium and blood pressure was INTERSALT, which studied more than 10 000 men and women in 32 countries. Both cross-population and within-population analyses supported the same conclusions, that sodium intake, measured by 24-hour urine collections, was associated with blood pressure.[27] Subsequent analyses that used more sophisticated statistical techniques made the relationships even stronger than previously reported.[28]

Clinical trials and meta-analyses. Many randomized clinical trials have examined the effect of dietary salt reduction on blood pressure in hypertensive and nonhypertensive people (please note that nonhypertensive does not necessarily mean normotensive [normal blood pressure] because the nonhypertensive blood pressure range could encompass what is now called prehypertensive). Several investigators have used a technique called meta-analysis to analyze the pooled data from many different trials to estimate the magnitude of the effect of dietary salt reduction on blood pressure.[29–34] Estimates of the magnitude of the effect of dietary salt reduction on blood pressure did not differ substantially among the analyses, although the number and types of trials that were included in the various meta-analyses differed substantially. The Cochrane meta-analysis assessed the results of modest salt reduction from 20 trials in participants with high blood pressure and 11 trials in participants without high blood pressure. Modest salt reduction (by 1.7–1.8 g/day of sodium, based on 24-hour urinary sodium excretions) decreased systolic and diastolic blood pressure by an average of 5.1/2.7 mmHg in participants with hypertension and 2.0/1.0 mmHg in participants without hypertension.[34]

Of particular importance are the results of two large, long-term trials (more than 2 years in duration) that are the most relevant to clinical and public health practice, called TONE[35] and TOHP-Phase II.[36] TONE showed that modest reduction in sodium intake by about 1.0 g/day resulted in better control of hypertension in older adults who initially were on blood pressure medication. TOHP-Phase II (the second of two hypertension prevention trials) showed that a similar level of sodium reduction not only reduced systolic and diastolic blood pressure by 1.2/1.6 mmHg in overweight participants who did not have hypertension, but also reduced the onset of hypertension by 14% after 4 years.[36] Although some clinicians have questioned the value of modest blood pressure reductions in hypertensive patients, overviews of observational studies and randomized trials suggest that reducing diastolic blood pressure by an average of 2 mmHg in the US population would reduce the prevalence of hypertension by 17%, the risk of a heart attack by 5%, and the risk of stroke by 15%.[37] Thus, modest mean reductions in blood pressure may translate into significant public health benefits for the overall US population.

Salt sensitivity (variation in response to dietary sodium changes). There is a considerable literature on variation in response of blood pressure to short-term changes in sodium intake.[38,39] However, classifying individuals based on their blood pressure response to salt changes, usually from an experimental protocol conducted just once, is extremely problematic. Similar to most physiological responses, there is a continuous, approximately normal distribution of responses of blood pressure to changes in salt intake.[40] There is also variation in blood pressure from day to day, even when there is no change in diet.[40] The classification of individuals as salt sensitive or salt resistant has thus far not been based on population samples and has not yet been shown to be highly reproducible over time. In addition, most of the protocols used in "salt sensitivity" studies involved extreme manipulations of sodium intake (sodium loading and sodium depletion) over a short time span of a few days or up to a week.

There is no evidence that these very short-term studies have relevance to blood pressure changes occurring from long-term, gradual, and moderate changes in salt intake.

Nevertheless, it is well known that certain subgroups of the population tend to have greater average blood pressure responses to changes in sodium intake. These include people who already have hypertension, older individuals, and African–American individuals.[41] Research examining a genetic basis for salt sensitivity may eventually lead to better and more reliable classification of individuals for salt sensitivity. Common variations in specific genes, known as *polymorphisms*, are currently under investigation and include those of genes with products that function prominently in the renin–angiotensin–aldosterone system.[42] In addition, diet quality (e.g., the DASH diet—see below) and weight loss reduce blood pressure.[43–45] Thus, environmental influences, in addition to genetic factors, likely contribute to salt sensitivity.

Dietary patterns and blood pressure (the DASH trials). A multicenter, randomized feeding study, called the Dietary Approaches to Stop Hypertension (DASH) trial, demonstrated that a diet emphasizing fruit, vegetables, whole grains, poultry, fish, nuts, and low-fat dairy products substantially lowered blood pressure in hypertensive (systolic BP/diastolic BP: 11.4/5.5 mmHg) and normotensive people (3.5/2.1 mmHg) compared with a typical US diet.[46] The DASH diet was markedly higher in potassium and calcium, modestly higher in protein, and lower in total fat, saturated fat, and cholesterol than the typical US diet. However, sodium levels were kept constant throughout the study in order to better evaluate the effects of other dietary components. Subsequently, the DASH-sodium trial compared the DASH diet with a typical US (control) diet at three levels of salt intake: low (2.9 g/day), medium (5.8 g/day—recommended as an upper limit by US dietary guidelines), and high (8.7 g/day—typical US intake).[47]

The DASH diet significantly lowered systolic and diastolic blood pressures in hypertensive and normotensive people at each level of salt intake compared with the control diet. Reduction of salt intake resulted in an additional lowering of systolic and diastolic blood pressures. The combination of the DASH diet and reduced salt intake lowered blood pressure more than either intervention alone. Compared with the high-salt control diet, average blood pressure on the low-sodium DASH diet was decreased 8.9/4.5 mmHg. The effect of salt reduction was greater in the control diet than in the DASH diet, suggesting that salt reduction may be more beneficial in those who consume typical US diets. The results of the DASH trials support the idea that healthy dietary patterns offer an effective approach to the prevention and treatment of hypertension.[48] Furthermore, a prospective cohort study in 88 517 middle-aged women followed for 24 years found that adherence to a DASH-style diet significantly lowered risk for coronary heart disease and stroke.[49]

The National High Blood Pressure Education Program and the National Heart, Lung, and Blood Institute of the National Institutes of Health (NIH) recommend consuming no more than 6 g/day of salt,[50] and the FNB recently recommended that adults consume no more than 5.8 g/day of salt.[5]

Target organ damage. Chronic hypertension damages the heart, blood vessels, and kidneys, thereby increasing the risk of heart disease and stroke, as well as hypertensive kidney disease. In a number of clinical studies, salt intake correlated significantly with left ventricular hypertrophy, an abnormal thickening of the heart muscle, which is associated with increased mortality from cardiovascular diseases.[51] Research indicates that a high salt intake may contribute to organ damage in ways that are independent of its effects on blood pressure.[52–54] For example, studies in animals and humans have found increased salt intake to be associated with pathological changes in the structure and function of large elastic arteries that are independent of changes in blood pressure.[55]

Cardiovascular Diseases

Only a few studies have investigated the effects of sodium reduction on cardiovascular disease and on mortality, with mixed results.[56–61] In general, the studies suggest a direct association, particularly the studies that used urinary sodium as a measure of sodium intake.[56–58] In the TONE study, there was a trend toward reduced cardiovascular disease in participants assigned to the sodium

reduction intervention.[35] Importantly, a recent study found that participants initially without hypertension, who were enrolled in the sodium interventions in the two previous TOHP trials, had a 25% reduction in cardiovascular events 10–15 years later compared with the control groups.[62] Subsequent analyses from this TOHP follow-up study showed that the sodium: potassium ratio was associated with increased risk of cardiovascular disease in a dose–response relationship,[63] providing complementary evidence for the adverse association between salt intake and cardiovascular disease.

Sources

Most of the sodium and chloride in the diet comes from salt. It has been estimated that 75% of the salt intake in the United States is derived from salt added during food processing or manufacturing, rather than from salt added at the table or during cooking. The lowest salt intakes are associated with diets that emphasize unprocessed foods, especially fruit, vegetables, and legumes. Recent surveys have found that the average dietary salt intake in the United States is 7.8–11.8 g/day for men and 5.8–7.8 g/day for women.[5] These figures could be underestimations because they did not include salt added to food at the table.

Table 26.2 lists the sodium content of some foods that are high in salt, and **Table 26.3** lists the sodium content of some foods that are relatively low in salt. Since most of the sodium and chloride intake comes from salt, dietary salt content can be estimated by multiplying sodium content by 2.5:

2000 mg sodium × 2.5 = 5000 mg (5 g) salt.

Safety

Toxicity

Excessive intakes of sodium chloride lead to an increase in extracellular fluid volume as water is pulled from cells to maintain normal sodium concentrations. However, as long as water needs can be met, normally functioning kidneys can excrete the excess sodium and restore the system to normal.[50] Ingestion of large amounts of salt may lead to nausea, vomiting, diarrhea, and abdominal cramps.[64] Abnormally high plasma sodium

Table 26.2 Foods that are high in salt

Food	Serving	Sodium (mg)	Salt (mg)
Canned, chicken noodle soup	1 cup	1400	3400
Macaroni and cheese, canned	1 cup	1300	3300
Potato chips, salted	8 ounces (1 bag)	1200	3000
Ham	3 ounces	1000	2500
Corned beef hash	1 cup	1000	2500
Pretzels, salted	2 ounces (10 pretzels)	1000	2500
Fish sandwich with tartar sauce and cheese	1 sandwich	940	2400
Tomato juice, canned (salt added)	1 cup (8 fluid ounces)	650	1600
Hot dog (beef)	1	510	1300
Bread, white	2 slices	340	850
Dill pickle	1 spear	300	800
Cereal, bran flakes	1 cup	293	733
Cereal, corn flakes	1 cup	266	665
Bread, whole-wheat	2 slices	264	660

Table 26.3 Foods that are low in salt

Food	Serving	Sodium (mg)	Salt (mg)
Olive oil	1 tablespoon	0	0
Orange juice (frozen)	1 cup (8 fluid ounces)	0	0
Popcorn, air-popped (unsalted)	1 cup	1	3
Almonds (unsalted)	1 cup	1	3
Pear, raw	1 medium	2	5
Mango	1 fruit	4	10
Tomato	1 medium	6	15
Fruit cocktail, canned	1 cup	9	23
Brown rice	1 cup, cooked	10	25
Potato chips, unsalted	8 ounces (1 bag)	18	45
Tomato juice, canned (no salt added)	1 cup (8 fluid ounces)	24	60
Carrot	1 medium	42	105

concentrations (hypernatremia) generally develop from excess water loss, frequently accompanied by an impaired thirst mechanism or lack of access to water. Symptoms of hypernatremia in the presence of excess fluid loss may include dizziness or fainting, low blood pressure, and diminished urine production. Severe hypernatremia may result in edema (swelling), hypertension, rapid heart rate, difficulty breathing, convulsions, coma, and death. Hypernatremia is rarely caused by excessive sodium intake (e.g., the ingestion of large amounts of seawater or intravenous infusion of concentrated saline solution). In end-stage renal failure (kidney failure), impaired urinary sodium excretion may lead to fluid retention, resulting in edema, high blood pressure, or congestive heart failure if salt and water intake are not restricted.[2,65]

Adverse Effects

In 2004, the FNB established a tolerable upper intake level (UL) for sodium at 2.3 g/day for adults based on the adverse effects of high sodium intakes on blood pressure, a major risk factor for cardiovascular and kidney diseases.[5] It should be

Table 26.4 Tolerable upper intake level for sodium, with estimated sodium chloride (salt) equivalence

Life stage	Age	Sodium (g/day)	Salt (g/day)
Infants	0–12 months	Not determined[a]	Not determined[a]
Children	1–3 years	1.5	3.8
Children	4–8 years	1.9	4.8
Children	9–13 years	2.2	5.5
Adolescents	14–18 years	2.3	5.8
Adults	≥19 years	2.3	5.8

[a]Intake should be from food and formula only.

Table 26.5 Medications associated with hyponatremia[6]

Medication class	Examples
Classes of medications associated with hyponatremia	
Diuretics	Hydrochlorthiazide, furosemide
Nonsteroidal anti-inflammatory drugs	Ibuprofen, naproxen sodium
Opiate derivatives	Codeine, morphine
Phenothiazines	Prochlorperazine, promethazine
Selective serotonin reuptake inhibitors	Fluoxetine, paroxetine
Tricyclic antidepressants	Amitriptyline, imipramine
Individual medications associated with hyponatremia	
Anticonvulsant	Carbamazepine
Antilipidemic	Clofibrate
Antineoplastics	Cyclophosphamide, vincristine
Hormones	Desmopressin, oxytocin
Oral hypoglycemic	Chlorpropamide

noted that the UL for sodium may be lower for those who are most sensitive to the blood pressure effects of sodium, including older people, African–American individuals, and individuals with hypertension, diabetes, or chronic kidney disease. The UL values for sodium and salt in different age groups are listed in **Table 26.4**.

Drug Interactions

The medications listed in **Table 26.5** increase the risk of hyponatremia (abnormally low blood sodium concentration).[6]

LPI Recommendation

There is strong and consistent evidence that diets relatively low in salt (5.8 g/day or less) and high in potassium (at least 4.7 g/day) are associated with decreased risk of high blood pressure and the associated risks of cardiovascular and kidney diseases. Moreover, the DASH trial demonstrated that a diet emphasizing fruit, vegetables, whole grains, nuts, and low-fat dairy products substantially lowered blood pressure, an effect that was enhanced by reducing salt intake to 5.8 g/day or less. A lower salt intake of 3.8 g/day should be the aim. The Linus Pauling Institute recommends a diet that is rich in fruit and vegetables (at least five servings per day) and limits processed foods that are high in salt.

Older Adults

Diets low in salt (3.8 g/day or less) and rich in potassium (at least 4.7 g/day) are likely to be of particular benefit for older adults, who are at increased risk of high blood pressure along with its associated risks of cardiovascular and kidney diseases. Because sensitivity to the blood pressure-raising effects of salt increases with age, diets that are low in salt and high in potassium may especially benefit older adults.

References

1. Taubes G. The (political) science of salt. Science 1998;281(5379):898–901, 903–897
2. Harper ME, Willis JS, Patrick J. Sodium and chloride in nutrition. In: O'Dell BL, Sunde RA, eds. Handbook of Nutritionally Essential Minerals. New York: Marcel Dekker; 1997:93–116
3. Brody T. Nutritional Biochemistry. 2nd ed. San Diego, CA: Academic Press; 1999
4. Sheng H-W. Sodium, chloride and potassium. In: Stipanuk M, ed. Biochemical and Physiological Aspects of Human Nutrition. Philadelphia, PA: WB Saunders Co.; 2000:686–710
5. Food and Nutrition Board, Institute of Medicine. Sodium and Chloride. Dietary Reference Intakes for Water, Potassium, Sodium, Chloride, and Sulfate. Washington, DC: National Academies Press; 2005: 269–423
6. Adrogué HJ, Madias NE. Hyponatremia. N Engl J Med 2000;342(21):1581–1589

7. Speedy DB, Rogers IR, Noakes TD, et al. Diagnosis and prevention of hyponatremia at an ultradistance triathlon. Clin J Sport Med 2000;10(1):52–58

8. Speedy DB, Noakes TD, Kimber NE, et al. Fluid balance during and after an ironman triathlon. Clin J Sport Med 2001;11(1):44–50

9. Ayus JC, Varon J, Arieff AI. Hyponatremia, cerebral edema, and noncardiogenic pulmonary edema in marathon runners. Ann Intern Med 2000;132(9): 711–714

10. Palli D. Epidemiology of gastric cancer: an evaluation of available evidence. J Gastroenterol 2000;35(Suppl 12):84–89

11. Tsugane S. Salt, salted food intake, and risk of gastric cancer: epidemiologic evidence. Cancer Sci 2005; 96(1):1–6

12. Liu C, Russell RM. Nutrition and gastric cancer risk: an update. Nutr Rev 2008;66(5):237–249

13. Cohen AJ, Roe FJ. Evaluation of the aetiological role of dietary salt exposure in gastric and other cancers in humans. Food Chem Toxicol 1997;35(2):271–293

14. Hirohata T, Kono S. Diet/nutrition and stomach cancer in Japan. Int J Cancer 1997;(Suppl 10):34–36

15. Weaver CM, Heaney RP. Calcium. In: Shils M, Olson JA, Shike M, Ross AC, eds. Modern Nutrition in Health and Disease. 9th ed. Baltimore, MD: Lippincott Williams & Wilkins; 1999:141–155

16. Cohen AJ, Roe FJ. Review of risk factors for osteoporosis with particular reference to a possible aetiological role of dietary salt. Food Chem Toxicol 2000;38 (2-3):237–253

17. Devine A, Criddle RA, Dick IM, Kerr DA, Prince RL. A longitudinal study of the effect of sodium and calcium intakes on regional bone density in postmenopausal women. Am J Clin Nutr 1995;62(4):740–745

18. Carbone LD, Barrow KD, Bush AJ, et al. Effects of a low sodium diet on bone metabolism. J Bone Miner Metab 2005;23(6):506–513

19. Heller HJ. The role of calcium in the prevention of kidney stones. J Am Coll Nutr 1999; 18(5, Suppl): 373S–378S

20. Audran M, Legrand E. Hypercalciuria. Joint Bone Spine 2000;67(6):509–515

21. Curhan GC, Willett WC, Speizer FE, Spiegelman D, Stampfer MJ. Comparison of dietary calcium with supplemental calcium and other nutrients as factors affecting the risk for kidney stones in women. Ann Intern Med 1997;126(7):497–504

22. Curhan GC, Willett WC, Rimm EB, Stampfer MJ. A prospective study of dietary calcium and other nutrients and the risk of symptomatic kidney stones. N Engl J Med 1993;328(12):833–838

23. Assimos DG, Holmes RP. Role of diet in the therapy of urolithiasis. Urol Clin North Am 2000;27(2):255–268

24. Borghi L, Schianchi T, Meschi T, et al. Comparison of two diets for the prevention of recurrent stones in idiopathic hypercalciuria. N Engl J Med 2002;346(2): 77–84

25. Denton D, Weisinger R, Mundy NI, et al. The effect of increased salt intake on blood pressure of chimpanzees. Nat Med 1995;1(10):1009–1016

26. Elliott P. Observational studies of salt and blood pressure. Hypertension 1991; 17(1, Suppl):I3–I8

27. Intersalt Cooperative Research Group. Intersalt: an international study of electrolyte excretion and blood pressure. Results for 24 hour urinary sodium and potassium excretion. BMJ 1988;297(6644):319–328

28. Elliott P, Stamler J, Nichols R, et al; Intersalt Cooperative Research Group. Intersalt revisited: further analyses of 24 hour sodium excretion and blood pressure within and across populations. BMJ 1996;312(7041): 1249–1253

29. He FJ, MacGregor GA. Importance of salt in determining blood pressure in children: meta-analysis of controlled trials. Hypertension 2006;48(5):861–869

30. Dickinson HO, Mason JM, Nicolson DJ, et al. Lifestyle interventions to reduce raised blood pressure: a systematic review of randomized controlled trials. J Hypertens 2006;24(2):215–233

31. Graudal NA, Galløe AM, Garred P. Effects of sodium restriction on blood pressure, renin, aldosterone, catecholamines, cholesterols, and triglyceride: a meta-analysis. JAMA 1998;279(17):1383–1391

32. Cutler JA, Follmann D, Allender PS. Randomized trials of sodium reduction: an overview. Am J Clin Nutr 1997; 65(2, Suppl):643S–651S

33. Midgley JP, Matthew AG, Greenwood CM, Logan AG. Effect of reduced dietary sodium on blood pressure: a meta-analysis of randomized controlled trials. JAMA 1996;275(20):1590–1597

34. He FJ, MacGregor GA. Effect of longer-term modest salt reduction on blood pressure. Cochrane Database Syst Rev 2004; (3):CD004937

35. Whelton PK, Appel LJ, Espeland MA, et al; TONE Collaborative Research Group. Sodium reduction and weight loss in the treatment of hypertension in older persons: a randomized controlled trial of nonpharmacologic interventions in the elderly (TONE). JAMA 1998;279(11):839–846

36. The Trials of Hypertension Prevention Collaborative Research Group. Effects of weight loss and sodium reduction intervention on blood pressure and hypertension incidence in overweight people with high-normal blood pressure. The Trials of Hypertension Prevention, phase II. Arch Intern Med 1997;157(6): 657–667

37. Cook NR, Cohen J, Hebert PR, Taylor JO, Hennekens CH. Implications of small reductions in diastolic blood pressure for primary prevention. Arch Intern Med 1995;155(7):701–709

38. Luft FC, Weinberger MH. Heterogeneous responses to changes in dietary salt intake: the salt-sensitivity paradigm. Am J Clin Nutr 1997; 65(2, Suppl):612S–617S

39. Weinberger MH. Salt sensitivity of blood pressure in humans. Hypertension 1996;27(3 Pt 2):481–490

40. Obarzanek E, Proschan MA, Vollmer WM, et al. Individual blood pressure responses to changes in salt intake: results from the DASH-Sodium trial. Hypertension 2003;42(4):459–467

41. Vollmer WM, Sacks FM, Ard J, et al; DASH-Sodium Trial Collaborative Research Group. Effects of diet and sodium intake on blood pressure: subgroup analysis of the DASH-sodium trial. Ann Intern Med 2001; 135(12):1019–1028

42. Giner V, Poch E, Bragulat E, et al. Renin-angiotensin system genetic polymorphisms and salt sensitivity in essential hypertension. Hypertension 2000;35(1 Pt 2): 512–517

43. Neter JE, Stam BE, Kok FJ, Grobbee DE, Geleijnse JM. Influence of weight reduction on blood pressure: a meta-analysis of randomized controlled trials. Hypertension 2003;42(5):878–884

44. Franco V, Oparil S. Salt sensitivity, a determinant of blood pressure, cardiovascular disease and survival. J Am Coll Nutr 2006; 25(3, Suppl):247S–255S

45. Akita S, Sacks FM, Svetkey LP, Conlin PR, Kimura G; DASH-Sodium Trial Collaborative Research Group. Effects of the Dietary Approaches to Stop Hypertension (DASH) diet on the pressure-natriuresis relationship. Hypertension 2003;42(1):8–13

46. Appel LJ, Moore TJ, Obarzanek E, et al; DASH Collaborative Research Group. A clinical trial of the effects of dietary patterns on blood pressure. N Engl J Med 1997;336(16):1117–1124

47. Sacks FM, Svetkey LP, Vollmer WM, et al; DASH-Sodium Collaborative Research Group. Effects on blood pressure of reduced dietary sodium and the Dietary Approaches to Stop Hypertension (DASH) diet. N Engl J Med 2001;344(1):3–10

48. Greenland P. Beating high blood pressure with low-sodium DASH. N Engl J Med 2001;344(1):53–55

49. Fung TT, Chiuve SE, McCullough ML, Rexrode KM, Logroscino G, Hu FB. Adherence to a DASH-style diet and risk of coronary heart disease and stroke in women. Arch Intern Med 2008;168(7):713–720

50. Chobanian AV, Hill M. National Heart, Lung, and Blood Institute Workshop on Sodium and Blood Pressure: a critical review of current scientific evidence. Hypertension 2000;35(4):858–863

51. Chrysant GS. High salt intake and cardiovascular disease: is there a connection? Nutrition 2000;16 (7-8):662–664

52. du Cailar G, Ribstein J, Mimran A. Dietary sodium and target organ damage in essential hypertension. Am J Hypertens 2002;15(3):222–229

53. Perry IJ, Beevers DG. Salt intake and stroke: a possible direct effect. J Hum Hypertens 1992;6(1):23–25

54. Aviv A. Salt and hypertension: the debate that begs the bigger question. Arch Intern Med 2001;161(4):507–510

55. Safar ME, Thuilliez C, Richard V, Benetos A. Pressure-independent contribution of sodium to large artery structure and function in hypertension. Cardiovasc Res 2000;46(2):269–276

56. Nagata C, Takatsuka N, Shimizu N, Shimizu H. Sodium intake and risk of death from stroke in Japanese men and women. Stroke 2004;35(7):1543–1547

57. Tuomilehto J, Jousilahti P, Rastenyte D, et al. Urinary sodium excretion and cardiovascular mortality in Finland: a prospective study. Lancet 2001;357(9259):848–851

58. Tunstall-Pedoe H, Woodward M, Tavendale R, A'Brook R, McCluskey MK. Comparison of the prediction by 27 different factors of coronary heart disease and death in men and women of the Scottish Heart Health Study: cohort study. BMJ 1997;315(7110):722–729

59. He J, Ogden LG, Vupputuri S, Bazzano LA, Loria C, Whelton PK. Dietary sodium intake and subsequent risk of cardiovascular disease in overweight adults. JAMA 1999;282(21):2027–2034

60. Cohen HW, Hailpern SM, Fang J, Alderman MH. Sodium intake and mortality in the NHANES II follow-up study. Am J Med 2006;119(3):275.e7–14

61. Alderman MH, Cohen H, Madhavan S. Dietary sodium intake and mortality: the National Health and Nutrition Examination Survey (NHANES I). Lancet 1998;351(9105):781–785

62. Cook NR, Cutler JA, Obarzanek E, et al. Long term effects of dietary sodium reduction on cardiovascular disease outcomes: observational follow-up of the trials of hypertension prevention (TOHP). BMJ 2007;334(7599):885–888

63. Cook NR, Obarzanek E, Cutler JA, et al; Trials of Hypertension Prevention Collaborative Research Group. Joint effects of sodium and potassium intake on subsequent cardiovascular disease: the Trials of Hypertension Prevention follow-up study. Arch Intern Med 2009;169(1):32–40

64. Electrolytes. Drug Facts and Comparisons; 54th ed. St. Louis: Facts and Comparisons; 2000:46

65. Okuda T. Fluid and electrolyte disorders. In: Tierney LM, McPhee SJ, Papadakis MA, eds. Current Medical Diagnosis and Treatment. 37th ed. Stamford, CA: Appleton & Lange; 1998:824–849

27 Zinc

Zinc is an essential trace element for all forms of life. The significance of zinc in human nutrition and public health was recognized relatively recently. Clinical zinc deficiency in humans was first described in 1961, when the consumption of diets with low zinc bioavailability due to high phytic acid content was associated with "adolescent nutritional dwarfism" in the Middle East.[1] Since then, zinc insufficiency has been recognized by a number of experts as an important public health issue, especially in developing countries.[2]

Function

Numerous aspects of cellular metabolism are zinc dependent. Zinc plays important roles in growth and development, the immune response, neurological function, and reproduction. On the cellular level, the function of zinc can be divided into three categories: (1) catalytic, (2) structural, and (3) regulatory.[3]

Catalytic Role

Nearly 100 different enzymes depend on zinc for their ability to catalyze vital chemical reactions. Zinc-dependent enzymes can be found in all known classes of enzymes.[4]

Structural Role

Zinc plays an important role in the structure of proteins and cell membranes. A fingerlike structure, known as a *zinc finger motif*, stabilizes the structure of a number of proteins. For example, copper provides the catalytic activity for the antioxidant enzyme copper–zinc superoxide dismutase (CuZnSOD), while zinc plays a critical structural role.[4,5] The structure and function of cell membranes are also affected by zinc. Loss of zinc from biological membranes increases their susceptibility to oxidative damage and impairs their function.[6]

Regulatory Role

Zinc finger proteins have been found to regulate gene expression by acting as transcription factors (binding to DNA and influencing the transcription of specific genes). Zinc also plays a role in cell signaling and has been found to influence hormone release and nerve impulse transmission. More recently, zinc has been found to play a role in apoptosis (gene-directed cell death), a critical cellular regulatory process with implications for growth and development, as well as a number of chronic diseases.[7]

Nutrient Interactions

Copper. Taking large quantities of zinc (50 mg/day or more) over a period of weeks can interfere with copper bioavailability. High intake of zinc induces the intestinal synthesis of a copper-binding protein called *metallothionein*. Metallothionein traps copper within intestinal cells and prevents its systemic absorption. More typical intakes of zinc do not affect copper absorption and high copper intakes do not affect zinc absorption.[5]

Iron. Supplemental (38–65 mg/day of elemental iron) but not dietary levels of iron may decrease zinc absorption.[8] This interaction is of concern in the management of iron supplementation during pregnancy and lactation, and has led some experts to recommend zinc supplementation for pregnant and lactating women taking more than 60 mg/day of elemental iron.[9,10]

Calcium. High levels of dietary calcium impair zinc absorption in animals, but it is uncertain whether this occurs in humans. One study showed that increasing the calcium intake of postmenopausal women by 890 mg/day in the form of milk or calcium phosphate (total calcium intake, 1360 mg/day) reduced zinc absorption and zinc balance in postmenopausal women,[11] but increasing the calcium intake of adolescent girls by 1000 mg/day in the form of calcium citrate malate (total calcium intake, 1667 mg/day) did not affect zinc absorption or balance.[12] Calcium in combination with phytic acid reduces zinc absorption. This effect is particularly relevant to individuals who very frequently consume tortillas made with lime (i.e., calcium oxide). For more information on phytic acid, see "Food Sources," p. 229.

Folic acid. The bioavailability of dietary folate is increased by the action of a zinc-dependent enzyme, suggesting a possible interaction between zinc and folate. In the past, some studies found that low zinc intake decreased folate absorption, whereas other studies found that folic acid supplementation impaired zinc utilization in individuals with marginal zinc status.[4,5] However, a more recent study reported that supplementation with a relatively high dose of folic acid (800 µg/day) for 25 days did not alter zinc status in a group of students being fed low-zinc diets (3.5 mg/day); the level of zinc intake did not impair folate utilization in this study.[13]

Vitamin A. Zinc and vitamin A interact in several ways. Zinc is a component of retinol-binding protein, a protein necessary for transporting vitamin A in the blood. Zinc is also required for the enzyme that converts retinol (vitamin A) to retinal. This latter form of vitamin A is necessary for the synthesis of rhodopsin, a protein in the eye that absorbs light and thus is involved in dark adaptation. Zinc deficiency is associated with a decreased release of vitamin A from the liver, which may contribute to symptoms of night blindness that are seen with zinc deficiency.[14,15]

Deficiency

Severe Zinc Deficiency

Much of what is known about severe zinc deficiency has been derived from the study of individuals born with acrodermatitis enteropathica, a genetic disorder resulting from the impaired uptake and transport of zinc. The symptoms of severe zinc deficiency include the slowing or cessation of growth and development, delayed sexual maturation, characteristic skin rashes, chronic and severe diarrhea, immune system deficiencies, impaired wound healing, diminished appetite, impaired taste sensation, night blindness,

swelling and clouding of the corneas, and behavioral disturbances. Before the cause of acrodermatitis enteropathica was known, patients typically died in infancy. Oral zinc therapy results in the complete remission of symptoms, although it must be maintained indefinitely in individuals with the genetic disorder.[5,16] Although dietary zinc deficiency is unlikely to cause severe zinc deficiency in individuals without a genetic disorder, zinc malabsorption or conditions of increased zinc loss, such as severe burns or prolonged diarrhea, may also result in severe zinc deficiency.

Mild Zinc Deficiency

It has recently become apparent that milder zinc deficiency contributes to a number of health problems, especially common in children who live in developing countries. The lack of a sensitive indicator of mild zinc deficiency hinders the scientific study of its health implications. However, controlled trials of moderate zinc supplementation have demonstrated that mild zinc deficiency contributes to impaired physical and neuropsychological development and increased susceptibility to life-threatening infections in young children.[16]

Individuals at risk of zinc deficiency. Populations at increased risk of zinc deficiency include: infants and children; pregnant and lactating women, especially teenagers; patients receiving total parenteral nutrition (intravenous feeding); malnourished individuals, including those with protein–energy malnutrition and anorexia nervosa; individuals with severe or persistent diarrhea; individuals with malabsorption syndromes, including celiac disease and short bowel syndrome; individuals with inflammatory bowel disease, including Crohn disease and ulcerative colitis; individuals with alcoholic liver disease; individuals with sickle cell anemia; and older adults (65 years and older).[5]

Strict vegetarians. The requirement for dietary zinc may be as much as 50% greater for strict vegetarians whose major food staples are grains and legumes, because high levels of phytic acid in these foods reduce zinc absorption.[4]

Table 27.1 Recommended dietary allowance for zinc

Life stage	Age	Males (mg/day)	Females (mg/day)
Infants	0–6 months	2 (AI)	2 (AI)
Infants	7–12 months	3	3
Children	1–3 years	3	3
Children	4–8 years	5	5
Children	9–13 years	8	8
Adolescents	14–18 years	11	9
Adults	≥19 years	11	8
Pregnancy	≤18 years	–	12
Pregnancy	≥19 years	–	11
Breast-feeding	≤18 years	–	13
Breast-feeding	≥19 years	–	12

AI, adequate intake.

Recommended Dietary Allowance

The US recommended dietary allowance (RDA) for zinc is listed in **Table 27.1** by life stage and gender. Infants, children, and pregnant and lactating women are at increased risk of zinc deficiency. As a sensitive indicator of zinc nutritional status is not readily available, the RDA for zinc is based on a number of different indicators of zinc nutritional status and represents the daily intake likely to prevent deficiency in nearly all individuals in a specific age and gender group.[4]

Disease Prevention

The following health problems and diseases may be avoided by addressing zinc deficiency.

Impaired Growth and Development

Growth retardation. Significant delays in linear growth and weight gain, known as *growth retardation* or *failure to thrive*, are common features of mild zinc deficiency in children. In the 1970s and 1980s, several randomized, placebo-controlled studies of zinc supplementation in young children with significant growth delays were conducted in Denver, Colorado. Modest zinc supplementation (5.7 mg/day) resulted in increased growth rates compared with placebo.[17] More recently, a number of larger studies in developing countries observed similar results with modest zinc supplementation. A meta-analysis of growth data from zinc intervention trials recently con-firmed the widespread occurrence of growth-limiting zinc deficiency in young children, especially in developing countries.[18] Although the exact mechanism for the growth-limiting effects of zinc deficiency are not known, research indicates that zinc availability affects cell-signaling systems that coordinate the response to the growth-regulating hormone, insulin-like growth factor-1 (IGF-1).[19]

Delayed neurological and behavioral development in young children. Low maternal zinc nutritional status has been associated with diminished attention in newborn infants and poorer motor function at 6 months of age. Zinc supplementation has been associated with improved motor development in very low-birth-weight infants, more vigorous activity in Indian infants and toddlers, and more functional activity in Guatemalan infants and toddlers.[20] In addition, zinc supplementation was associated with better neuropsychological functioning (e.g., attention) in Chinese first-grade students, but this was observed only when zinc was provided with other micronutrients.[21] Two other studies failed to find an association between zinc supplementation and measures of attention in children diagnosed with growth retardation. Although initial studies suggest that zinc deficiency may depress cognitive development in young children, more controlled research is required to determine the nature of the effect and whether zinc supplementation is beneficial.[22]

Increased Susceptibility to Infectious Disease in Children

Adequate zinc intake is essential in maintaining the integrity of the immune system,[23] and zinc-deficient individuals are known to experience increased susceptibility to a variety of infectious agents.[24]

Diarrhea. It is estimated that diarrheal diseases result in the deaths of over 3 million children in developing countries each year. The adverse effects of zinc deficiency on immune system function are likely to increase the susceptibility of children to infectious diarrhea, and persistent diarrhea contributes to zinc deficiency and malnutrition. Research indicates that zinc deficiency may also potentiate the effects of toxins produced by diarrhea-causing bacteria such as *Escherichia coli*.[25] Zinc supplementation in combination with oral rehydration therapy has been shown to significantly reduce the duration and severity of acute and persistent childhood diarrhea and to increase survival in a number of randomized controlled trials.[26,27] Recently, a meta-analysis of randomized controlled trials concluded that zinc supplementation reduces the frequency, severity, and duration of diarrheal episodes in children aged under 5 years.[28] The World Health Organization and the United Nations Children's Fund currently recommend zinc supplementation as part of the treatment for diarrheal diseases in young children.[29]

Pneumonia. Zinc supplementation may also reduce the incidence of lower respiratory infections, such as pneumonia. A pooled analysis of a number of studies in developing countries demonstrated a substantial reduction in the prevalence of pneumonia in children supplemented with zinc.[30] A recent meta-analysis found that zinc supplementation reduced the incidence but not duration of pneumonia or respiratory tract illnesses in children aged under 5 years.[28]

Malaria. Some studies have indicated that zinc supplementation may reduce the incidence of clinical attacks of malaria in children.[31] A placebo-controlled trial in preschool-aged children in Papua New Guinea found that zinc supplementation reduced the frequency of health center attendance due to *Plasmodium falciparum* malaria by 38%.[32] In addition, the number of malaria episodes accompanied by high blood levels of this malaria-causing parasite was reduced by 68%, suggesting that zinc supplementation may be of benefit in preventing more severe episodes of malaria. However, a 6-month trial in more than 700 West African children did not find the frequency or severity of malaria episodes caused by *P. falciparum* to be different in children supplemented with zinc compared with those given a placebo.[33] In addition, a randomized controlled trial reported that zinc supplementation did not benefit preschool-aged children with acute, uncomplicated *P. falciparum* malaria.[34] Further, a randomized controlled trial in over 42 000 children aged 1–48 months found that zinc supplementation did not significantly reduce mortality associated with malaria and other infections.[35] Due to conflicting reports, it is not yet clear whether zinc supplementation has any utility in treating childhood malaria.

Impaired Immune Response in Elderly People

Age-related declines in immune function are similar to those associated with zinc deficiency, and elderly people are vulnerable to mild zinc deficiency. However, the results of zinc supplementation trials on immune function in elderly people have been mixed. Certain aspects of immune function in elderly people have been found to improve with zinc supplementation.[36] For example, a randomized placebo-controlled study in men and women aged over 65 years found that a zinc supplement of 25 mg/day for 3 months increased levels of some circulating immune cells (i.e., CD4 T cells and cytotoxic T lymphocytes) compared with placebo.[37] However, other studies have reported that zinc supplementation does not improve parameters of immune function, indicating that more research is required before any recommendations can be made about zinc and immune system response in elderly people.

Pregnancy Complications

It has been estimated that 82% of pregnant women worldwide are likely to have inadequate zinc intakes. Poor maternal zinc nutritional status has been associated with a number of adverse outcomes of pregnancy, including low birth weight, premature delivery, labor and delivery complications, and congenital anomalies.[38] However, the results of maternal zinc supplementation trials in the United States and developing countries have been mixed.[20] Although some studies have found maternal zinc supplementation to increase birth weight and decrease the likelihood of premature delivery, two placebo-controlled studies in Peruvian and Bangladeshi women found that zinc supplementation did not affect the incidence of low birth weight or premature delivery.[39,40] Supplementation studies designed to examine the effect of zinc supplementation on labor and delivery complications have also generated mixed results, although few have been conducted in zinc-deficient populations.[20] A recent systematic review of 17 randomized controlled trials found that zinc supplementation during pregnancy was associated with a 14% reduction in premature deliveries; the lower incidence of preterm births was observed mainly in low-income women.[41] This analysis did not, however, find zinc supplementation to benefit other indicators of maternal or infant health.[41]

Disease Treatment

Common Cold

Zinc lozenges. The use of zinc lozenges within 24 hours of the onset of cold symptoms, and continued every 2–3 hours while awake until symptoms resolve, has been advocated for reducing the duration of the common cold. At least 10 controlled trials of zinc gluconate lozenges for the treatment of common colds in adults have been published. Five studies found that zinc lozenges reduced the duration of cold symptoms, whereas five studies found no difference between zinc lozenges and placebo lozenges with respect to the duration or severity of cold symptoms. A meta-analysis of published randomized controlled trials on the use of zinc gluconate lozenges in colds found that evidence for their effectiveness in reducing the duration of common colds was still lacking.[42] Two clinical trials examined the effect of zinc acetate lozenges on cold symptoms. Although one of the trials found that zinc acetate lozenges (12.8 mg zinc per lozenge) taken every 2–3 hours while awake reduced the duration of overall cold symptoms (4.5 vs. 8.1 days) compared with placebo,[43] the other study found that zinc acetate lozenges were no different from placebo in reducing the duration or severity of cold symptoms.[44]

Despite numerous well-controlled trials, the efficacy of zinc lozenges in treating common cold symptoms remains questionable, although a recent Cochrane review of 13 therapeutic trials found that, when taken within 24 hours of the onset of cold symptoms, zinc supplementation in the form of lozenges or syrup reduced the severity and duration of cold symptoms.[70] The physiological basis for a beneficial effect of high-dose zinc supplementation on cold symptoms is not known. Taking zinc lozenges every 2–3 hours while awake often results in daily zinc intakes well above the tolerable upper intake level (UL) of 40 mg/day. Short-term use of zinc lozenges (e.g., less than 5 days) has not resulted in serious side effects, although some individuals experienced gastrointestinal disturbances and mouth irritation. Use of zinc lozenges for prolonged periods (e.g., 6–8 weeks) is likely to result in copper deficiency. For this reason, some experts have recommended that a person who does not show clear evidence of improvement of cold symptoms after 3–5 days of zinc lozenge treatment seek medical evaluation.[43]

Intranasal zinc (zinc nasal gels and nasal sprays). Intranasal zinc preparations, designed to be applied directly to the nasal epithelium (cells lining the nasal passages), are also marketed as over-the-counter cold remedies. Although two placebo-controlled trials found that intranasal zinc gluconate modestly shortened the duration of cold symptoms,[45,46] three other placebo-controlled studies found intranasal zinc to be of no benefit.[47–49] In the most rigorously controlled of these studies, intranasal zinc gluconate did not affect the severity or duration of cold symptoms in volunteers inoculated with rhinovirus, a common cause of colds.[47] Of serious concern are several case reports of individuals experiencing loss of the sense of smell (anosmia) after using intranasal zinc as a cold remedy.[50,51] Because zinc-associated anosmia may be irreversible, intranasal zinc preparations should be avoided.

Age-related Macular Degeneration

A leading cause of blindness in people over the age of 65 in the United States is a degenerative disease of the macula, known as age-related macular degeneration (ARMD). The macula is the portion of the retina in the back of the eye involved with central vision. Zinc is hypothesized to play a role in the development of ARMD for several reasons:

- Zinc is found at high concentrations in the part of the retina affected by ARMD.
- Retinal zinc content has been shown to decline with age.
- The activities of some zinc-dependent retinal enzymes have been shown to decline with age.

However, scientific evidence that zinc intake is associated with the development or progression of ARMD is limited. Observational studies have not demonstrated clear associations between dietary zinc intake and the incidence of ARMD.[52–54] A randomized controlled trial provoked interest when it found that 200 mg/day of zinc sulfate (81 mg/day of elemental zinc) over 2 years reduced the loss of vision in patients with ARMD.[55] However, a later trial using the same dose and duration found no beneficial effect in patients with a more advanced form of ARMD in one eye.[56] A large randomized controlled trial of daily supplementation with antioxidants (500 mg vitamin C, 400 IU vitamin E, and 15 mg β-carotene) and high-dose zinc (80 mg zinc and 2 mg copper) found that the antioxidant combination plus high-dose zinc, and high-dose zinc alone, both significantly reduced the risk of advanced macular degeneration compared with placebo in individuals with signs of moderate-to-severe macular degeneration in at least one eye.[57] Data from smaller trials have generally not observed a protective effect of vitamin and mineral supplementation on ARMD.[58] At present, there is little evidence that zinc supplementation would be beneficial to people with early signs of macular degeneration, but further randomized controlled trials are warranted.[59]

Diabetes Mellitus

Moderate zinc deficiency may be relatively common in individuals with diabetes mellitus. Increased loss of zinc by frequent urination appears to contribute to the marginal zinc nutritional status that has been observed in people with diabetes.[60] Although zinc supplementation reportedly improves immune function in people with diabetes, zinc supplementation of 50 mg/day adversely affected control of blood glucose in type 1 diabetes in one study.[61] In a more recent study, supplementation of people with type 2 diabetes with 30 mg/day of zinc for 6 months reduced a nonspecific measure of oxidative stress (plasma TBARS) without significantly affecting blood glucose control.[62] Currently, the influence of zinc on glucose metabolism requires further study before high-dose zinc supplementation can be advocated for people with diabetes.[5]

HIV/AIDS

Sufficient zinc is essential in maintaining immune system function and human immunodeficiency virus (HIV)-infected individuals are particularly susceptible to zinc deficiency. In HIV-infected patients, low serum levels of zinc have been associated with a more advanced stage of the disease and also with increased mortality.[63,64] In one of the few zinc supplementation studies conducted in patients with acquired immune deficiency syndrome (AIDS), 45 mg/day of zinc for 1 month resulted in a decreased incidence in opportunistic infections compared with placebo.[65] However, HIV also requires zinc, and excessive zinc intake may stimulate the progression of HIV infection. In an observational study of HIV-infected men, increased zinc intake was associated with more rapid disease progression, and any intake of zinc supplements was associated with poorer survival.[66] These results indicate that further research is necessary to determine optimal zinc intakes for HIV-infected individuals.[23,67]

Sources

Food Sources

Shellfish, beef, and other red meats are rich sources of zinc. Nuts and legumes are relatively good plant sources of zinc. Zinc bioavailability (the fraction of zinc retained and used by the body) is relatively high in meat, eggs, and seafood because of the relative absence of compounds that inhibit zinc absorption and the presence of certain amino acids (cysteine and methionine)

Table 27.2 Food sources of zinc

Food	Serving	Zinc (mg)
Oysters, cooked	6 medium	76.3
Beef, cooked	3 ounces[a]	6.0
Crab, Dungeness, cooked	3 ounces[a]	4.7
Turkey, dark meat, cooked	3 ounces[a]	3.8
Pork, cooked	3 ounces[a]	2.2
Chicken, dark meat, cooked	3 ounces[a]	1.8
Beans, baked	½ cup	1.8
Yogurt, fruit	1 cup (8 ounces)	1.8
Milk	1 cup (8 ounces)	1.8
Cashews	1 ounce	1.6
Chickpeas (garbanzo beans)	½ cup	1.3
Almonds	1 ounce	1.0
Peanuts	1 ounce	0.9
Cheese, cheddar	1 ounce	0.9

[a]A three-ounce serving of meat or seafood is about the size of a deck of cards.

that improve zinc absorption. The zinc in whole-grain products and plant proteins is less bioavailable due to their relatively high content of phytic acid, a compound that inhibits zinc absorption.[5] The enzymatic action of yeast reduces the level of phytic acid in foods. Therefore, leavened whole-grain breads have more bioavailable zinc than unleavened whole-grain breads. National dietary surveys in the United States estimate that average dietary zinc intake is 9 mg/day for women and 13 mg/day for men.[4] The zinc content of some relatively zinc-rich foods is listed in **Table 27.2**.

Supplements

A number of zinc supplements are available, including zinc acetate, zinc gluconate, zinc picolinate, and zinc sulfate. Zinc picolinate has been promoted as a more absorbable form of zinc, but there are few data to support this idea in humans. Limited work in animals suggests that increased intestinal absorption of zinc picolinate may be offset by increased elimination.[4]

Safety

Toxicity

Acute toxicity. Isolated outbreaks of acute zinc toxicity have occurred as a result of the consumption of food or beverages contaminated with zinc released from galvanized containers. Signs of acute zinc toxicity are abdominal pain, diarrhea, nausea, and vomiting. Single doses of 225–450 mg zinc usually induce vomiting. Milder gastrointestinal distress has been reported at doses of 50–150 mg/day of supplemental zinc. Metal fume fever has been reported after the inhalation of zinc oxide fumes. Specifically, profuse sweating, weakness, and rapid breathing may develop within 8 hours of zinc oxide inhalation and persist 12–24 hours after exposure is terminated.[4,5]

Chronic toxicity. The major consequence of long-term consumption of excessive zinc is copper deficiency. Total zinc intakes of 60 mg/day (50 mg supplemental and 10 mg dietary zinc) have been found to result in signs of copper deficiency. To prevent copper deficiency, the US Food and Nutrition Board set a UL for adults at 40 mg/day, including dietary and supplemental zinc (**Table 27.3**).[4]

Intranasal zinc. Intranasal zinc is known to cause a loss of the sense of smell (anosmia) in laboratory animals,[68] and there have been several case reports of individuals who developed anosmia after using intranasal zinc gluconate.[50,51] Because zinc-associated anosmia may be irreversible, zinc nasal gels and sprays should be avoided.

Drug Interactions

Concomitant administration of zinc supplements and certain antibiotics, specifically tetracyclines and quinolones, may decrease absorption of the antibiotic and potentially reduce its efficacy. Taking zinc supplements and these antibiotics at least 2 hours apart should prevent this interaction.[69] In addition, the therapeutic use of metal-chelating (binding) agents such as penicillamine (used to treat copper overload in Wilson disease) and diethylenetriamine pentaacetate or DTPA (used to treat iron overload) has resulted in severe zinc deficiency. Anticonvulsant drugs, espe-

Table 27.3 Tolerable upper intake level (UL) for zinc

Life stage	Age	UL (mg/day)
Infants	0–6 months	4
Infants	7–12 months	5
Children	1–3 years	7
Children	4–8 years	12
Children	9–13 years	23
Adolescents	14–18 years	34
Adults	≥19 years	40

cially sodium valproate, may also precipitate zinc deficiency. Prolonged use of diuretics may increase urinary zinc excretion, resulting in increased loss of zinc. Further, the tuberculosis medication, ethambutol, has metal-chelating properties and has been shown to increase zinc loss in rats.[5]

LPI Recommendation

The RDA for zinc (8 mg/day for women and 11 mg/day for men) appears sufficient to prevent deficiency in most individuals, but the lack of sensitive indicators of zinc nutritional status in humans makes it difficult to determine the level of zinc intake most likely to promote optimum health. Following the Linus Pauling Institute recommendation to take a multivitamin/mineral supplement containing 100% of the daily values of most nutrients will generally provide 15 mg/day of zinc.

Older Adults

Although the requirement for zinc is not known to be higher for older adults, their average zinc intake tends to be considerably less than the RDA. A reduced capacity to absorb zinc, increased likelihood of disease states that alter zinc utilization, and increased use of drugs that increase zinc excretion may all contribute to an increased risk of mild zinc deficiency in older adults. Because the consequences of mild zinc deficiency, such as impaired immune system function, are particularly relevant to the health of older adults, they should pay particular attention to maintaining adequate zinc intake.

References

1. Prasad AS, Halsted JA, Nadimi M. Syndrome of iron deficiency anemia, hepatosplenomegaly, hypogonadism, dwarfism and geophagia. Am J Med 1961;31: 532–546
2. Prasad AS. Zinc deficiency in humans: a neglected problem. J Am Coll Nutr 1998;17(6):542–543
3. Cousins RJ. Zinc. In: Bowman BA, Russell RM, eds. Present Knowledge in Nutrition, Vol. 1. 9th ed. Washington, DC: ILSI Press, 2006:445–457
4. Food and Nutrition Board, Institute of Medicine. Zinc. In: Dietary Reference Intakes for Vitamin A, Vitamin K, Boron, Chromium, Copper, Iodine, Iron, Manganese, Molybdenum, Nickel, Silicon, Vanadium, and Zinc. Washington, DC: National Academy Press, 2001: 442–501
5. King JC, Cousins RJ. Zinc. In: Shils ME, Shike M, Ross AC, Caballero B, Cousins RJ, eds. Modern Nutrition in Health and Disease. 10th ed. Baltimore, MD: Lippincott Williams & Wilkins, 2006: 271–285
6. O'Dell BL. Role of zinc in plasma membrane function. J Nutr 2000;130(5S, Suppl):1432S–1436S
7. Truong-Tran AQ, Ho LH, Chai F, Zalewski PD. Cellular zinc fluxes and the regulation of apoptosis/gene-directed cell death. J Nutr 2000;130(5S, Suppl):1459S–1466S
8. Sandström B. Micronutrient interactions: effects on absorption and bioavailability. Br J Nutr 2001;85(Suppl 2):S181–S185
9. O'Brien KO, Zavaleta N, Caulfield LE, Wen J, Abrams SA. Prenatal iron supplements impair zinc absorption in pregnant Peruvian women. J Nutr 2000;130(9): 2251–2255
10. Fung EB, Ritchie LD, Woodhouse LR, Roehl R, King JC. Zinc absorption in women during pregnancy and lactation: a longitudinal study. Am J Clin Nutr 1997; 66(1):80–88
11. Wood RJ, Zheng JJ. High dietary calcium intakes reduce zinc absorption and balance in humans. Am J Clin Nutr 1997;65(6):1803–1809
12. McKenna AA, Ilich JZ, Andon MB, Wang C, Matkovic V. Zinc balance in adolescent females consuming a low- or high-calcium diet. Am J Clin Nutr 1997;65(5): 1460–1464
13. Kauwell GP, Bailey LB, Gregory JF III, Bowling DW, Cousins RJ. Zinc status is not adversely affected by folic acid supplementation and zinc intake does not impair folate utilization in human subjects. J Nutr 1995;125(1):66–72
14. Boron B, Hupert J, Barch DH, et al. Effect of zinc deficiency on hepatic enzymes regulating vitamin A status. J Nutr 1988;118(8):995–1001
15. Christian P, West KP Jr. Interactions between zinc and vitamin A: an update. Am J Clin Nutr 1998;68(2, Suppl):435S–441S
16. Hambidge M. Human zinc deficiency. J Nutr 2000;130(5S, Suppl)1344S–1349S
17. Walravens PA, Hambidge KM, Koepfer DM. Zinc supplementation in infants with a nutritional pattern of failure to thrive: a double-blind, controlled study. Pediatrics 1989;83(4):532–538
18. Hambidge M, Krebs N. Zinc and growth. In: Roussel AM, ed. Trace Elements in Man and Animals 10: Proceedings of the Tenth International Symposium on Trace Elements in Man and Animals. New York: Plenum Press, 2000: 977–980
19. MacDonald RS. The role of zinc in growth and cell proliferation. J Nutr 2000;130(5S, Suppl):1500S–1508S
20. Caulfield LE, Zavaleta N, Shankar AH, Merialdi M. Potential contribution of maternal zinc supplementation during pregnancy to maternal and child survival. Am J Clin Nutr 1998;68(2, Suppl):499S–508S
21. Sandstead HH, Penland JG, Alcock NW, et al. Effects of repletion with zinc and other micronutrients on neuropsychologic performance and growth of Chinese children. Am J Clin Nutr 1998;68(2, Suppl):470S–475S

22. Black MM. Zinc deficiency and child development. Am J Clin Nutr 1998;68(2, Suppl):464S–469S
23. Baum MK, Shor-Posner G, Campa A. Zinc status in human immunodeficiency virus infection. J Nutr 2000;130(5S, Suppl):1421S–1423S
24. Shankar AH, Prasad AS. Zinc and immune function: the biological basis of altered resistance to infection. Am J Clin Nutr 1998;68(2, Suppl):447S–463S
25. Wapnir RA. Zinc deficiency, malnutrition and the gastrointestinal tract. J Nutr 2000;130(5S, Suppl):1388S–1392S
26. Bhutta ZA, Bird SM, Black RE, et al. Therapeutic effects of oral zinc in acute and persistent diarrhea in children in developing countries: pooled analysis of randomized controlled trials. Am J Clin Nutr 2000; 72(6):1516–1522
27. Fischer Walker CL, Black RE. Micronutrients and diarrheal disease. Clin Infect Dis 2007;45(Suppl 1): S73–S77
28. Aggarwal R, Sentz J, Miller MA. Role of zinc administration in prevention of childhood diarrhea and respiratory illnesses: a meta-analysis. Pediatrics 2007; 119(6):1120–1130
29. The United Nations Children's Fund/World Health Organization. WHO/UNICEF Joint Statement: Clinical Management of Acute Diarrhoea. Geneva: Unicef, 2004: 1–8. Available at: www.unicef.org/publications/index_21433.html
30. Bhutta ZA, Black RE, Brown KH, et al. Prevention of diarrhea and pneumonia by zinc supplementation in children in developing countries: pooled analysis of randomized controlled trials. Zinc Investigators' Collaborative Group. J Pediatr 1999;135(6):689–697
31. Black RE. Therapeutic and preventive effects of zinc on serious childhood infectious diseases in developing countries. Am J Clin Nutr 1998;68(2, Suppl):476S–479S
32. Shankar AH. Nutritional modulation of malaria morbidity and mortality. J Infect Dis 2000;182 (Suppl 1):S37–S53
33. Müller O, Becher H, van Zweeden AB, et al. Effect of zinc supplementation on malaria and other causes of morbidity in west African children: randomised double blind placebo controlled trial. BMJ 2001; 322(7302):1567
34. Zinc Against Plasmodium Study Group. Effect of zinc on the treatment of Plasmodium falciparum malaria in children: a randomized controlled trial. Am J Clin Nutr 2002;76(4):805–812
35. Sazawal S, Black RE, Ramsan M, et al. Effect of zinc supplementation on mortality in children aged 1-48 months: a community-based randomised placebo-controlled trial. Lancet 2007;369(9565):927–934
36. Salgueiro MJ, Zubillaga M, Lysionek A, et al. Zinc status and immune system relationship: a review. Biol Trace Elem Res 2000;76(3):193–205
37. Fortes C, Forastiere F, Agabiti N, et al. The effect of zinc and vitamin A supplementation on immune response in an older population. J Am Geriatr Soc 1998;46(1):19–26
38. Shah D, Sachdev HP. Zinc deficiency in pregnancy and fetal outcome. Nutr Rev 2006;64(1):15–30
39. Caulfield LE, Zavaleta N, Figueroa A, Leon Z. Maternal zinc supplementation does not affect size at birth or pregnancy duration in Peru. J Nutr 1999;129(8): 1563–1568
40. Osendarp SJ, van Raaij JM, Arifeen SE, Wahed M, Baqui AH, Fuchs GJ. A randomized, placebo-controlled trial

of the effect of zinc supplementation during pregnancy on pregnancy outcome in Bangladeshi urban poor. Am J Clin Nutr 2000;71(1):114–119
41. Mahomed K, Bhutta Z, Middleton P. Zinc supplementation for improving pregnancy and infant outcome. Cochrane Database Syst Rev 2007;(2):CD000230
42. Jackson JL, Lesho E, Peterson C. Zinc and the common cold: a meta-analysis revisited. J Nutr 2000;130(5S, Suppl):1512S–1515S
43. Prasad AS, Fitzgerald JT, Bao B, Beck FW, Chandrasekar PH. Duration of symptoms and plasma cytokine levels in patients with the common cold treated with zinc acetate. A randomized, double-blind, placebo-controlled trial. Ann Intern Med 2000;133(4): 245–252
44. Turner RB, Cetnarowski WE. Effect of treatment with zinc gluconate or zinc acetate on experimental and natural colds. Clin Infect Dis 2000;31(5):1202–1208
45. Mossad SB. Effect of zincum gluconicum nasal gel on the duration and symptom severity of the common cold in otherwise healthy adults. QJM 2003;96(1): 35–43
46. Hirt M, Nobel S, Barron E. Zinc nasal gel for the treatment of common cold symptoms: a double-blind, placebo-controlled trial. Ear Nose Throat J 2000; 79(10):778–780, 782
47. Turner RB. Ineffectiveness of intranasal zinc gluconate for prevention of experimental rhinovirus colds. Clin Infect Dis 2001;33(11):1865–1870
48. Belongia EA, Berg R, Liu K. A randomized trial of zinc nasal spray for the treatment of upper respiratory illness in adults. Am J Med 2001;111(2):103–108
49. Eby GA, Halcomb WW. Ineffectiveness of zinc gluconate nasal spray and zinc orotate lozenges in common-cold treatment: a double-blind, placebo-controlled clinical trial. Altern Ther Health Med 2006; 12(1):34–38
50. Jafek BW, Linschoten M, Murrow BW. Zicam Induced Anosmia. American Rhinologic Society 49th Annual Fall Scientific Meeting, 48–49. Available at: http://app.american-rhinologic.org/programs/2003ARSFall Program071503.pdf (accessed 4 Jan 2011)
51. DeCook CA, Hirsch AR. Anosmia due to inhalational zinc: a case report. Chem Senses 2000;25(5):659
52. VandenLangenberg GM, Mares-Perlman JA, Klein R, Klein BE, Brady WE, Palta M. Associations between antioxidant and zinc intake and the 5-year incidence of early age-related maculopathy in the Beaver Dam Eye Study. Am J Epidemiol 1998;148(2):204–214
53. Smith W, Mitchell P, Webb K, Leeder SR. Dietary antioxidants and age-related maculopathy: the Blue Mountains Eye Study. Ophthalmology 1999;106(4): 761–767
54. Cho E, Stampfer MJ, Seddon JM, et al. Prospective study of zinc intake and the risk of age-related macular degeneration. Ann Epidemiol 2001;11(5):328–336
55. Newsome DA, Swartz M, Leone NC, Elston RC, Miller E. Oral zinc in macular degeneration. Arch Ophthalmol 1988;106(2):192–198
56. Stur M, Tittl M, Reitner A, Meisinger V. Oral zinc and the second eye in age-related macular degeneration. Invest Ophthalmol Vis Sci 1996;37(7):1225–1235
57. Age-Related Eye Disease Study Research Group. A randomized, placebo-controlled, clinical trial of high-dose supplementation with vitamins C and E, beta carotene, and zinc for age-related macular degenera-

tion and vision loss: AREDS report no. 8. Arch Ophthalmol 2001;119(10):1417–1436

58. Evans JR. Antioxidant vitamin and mineral supplements for slowing the progression of age-related macular degeneration. Cochrane Database Syst Rev 2006;(2):CD 000254

59. Evans JR. Antioxidant vitamin and mineral supplements for age-related macular degeneration. Cochrane Database Syst Rev 2002; (1):CD 000254

60. Blostein-Fujii A, DiSilvestro RA, Frid D, Katz C, Malarkey W. Short-term zinc supplementation in women with non-insulin-dependent diabetes mellitus: effects on plasma 5′-nucleotidase activities, insulin-like growth factor I concentrations, and lipoprotein oxidation rates in vitro. Am J Clin Nutr 1997;66(3):639–642

61. Cunningham JJ, Fu A, Mearkle PL, Brown RG. Hyperzincuria in individuals with insulin-dependent diabetes mellitus: concurrent zinc status and the effect of high-dose zinc supplementation. Metabolism 1994; 43(12):1558–1562

62. Anderson RA, Roussel AM, Zouari N, Mahjoub S, Matheau JM, Kerkeni A. Potential antioxidant effects of zinc and chromium supplementation in people with type 2 diabetes mellitus. J Am Coll Nutr 2001;20(3):212–218

63. Lai H, Lai S, Shor-Posner G, Ma F, Trapido E, Baum MK. Plasma zinc, copper, copper:zinc ratio, and survival in a cohort of HIV-1-infected homosexual men. J Acquir Immune Defic Syndr 2001;27(1):56–62

64. Wellinghausen N, Kern WV, Jöchle W, Kern P. Zinc serum level in human immunodeficiency virus-infected patients in relation to immunological status. Biol Trace Elem Res 2000;73(2):139–149

65. Mocchegiani E, Muzzioli M. Therapeutic application of zinc in human immunodeficiency virus against opportunistic infections. J Nutr 2000;130(5S, Suppl):1424S–1431S

66. Tang AM, Graham NM, Saah AJ. Effects of micronutrient intake on survival in human immunodeficiency virus type 1 infection. Am J Epidemiol 1996;143(12):1244–1256

67. Kupka R, Fawzi W. Zinc nutrition and HIV infection. Nutr Rev 2002;60(3):69–79

68. McBride K, Slotnick B, Margolis FL. Does intranasal application of zinc sulfate produce anosmia in the mouse? An olfactometric and anatomical study. Chem Senses 2003;28(8):659–670

69. Trace elements. Drug Facts and Comparisons, 54th ed. St. Louis: Facts and Comparisons; 2000:43

70. Singh M.Dag RR. Zinc for the common cold. Cochrane Database Syst Rev 2011; 2:CD001364

Appendix

Nutrient–Nutrient Interactions

Nutrient	Nutrient	Interaction
Biotin	Pantothenic acid	High doses of pantothenic acid may compete with biotin for absorption
Folic acid	Riboflavin	Works synergistically with folate to lower homocysteine levels
	Vitamin B_6	Works synergistically with folate to lower homocysteine levels
	Vitamin B_{12}	Works synergistically with folate to lower homocysteine levels High-dose folic acid therapy may mask the symptoms of vitamin B_{12} deficiency
Niacin	Riboflavin	Riboflavin deficiency may increase the risk of niacin deficiency by decreasing niacin synthesis from tryptophan
	Tryptophan	Niacin can be synthesized from tryptophan, reducing the dietary niacin requirement
Pantothenic acid	Biotin	High doses of pantothenic acid may compete with biotin for absorption
Riboflavin	Folic acid	Works synergistically with riboflavin to lower homocysteine levels
	Iron	Riboflavin deficiency may impair iron absorption or utilization
	Niacin	Riboflavin deficiency may increase the risk of niacin deficiency by decreasing niacin synthesis from tryptophan
	Vitamin B_6	Riboflavin deficiency may decrease conversion of vitamin B_6 to its coenzyme form
Vitamin A	Iodine	Vitamin A deficiency may exacerbate the effects of iodine deficiency
	Iron	Vitamin A deficiency may exacerbate iron deficiency
	Vitamin K	High doses of vitamin A may decrease vitamin K absorption
	Zinc	Zinc deficiency may interfere with vitamin A metabolism
Vitamin B_6	Folic acid	Works synergistically with vitamin B_6 to lower homocysteine levels
	Riboflavin	Riboflavin deficiency may decrease conversion of vitamin B_6 to its coenzyme form
	Vitamin B_{12}	Works synergistically with vitamin B_6 to lower homocysteine levels
Vitamin B_{12}	Folic acid	Works synergistically with vitamin B_{12} to lower homocysteine levels High-dose folic acid therapy may mask the symptoms of vitamin B_{12} deficiency
	Riboflavin	Works synergistically with vitamin B_{12} to lower homocysteine levels
	Vitamin B_6	Works synergistically with vitamin B_{12} to lower homocysteine levels
Vitamin C	Chromium	Concomitant intake may enhance the absorption of chromium
	Iron	Concomitant intake increases the absorption of nonheme iron
	Selenium	Selenium-dependent enzymes catalyze the regeneration of vitamin C and function synergistically in antioxidant system
	Vitamin E	Vitamin C may regenerate vitamin E
Vitamin D	Calcium	Active form of vitamin D increases intestinal calcium absorption and decreases urinary calcium excretion
	Magnesium	Active form of vitamin D (calcitriol) may slightly increase intestinal absorption of magnesium

Nutrient	Nutrient	Interaction
Vitamin E	Selenium	Selenium-dependent enzymes function synergistically in antioxidant system
	Vitamin C	Vitamin C may regenerate vitamin E
	Vitamin K	High doses of vitamin E may inhibit activity of vitamin K-dependent enzymes, resulting in functional vitamin K deficiency
Vitamin K	Vitamin A	High doses of vitamin A may decrease vitamin K absorption
	Vitamin E	High doses of vitamin E may inhibit activity of vitamin K-dependent enzymes, resulting in functional vitamin K deficiency
Calcium	Fluoride	Supplemental use may decrease fluoride absorption
	Iron	Concomitant intake decreases nonheme iron absorption calcium and iron supplements should not be taken together
	Manganese	Concomitant intake may decrease manganese absorption
	Protein	Increases urinary calcium excretion
	Sodium	Increases urinary calcium excretion
	Vitamin D	Active form of vitamin D increases intestinal calcium absorption and decreases urinary calcium excretion
	Zinc	High calcium intakes may decrease zinc absorption
Chromium	Vitamin C	Concomitant intake may enhance the absorption of chromium
Copper	Iron	Copper deficiency may interfere with iron transport High-iron formula may decrease infant copper absorption
	Zinc	High supplemental zinc intakes may cause copper deficiency by decreasing intestinal copper absorption
Fluoride	Calcium	Concomitant intake of calcium may decrease absorption of sodium fluoride
	Magnesium	Concomitant intake of magnesium may decrease absorption of sodium fluoride
Iodine	Selenium	Selenium deficiency can exacerbate the effects of iodine deficiency
	Vitamin A	Vitamin A deficiency may exacerbate the effects of iodine deficiency
Iron	Calcium	Concomitant intake decreases nonheme iron absorption; iron and calcium supplements should not be taken together
	Copper	Copper deficiency may interfere with iron transport High-iron formula may decrease infant copper absorption
	Iodine	Iron deficiency may exacerbate the effects of iodine deficiency
	Magnesium	Concomitant intake may decrease nonheme iron absorption
	Manganese	Concomitant iron intake may decrease manganese absorption Manganese absorption is increased in iron-deficient individuals
	Riboflavin	Riboflavin deficiency may impair iron absorption or utilization
	Vitamin A	Vitamin A deficiency may exacerbate iron deficiency
	Vitamin C	Concomitant intake increases nonheme iron absorption
	Zinc	Supplemental doses of iron may decrease zinc absorption

Nutrient	Nutrient	Interaction
Magnesium	Fluoride	Concomitant intake of magnesium and sodium fluoride may decrease absorption of sodium fluoride
	Iron	Concomitant intake may decrease nonheme iron absorption
	Manganese	Supplemental magnesium may decrease manganese absorption
	Vitamin D	Active form of vitamin D (calcitriol) may slightly increase intestinal absorption
	Zinc	High-dose zinc supplement intake may decrease magnesium absorption
Manganese	Calcium	Concomitant intake may decrease manganese absorption
	Iron	Concomitant iron intake may decrease manganese absorption. Manganese absorption is increased in iron-deficient individuals
	Magnesium	Supplemental magnesium may decrease manganese absorption
Phosphorus	Potassium	Taking potassium supplements together with phosphate may cause hyperkalemia
Potassium	Phosphorus	Taking phosphates together with potassium supplements may cause hyperkalemia
Selenium	Iodine	Selenium deficiency can exacerbate the effects of iodine deficiency
	Vitamin C	Selenium-dependent enzymes catalyze the regeneration of vitamin C and function synergistically in antioxidant system
	Vitamin E	Selenium-dependent enzymes function synergistically in antioxidant system
Zinc	Calcium	High calcium intakes may decrease zinc absorption
	Copper	High supplemental zinc intakes may cause copper deficiency by decreasing intestinal copper absorption
	Iron	Supplemental doses of iron may decrease zinc absorption
	Vitamin A	Zinc deficiency may interfere with vitamin A metabolism

Drug–Nutrient Interactions

Drug classes are listed first, alphabetically, followed by specific drugs known to act with specific nutrients. As there may be drug–nutrient interactions that are not listed below, it is important to review the prescribing or patient information of any medication before its use for the possibility of clinically significant drug–nutrient interactions. This appendix does not address the potential for multiple drug–nutrient interactions in individuals taking more than one medication. Note: medications that increase the risk of hyperkalemia and hypokalemia are listed in **Tables 24.3** and **24.4**, respectively. Medications that increase the risk of hyponatremia are listed in **Table 26.5**.

Drug class	Nutrient	Interaction
Antacids	Copper	High doses may decrease copper absorption
	Fluoride	Concomitant intake may decrease fluoride absorption
	Iron	May decrease iron absorption
	Manganese	Concomitant intake of manganese and magnesium-containing antacids may decrease manganese absorption
	Phosphorus	Aluminum-containing antacids decrease phosphate absorption and may cause hypophosphatemia in high doses
Antibiotics	Biotin	Prolonged use of broad-spectrum antibiotics may decrease biotin synthesis by intestinal bacteria
	Vitamin B_{12}	May decrease the absorption of food-bound but not supplemental vitamin B_{12}
	Vitamin K	Prolonged use of broad-spectrum antibiotics may decrease vitamin K synthesis by intestinal bacteria Cephalosporins may decrease vitamin K recycling
	Calcium	Concomitant use of calcium and quinolone or tetracycline classes of antibiotics may decrease antibiotic absorption
	Iron	Concomitant intake of iron supplements may decrease the efficacy of quinolone and tetracycline classes of antibiotics
	Magnesium	Concomitant intake of magnesium supplements may decrease the absorption of nitrofurantoin and quinolone and tetracycline classes of antibiotics
	Manganese	Concomitant intake of manganese and tetracycline classes of antibiotics may decrease manganese absorption
	Zinc	Concomitant intake of zinc supplements may decrease the efficacy of quinolone and tetracycline classes of antibiotics
Anticonvulsants	Biotin	Long-term therapy may increase dietary biotin requirement
	Folic acid	May interfere with dietary folate absorption
	Riboflavin	Long-term therapy may increase riboflavin requirement by increasing hepatic metabolism
	Thiamin	Long-term therapy may increase dietary thiamin requirement
	Vitamin B_6	High doses of vitamin B_6 may decrease the efficacy of the anticonvulsants phenobarbital and phenytoin
	Vitamin D	May decrease plasma levels of calcidiol
	Vitamin E	May decrease plasma levels of vitamin E
	Vitamin K	May increase the risk of neonatal vitamin K deficiency and hemorrhagic disease of newborn infants when taken by pregnant women
	Selenium	Valproic acid use may decrease plasma selenium levels
	Zinc	Anticonvulsant use, especially valproic acid, may precipitate zinc deficiency

Drug class	Nutrient	Interaction
Antiplatelet drugs	Vitamin E	High doses of vitamin E may potentiate antiplatelet effects
Bisphosphonates	Calcium	Concomitant intake may decrease bisphosphonate absorption
	Iron	Concomitant intake of iron supplements may decrease bisphosphonate absorption
	Magnesium	Concomitant intake may decrease bisphosphonate absorption
	Zinc	Concomitant intake may decrease bisphosphonate and zinc absorption
Calcium channel blockers	Calcium	Calcium supplements may decrease the efficacy of calcium channel blockers
Diuretics	Thiamin	Loop diuretics may increase urinary thiamin excretion
	Calcium	Thiazide diuretics increase renal reabsorption of calcium
	Magnesium	Prolonged high doses of diuretics may result in magnesium depletion
	Phosphorus	Taking potassium-sparing diuretics together with phosphates may cause hyperkalemia
	Zinc	May increase urinary zinc excretion
H_2-receptor antagonists	Vitamin B_{12}	May decrease the absorption of food-bound but not supplemental vitamin B_{12}
	Calcium	May decrease the absorption of calcium salts (supplements)
	Iron	May decrease iron absorption
Laxatives	Manganese	Concomitant intake of manganese and magnesium-containing antacids may decrease manganese absorption
Nonsteroidal anti-inflammatory drugs	Folic acid	High doses may interfere with folate metabolism
	Vitamin E	Supplemental use could increase the risk of bleeding
Oral contraceptives (estrogen containing)	Pantothenic acid	May increase pantothenic acid requirement
	Vitamin C	May decrease plasma and leukocyte vitamin C levels
Phenothiazine derivatives	Riboflavin	May inhibit the incorporation of riboflavin into active coenzymes flavin adenine dinucleotide (FAD) and flavin mononucleotide (FMN)
	Magnesium	Magnesium supplements may decrease the efficacy of chlorpromazine
Proton pump inhibitors	Vitamin B_{12}	May decrease the absorption of food-bound but not supplemental vitamin B_{12}
	Calcium	May decrease the absorption of calcium salts (supplements)
	Iron	May decrease iron absorption
Retinoid drugs	Vitamin A	Supplemental vitamin A may add to the risk of toxicity of retinoid drugs
Tricyclic anti-depressants	Riboflavin	May inhibit the incorporation of riboflavin into active coenzymes FAD and FMN

Specific drug	Nutrient	Interaction
Alcohol	Thiamin	Chronic alcohol abuse is associated with thiamin deficiency due to low dietary intake, impaired absorption and utilization, and increased excretion of the vitamin
	Vitamin A	Chronic alcohol consumption increases the risk of vitamin A-induced hepatotoxicity
Allopurinol	Iron	May increase iron storage in the liver; should not be used in combination with iron supplements
Aspirin	Vitamin C	High doses of aspirin may increase urinary excretion of vitamin C
	Vitamin K	May decrease vitamin K recycling
	Vitamin E	High doses of vitamin E may potentiate antiplatelet effects
Calcitriol	Phosphorus	High doses of calcitriol and some vitamin D analogs may cause hyperphosphatemia
Chloramphenicol	Vitamin B_{12}	May decrease the absorption of food-bound but not supplemental vitamin B_{12}
Chlorpromazine	Magnesium	May reduce the efficacy of chlorpromazine
Cholestyramine and colestipol	Most vitamins and minerals	May decrease vitamin and mineral absorption when taken concomitantly
Colchicine	Vitamin B_{12}	May decrease the absorption of food-bound but not supplemental vitamin B_{12}
Cycloserine	Vitamin B_6	May cause functional vitamin B_6 deficiency by forming inactive complex with vitamin B_6
Digoxin	Calcium	High doses of supplemental calcium may increase the risk of arrhythmia
	Magnesium	Concomitant use may decrease the absorption of digoxin
Diethylenetriamine pentaacetate (DTPA)	Zinc	Treatment with DTPA has resulted in severe zinc deficiency
Doxorubicin (Adriamycin)	Riboflavin	May inhibit the incorporation of riboflavin into active coenzymes FAD and FMN
5-Fluorouracil (5-FU)	Niacin	Long-term therapy has resulted in niacin deficiency
	Thiamin	5-FU decreases phosphorylation of thiamin to its active form
	Iron	May decrease iron absorption
Isoniazid	Niacin	Niacin antagonist; niacin supplementation is recommended during long-term isoniazid treatment
	Vitamin B_6	May cause functional vitamin B_6 deficiency by forming inactive complex with vitamin B_6
	Vitamin E	May decrease absorption of vitamin E
	Vitamin K	May increase the risk of vitamin K deficiency and hemorrhagic disease of newborn infants when taken by pregnant women
Ketoconazole (oral)	Vitamin D	May decrease blood levels of calcitriol, the active form of vitamin D
Levodopa	Vitamin B_6	May cause functional vitamin B_6 deficiency by forming inactive complex with vitamin B_6 High doses of vitamin B_6 may decrease the efficacy of levodopa
	Iron	Concomitant intake of iron supplements may decrease the efficacy of levodopa
Levothyroxine	Calcium	Concomitant intake may decrease levothyroxine absorption
	Iron	Concomitant intake of iron supplements may decrease the efficacy of levothyroxine

Specific drug	Nutrient	Interaction
Lithium	Iodine	Concomitant use of lithium and pharmacological doses of potassium iodide may result in hypothyroidism
Lovastatin	Niacin	Coadministration of pharmacological doses of nicotinic acid and lovastatin has resulted in cases of rhabdomyolysis
Metformin	Vitamin B_{12}	Decreases vitamin B_{12} absorption; may be corrected by taking vitamin B_{12} supplements with milk or calcium supplements
Methyldopa	Iron	Concomitant intake of iron supplements may decrease the efficacy of methyldopa
Methotrexate	Folic acid	Folate antagonist; may require folic acid supplementation during methotrexate therapy
Neomycin	Vitamin B_{12}	May decrease the absorption of food-bound but not supplemental vitamin B_{12}
Nitrous oxide	Vitamin B_{12}	Inhalation of nitrous oxide may result in functional vitamin B_{12} deficiency
Olestra	Fat-soluble vitamins	Inhibits the absorption of fat-soluble vitamins; vitamins A, D, E, and K are added to olestra for this reason
Orlistat	Fat-soluble vitamins	May decrease the absorption of fat-soluble vitamins (vitamins A, D, E, and K); take orlistat and vitamin supplements at least 2 hours apart
Penicillamine	Vitamin B_6	May cause functional vitamin B_6 deficiency by forming inactive complex with vitamin B_6
	Copper	Increases urinary excretion of copper; used to treat copper overload in Wilson disease
	Iron	Concomitant intake of iron supplements may decrease the efficacy of penicillamine
	Magnesium	Concomitant intake may decrease the efficacy of penicillamine
	Zinc	Treatment with penicillamine has resulted in severe zinc deficiency
Phenytoin	Thiamin	Use may decrease blood levels of thiamin
Pyrimethamine	Folic acid	Folate antagonist; may increase folate requirement
Quinacrine	Riboflavin	May inhibit the incorporation of riboflavin into active coenzymes FAD and FMN
Rifampin	Vitamin K	May increase the risk of vitamin K deficiency and hemorrhagic disease of newborn infants when taken by pregnant women
Sucralfate	Vitamin E	May decrease vitamin E absorption
Sulfasalazine	Folic acid	Folate antagonist; may increase folate requirement
	Vitamin K	May decrease vitamin K recycling
Sulfinpyrazone	Niacin	Nicotinic acid may decrease the uricosuric effect of sulfinpyrazone
Triamterene	Folic acid	Folate antagonist; may increase folate requirement
Trimethoprim	Folic acid	Folate antagonist; may increase folate requirement
Warfarin	Vitamin C	High doses of vitamin C have been reported to decrease anticoagulant efficacy in a few cases
	Vitamin E	High doses of vitamin E may potentiate anticoagulant effects
	Vitamin K	High intake of dietary or supplemental vitamin K may decrease anticoagulant efficacy May increase the risk of neonatal vitamin K deficiency and hemorrhagic disease of newborn infants when taken by pregnant women
	Iodine	Pharmacological doses of potassium iodide may decrease the anticoagulant efficacy of warfarin
	Magnesium	Magnesium-containing antacids may decrease the anticoagulant efficacy of warfarin

Quick Reference to Diseases

Disease	Chapter section	Nutrient	Pages
Alzheimer disease	Prevention	Folic acid	13
		Vitamin B$_{12}$	65–66
	Treatment	Thiamin	38
		Vitamin E	100–101
	Safety	Iron	166
Asthma	Treatment	Magnesium	174
Autoimmune disease	Prevention	Vitamin D	89–90
Cancer (general)	Prevention	Folic acid	12
		Niacin	19–20
		Vitamin B$_{12}$	64
		Vitamin C	72–73
		Vitamin D	88–89
		Vitamin E	99
		Selenium	206–208
	Treatment	Thiamin	39
		Vitamin C	75
		Vitamin E	101
Breast cancer	Prevention	Folic acid	12
		Vitamin A	45–46
		Vitamin B$_{12}$	64–65
		Vitamin D	88–89
Colorectal cancer	Prevention	Folic acid	12
		Vitamin D	88
		Calcium	118
	Safety	Iron	165–166
Gastric cancer	Prevention	Sodium chloride	216
Gastroesophageal cancer	Prevention	Molybdenum	188–189
Leukemia (acute promyelotic)	Treatment	Vitamin A	46
Lung cancer	Prevention	Vitamin A	45
Prostate cancer	Prevention	Vitamin D	89
	Safety	Calcium	124
Thyroid cancer	Prevention	Iodine	152

Disease	Chapter section	Nutrient	Pages
Myocardial infarction	Prevention	Vitamin C	71
		Vitamin E	98
		Copper	138
		Selenium	208–209
	Treatment	Niacin	21
		Vitamin E	99–100
		Magnesium	173
	Safety	Iron	165
Stroke	Prevention	Vitamin C	72
		Potassium	197–198
Carpal tunnel syndrome	Treatment	Vitamin B_6	56
Cataracts	Prevention	Riboflavin	33
		Thiamin	38
		Vitamin C	73
		Vitamin E	98–99
Celiac disease	Deficiency	Vitamin B_{12}	62
		Copper	137
		Iron	160
		Magnesium	170
		Zinc	225
Common cold	Treatment	Vitamin C	76
		Zinc	228
Dementia	Deficiency	Vitamin B_{12}	62
	Prevention	Folic acid	13
		Vitamin B_{12}	65–66
	Treatment	Vitamin E	100–101
Dental caries (cavities)	Prevention	Fluoride	143
Depression	Deficiency	Vitamin B_6	52–53
	Prevention	Vitamin B_{12}	66
	Treatment	Vitamin B_6	56
Diabetes mellitus			
Type 1	Prevention	Niacin	20
		Vitamin D	89
	Treatment	Biotin	3
		Zinc	229
Type 2	Prevention	Chromium	130
		Manganese	181
		Selenium	209
	Treatment	Biotin	3
		Vitamin C	75–76
		Vitamin E	100
		Chromium	131
		Magnesium	173–174
		Zinc	229
	Safety	Iron	166

Disease	Chapter section	Nutrient	Pages
Gout	Prevention	Vitamin C	73
Growth/developmental delays	Prevention	Iron	161
		Zinc	226
HIV/AIDS	Treatment	Niacin	21
		Selenium	209
		Zinc	229
Hypercholesterolemia	Treatment	Niacin	21
		Pantothenic acid	27–28
Hypertension	Prevention	Magnesium	170–171
		Sodium chloride	217–219
		Vitamin D	90
	Treatment	Vitamin C	74–75
		Calcium	121
		Magnesium	172
		Potassium	199
		Sodium chloride	217–219
Immunity, impaired	Prevention	Vitamin B_6	54
		Vitamin E	99
		Copper	138–139
		Iron	161–162
		Selenium	206
		Zinc	227
Kidney stones (nephrolithiasis)	Prevention	Vitamin B_6	55
		Calcium	119–120
		Potassium	198–199
		Sodium chloride	217
	Safety	Vitamin C	78
Lead toxicity	Prevention	Vitamin C	73–74
		Calcium	120–121
		Iron	161
Macular degeneration	Treatment	Zinc	229
Migraine	Treatment	Riboflavin	33
		Magnesium	174
Osteoporosis	Prevention	Vitamin D	87–88
		Vitamin K	110–111
		Calcium	118–119
		Copper	139
		Fluoride	143–144
		Magnesium	171–172
		Manganese	181
		Potassium	198
		Sodium chloride	216–217
	Treatment	Fluoride	144

Disease	Chapter section	Nutrient	Pages
Pregnancy complications (general)	Prevention	Folic acid	10–11
		Iron	161
		Zinc	227–228
Gestational diabetes	Treatment	Chromium	131–132
Morning sickness	Treatment	Vitamin B_6	56
Multiple sclerosis	Prevention	Vitamin D	89–90
Neural tube defects	Prevention	Folic acid	10
		Vitamin B_{12}	65
Other birth defects	Prevention	Biotin	3
	Safety	Vitamin A	48–49
Pre-eclampsia–eclampsia	Prevention	Calcium	120
	Treatment	Magnesium	172–173
Premenstrual syndrome	Treatment	Calcium	121
		Vitamin B_6	55–56
Restless legs syndrome	Treatment	Iron	162
Retinitis pigmentosa	Treatment	Vitamin A	46
Rheumatoid arthritis	Prevention	Vitamin D	89–90
Seizure disorders (epilepsy)	Prevention	Manganese	181
Stroke	Prevention	Potassium	197–198
		Vitamin C	72

HDL, high-density lipoprotein; LDL, low-density lipoprotein.

Glossary

Acetylation: the addition of an acetyl group ($-COCH_3$) group to a molecule.

Acidic: having a pH of less than 7.

Acute: having a short and relatively severe course.

Adjunct therapy: a treatment or therapy used in addition to another, not alone.

Adrenal glands: a pair of small glands, located above the kidneys, consisting of an outer cortex and inner medulla. The adrenal cortex secretes cortisone-related hormones and the adrenal medulla secretes epinephrine (adrenaline) and nor-epinephrine (noradrenaline).

AI: adequate intake. Established by the Food and Nutrition Board of the US Institute of Medicine, the AI is a recommended intake value based on observed or experimentally determined estimates of nutrient intake by a group of healthy people that are assumed to be adequate. An AI is established when an RDA cannot be determined.

AIDS: acquired immune deficiency syndrome. AIDS is caused by the virus HIV (human immunodeficiency virus), which attacks the immune system, leaving the infected individual vulnerable to opportunistic infections.

Alkaline: basic; having a pH of more than 7.

Allele: one of a set of alternative forms of a gene. Diploid cells possess two homologous chromosomes (one derived from each parent) and therefore two copies of each gene. In a diploid cell, a gene will have two alleles, each occupying the same position on homologous chromosomes.

Alzheimer disease: the most common cause of dementia in older adults. Alzheimer disease is characterized by the formation of amyloid plaque in the brain and nerve cell degeneration. Symptoms include memory loss and confusion, which worsen over time.

Amino acids: organic (carbon-containing) molecules that serve as the building blocks of proteins.

Anaerobic: refers to the absence of oxygen or the absence of a need for oxygen.

Analog: a chemical compound that is structurally similar to another but differs slightly in composition (e.g., the replacement of one functional group by another).

Anaphylaxis: a rapidly developing and severe systemic allergic reaction. Symptoms may include swelling of the tongue, throat, and trachea, which can result in difficulty breathing, shock, and loss of consciousness. If not treated rapidly, anaphylaxis can be fatal.

Anemia: the condition of having less than the normal number of red blood cells or amount of hemoglobin in the blood, resulting in diminished oxygen transport. Anemia has many causes, including: iron, vitamin B_{12}, or folate deficiency, bleeding, abnormal hemoglobin formation (e.g., sickle cell anemia), rupture of red blood cells (hemolytic anemia), and bone marrow diseases.

Anencephaly: a birth defect, known as a neural tube defect, resulting from failure of the upper end of the neural tube to close during embryonic development. Anencephaly is a devastating and sometimes fatal birth defect resulting in the absence of most or all of the cerebral hemispheres of the brain.

Angina pectoris: pain generally experienced in the chest, but sometimes radiating to the arms or jaw, due to a lack of oxygen supply to the heart muscle.

Angiogenesis: the development of new blood vessels.

Angiography (coronary): imaging of the coronary arteries used to identify the location and severity of any obstructions. Coronary angiography typically involves the administration of a contrast medium and imaging of the coronary arteries using an X-ray-based technique.

Anion: a negatively charged ion.

Antagonist: a substance that counteracts or nullifies the biological effects of another, such as a compound that binds to a receptor but does not elicit a biological response.

Antibodies: specialized proteins produced by white blood cells (lymphocytes) that recognize and bind to foreign proteins or pathogens in order to neutralize them or mark them for destruction.

Anticoagulant: a class of compounds that inhibit blood clotting.

Anticonvulsant: a class of medication used to prevent seizures.

Antigen: a substance that is capable of eliciting an immune response.

Antihistamine: a chemical that blocks the affect of histamine in susceptible tissues. Histamine is released by immune cells during an allergic reaction and also during infection with viruses that cause the common cold. The interaction of histamine with the mucous membranes of the eyes and nose results in "watery eyes" and the "runny nose" often accompanying allergies and colds. Antihistamines can help alleviate such symptoms.

Antimicrobial: capable of killing or inhibiting the growth of microorganisms, such as bacteria.

Antioxidant: any substance that prevents or reduces damage caused by reactive oxygen species or reactive nitrogen species.

Antiresorptive agents: medications or hormones that inhibit bone resorption.

Apoptosis: gene-directed cell death or programmed cell death that occurs when age, condition, or state of cell health dictates. Cells that die by apoptosis do not usually elicit the inflammatory responses that are associated with necrosis. Cancer cells are resistant to apoptosis.

Arrhythmia: an abnormal heart rhythm. The heart rhythm may be too fast (tachycardia), too slow (bradycardia), or irregular. Some arrhythmias, such as ventricular fibrillation, may lead to cardiac arrest if not treated promptly.

Asthma: a chronic inflammatory disease of the airways, characterized by recurrent episodes of reversible airflow obstruction.

Ataxia: a lack of coordination or unsteadiness usually related to a disturbance in the cerebellum, a part of the brain that regulates coordination and equilibrium.

Atherogenic: capable of producing atherosclerosis.

Atherosclerosis: an inflammatory disease resulting in the accumulation of cholesterol-laden plaque in artery walls. Rupture of atherosclerotic plaque results in clot formation, which may cause myocardial infarction or ischemic stroke.

ATP: adenosine triphosphate. An important compound for the storage of energy in cells, as well as the synthesis of nucleic acids.

Atrial fibrillation: a cardiac arrhythmia, characterized by rapid, uncoordinated beating of the atria, which results in ineffective atrial contractions. Atrial fibrillation is known as a supraventricular arrhythmia because it originates above the ventricles.

Atrophic gastritis: a chronic inflammation of the lining of the stomach, which ultimately results in the loss of glands in the stomach (atrophy) and decreased stomach acid production.

Atrophy: decrease in size or wasting away of a body part or tissue.

Autoimmune disease: a condition in which the body's immune system reacts against its own tissues.

Bacteria: single-celled organisms that can exist independently, symbiotically (in cooperation with another organism), or parasitically (dependent on another organism, sometimes to the detriment of the other organism). Examples of bacteria include *Lactobacillus acidophilus* (found in yogurt), streptococci, the cause of a strep throat, and *Escherichia coli* (a normal intestinal bacterium, as well as a disease-causing agent).

Balance study: a nutritional balance study involves the measurement of the intake of a specific nutrient as well as the elimination of that nutrient in urine, feces, sweat, etc. If intake is greater than loss of a particular nutrient, the individual is said to be in "positive balance." If intake is less than loss, an individual is said to be in "negative balance" for the nutrient of interest.

Bias: any systematic error in an epidemiological study that results in an incorrect estimate of the association between an exposure and a disease risk.

Bile: a yellow, green fluid made in the liver and stored in the gallbladder. Bile may then pass through the common bile duct into the small intestine where some of its components aid in the digestion of fat.

Bile acids: components of bile, which are formed by the metabolism of cholesterol, and which aid in the digestion of fats.

Bioavailability: the fraction of an administered compound that reaches the systemic circulation and is transported to the site of action (target tissue).

Biomarker: a physical, functional, or biochemical indicator of a physiological or disease process.

Body mass index (BMI): body weight in kilograms divided by height in meters squared. In adults, BMI is a measure of body fat: underweight < 18.5; normal weight 18.5–24.9; overweight 25–29.9; obese ≥ 30.

Bone mineral density (BMD): the amount of mineral in a given area of bone. BMD is positively associated with bone strength and resistance to fracture, and measurements of BMD are used to diagnose osteoporosis.

Bone remodeling: the continuous turnover process of bone that includes bone resorption and bone formation. An imbalance in the regulation of the two contrasting events of bone remodeling (bone resorption and bone formation) increases the fragility of bone and may lead to osteoporosis.

Buffer: a chemical used to maintain the pH of a system by absorbing hydrogen ions (which would make it more acidic) or hydroxyl ions (which would make it more alkaline).

Calcification: the process of deposition of calcium salts. In the formation of bone this is a normal condition. In other organs, this could be an abnormal condition, for example, calcification of the aortic valve causes narrowing of the passage (aortic stenosis).

Cancer: refers to abnormal cells that have a tendency to grow uncontrollably and metastasize or spread to other areas of the body. Cancer can involve any tissue of the body and can have different forms in one tissue. Cancer is a group of more than 100 different diseases.

Carbohydrate: considered a macronutrient because carbohydrates provide a significant source of calories (energy) in the diet. Chemically, carbohydrates are neutral compounds composed of carbon, hydrogen, and oxygen. Carbohydrates come in simple forms known as sugars and complex forms, such as starches and fiber.

Carboxylation: the introduction of a carboxyl group (–COOH) or carbon dioxide into a compound.

Carcinogen: a cancer-causing agent; adjective: carcinogenic.

Carcinogenesis: the formation of cancer cells from normal cells.

Carcinoid syndrome: the pattern of symptoms exhibited by individuals with carcinoid tumors. Carcinoid tumors secrete excessive amounts of the neurotransmitter, serotonin. Symptoms may include flushing, diarrhea, and sometimes wheezing.

Cardiomyopathy: literally, disease of the heart muscle that often leads to abnormal function.

Cardiovascular: referring to the heart and blood vessels.

Cardiovascular diseases: literally, diseases affecting the heart and blood vessels. The term has come to encompass a number of conditions that result from atherosclerosis, including myocardial infarction (heart attack), congestive heart failure, and stroke.

Carnitine: a compound that is required to transport long chain fatty acids across the inner membrane of the mitochondria, in the form of acylcarnitine, where they can be metabolized for energy.

Carotid arteries: the left and right common carotid arteries are the principal blood vessels that supply oxygenated blood to the head and neck. Each has two main branches, the external and internal carotid arteries.

Cartilage: a soft, elastic tissue that composes most of the skeleton of vertebrate embryos and, except for a small number of structures, is replaced by bone during ossification in the higher vertebrates. Cartilage cushions joints, connects muscles with bones, and makes up other parts of the body such as the larynx (voice box) and the outside portion of the ears.

Case–control study: a study in which exposures of people who have been diagnosed with a disease (cases) are compared to those of people without the disease (controls). The results of case–control studies are more likely to be distorted by bias in the selection of cases and controls (selection bias) and dietary recall (recall bias) than prospective cohort studies.

Case reports: individual observations based on small numbers of individuals. This type of research cannot indicate causality but may indicate areas for further research.

Catabolism: the breakdown of complex molecules into smaller ones, accompanied by the release of energy.

Catalyze: increase the speed of a chemical reaction without the catalyst being changed in the overall reaction process (*see* Enzyme).

Cataract: clouding of the lens of the eye. As cataracts progress, they can impair vision.

Catecholamines: substances with a specific chemical structure (a benzene ring with two adjacent hydroxyl groups and a side chain of ethylamine) that function as hormones or neurotransmitters. Examples include epinephrine, norepinephrine, and dopamine.

Cation: a positively charged ion.

Celiac disease: also known as celiac sprue, celiac disease is an inherited disease in which the intestinal lining is inflamed in response to the ingestion of a protein known as gluten. Treatment of celiac disease involves the avoidance of gluten, which is present in many grains, including wheat, rye, oats, and barley. Inflammation and atrophy of the lining of the small intestine lead to impaired nutrient absorption.

Cell membrane: also called a plasma membrane, the barrier that separates the contents of a cell from its outside environment and controls what moves in and out of the cell. A mammalian cell membrane consists of a phospholipid bilayer with embedded proteins and cholesterol.

Cell signaling: communication among individual cells so as to coordinate their behavior to benefit the organism as a whole. Cell-signaling systems elucidated in animal cells include cell-surface and intracellular receptor proteins, GTP-binding proteins, as well as protein kinases and protein phosphatases (enzymes that phosphorylate and dephosphorylate proteins).

Central nervous system (CNS): the brain, spinal cord, and spinal nerves.

Cerebrospinal fluid: the fluid that bathes the brain and spinal cord.

Cerebrovascular disease: disease involving the blood vessels supplying the brain, including cerebrovascular accidents (CVAs), also known as strokes.

Cervical intraepithelial neoplasia (CIN): a term used to describe abnormal growth of cells on the surface of the uterine cervix. CIN1 is also known as low-grade squamous intraepithelial lesion (LSIL). CIN2 and CIN3 are also known as high-grade squamous intraepithelial lesions (HSILs). Although these abnormal cells are not cancerous, they may progress to cervical cancer.

Chelate: the combination of a metal with an organic molecule to form a ringlike structure known as a chelate. Chelation of a metal may inhibit or enhance its bioavailability.

Chemotaxis: movement of a cell or organism toward or away from a chemical stimulus.

Chemotherapy: literally, treatment with drugs. Commonly used to describe the systemic use of drugs to kill cancer cells, as a form of cancer treatment.

Cholestatic liver disease: liver disease resulting in the cessation of bile excretion. Cholestasis may occur in the liver, gallbladder, or bile duct (duct connecting the gallbladder to the small intestine).

Cholesterol: a compound that is an integral structural component of cell membranes and a precursor in the synthesis of steroid hormones. Dietary cholesterol is obtained from animal sources, but cholesterol is also synthesized by the liver. Cholesterol is carried in the blood by lipoproteins. In atherosclerosis, cholesterol accumulates in plaques on the walls of some arteries.

Cholinergic: resembling acetylcholine in action, a cholinergic drug, for example. Cholinergic nerve fibers liberate or are activated by the neurotransmitter, acetylcholine.

Chorionic villous sampling (CVS): a procedure for obtaining a small sample of tissue from the placenta (chorionic villi) for the purpose of prenatal diagnosis of genetic disorders. CVS can be performed between 9 and 12 weeks of pregnancy.

Chromatin: complex of DNA, RNA, and proteins that make up chromosomes.

Chromosome: a structure in the nucleus of a cell that contains genes. Chromosomes are composed of DNA and associated proteins. Normal human cells contain 46 chromosomes (22 pairs of autosomes and 2 sex chromosomes).

Chronic disease: an illness lasting a long time. By definition of the US Center for Health Statistics, a chronic disease is a disease lasting 3 months or more.

Cirrhosis: a condition characterized by irreversible scarring of the liver, leading to abnormal liver function. Cirrhosis has a number of different causes, including chronic alcohol use and viral hepatitis B and C.

Clinical trial: an intervention trial generally used to evaluate the efficacy and/or safety of a treatment or intervention in human participants.

Coagulation: the process involved in blood clot formation.

Coenzyme: a molecule that binds to an enzyme and is essential for its activity, but is not permanently altered by the reaction. Many coenzymes are derived from vitamins.

Cofactor: a compound that is essential for the activity of an enzyme.

Cognitive: an adjective referring to the processes of thinking, learning, perception, awareness, and judgment.

Cohort: a group of people who are followed over time as part of an epidemiological study.

Cohort study: a study that follows a large group of people over a long period of time, often 10 years or more. In cohort studies, dietary information is gathered before disease occurs, rather than relying on recall after disease develops.

Collagen: a fibrous protein that is the basis for the structure of skin, tendon, bone, cartilage and all other connective tissue.

Collagenous matrix (of bone): the organic (non-mineral) structural element of bone. Collagen is a fibrous protein that provides the organic matrix upon which bone minerals crystallize.

Colon: the portion of the large intestine that extends from the end of the small intestine to the rectum. The colon removes water from digested food after it has passed through the small intestine and stores the remaining stool until it can be evacuated.

Colorectal adenoma: a polyp or growth in the lining of the colon or rectum. Although they are not cancerous, colorectal adenomas may develop into colorectal cancer over time.

Colorectal cancer: cancer of the colon (large intestine) or rectum.

Complement: system of serum proteins that function to help destroy invading microorganisms.

Concomitant: accompanying. "Concomitant intake" refers to the intake of two compounds at the same time.

Congenital hypothyroidism: deficiency of thyroid gland activity in newborn infants.

Congestive heart failure (CHF): a condition, in which the heart loses the ability to pump blood efficiently enough to meet the demands of the body. Symptoms may include edema (swelling), shortness of breath, weakness, and exercise intolerance.

Cornea: the transparent covering of the front of the eye that transmits and focuses light into the eye.

Coronary artery: one of the vessels that supply oxygenated blood to the heart muscle itself. They are called coronary arteries because they encircle the heart in the form of a crown.

Coronary heart disease (CHD): also known as coronary artery disease and coronary disease, CHD is the result of atherosclerosis of the coronary arteries. Atherosclerosis may result in narrowing or blockage of the coronary arteries and is the underlying cause of myocardial infarction (heart attack).

Creatine phosphate: a high-energy compound found in muscle cells that is used to convert ADP into ATP by donating phosphate molecules to the ADP. ATP is the molecule that is converted into

ADP with release of energy that the body then uses.

Cretinism: a condition that can result from a severe form of congenital hypothyroidism. Cretinism occurs in two forms, although there is considerable overlap. The neurological form is characterized by learning disability, physical retardation, and deafness. It is the result of maternal iodine deficiency that affects the fetus before its own thyroid is functional. The myxedematous or hypothyroid form is characterized by short stature and learning disability. In addition to iodine deficiency, the hypothyroid form has been associated with selenium deficiency and the presence of goitrogens in the diet that interfere with thyroid hormone production.

Crohn disease: an inflammatory bowel disease that usually affects the lower part of the small intestine or upper part of the colon, but may affect any part of the gastrointestinal tract.

Crossover trial: a clinical trial in which at least two interventions or treatments are applied to the same individuals after an appropriate washout period. One of the treatments is often a placebo. In a randomized crossover design, interventions are applied in a randomized order to ensure that the order of treatments did not contribute to the outcome.

Cross-sectional study: a study of a group of people at one point in time to determine whether an exposure is associated with the occurrence of a disease. As the disease outcome and the exposure (e.g., nutrient intake) are measured at the same time, a cross-sectional study provides a "snapshot" view of their relationship. Cross-sectional studies cannot provide information about causality.

Cystic fibrosis (CF): a hereditary disease caused by mutations in the cystic fibrosis transmembrane conductance regulator (*CFTCR*) gene. Cystic fibrosis is characterized by the production of abnormal secretions, leading to the accumulation of mucus in the lungs, pancreas, and intestine. This build-up of mucus causes difficulty breathing and recurrent lung infections, as well as problems with nutrient absorption due to problems in the pancreas and intestines.

Cytochrome P450 (CYP): a family of phase I biotransformation enzymes that play an important role in the metabolism and elimination of drugs, toxins, carcinogens, and endogenous compounds, such as steroid hormones.

Cytokine: a protein made by cells that affects the behavior of other cells. Cytokines act on specific cytokine receptors in the cells that they affect.

Cytoplasm: the contents of a cell, excluding the nucleus.

Cytosol: the water-soluble contents of a cell's cytoplasm, excluding the organelles.

Decarboxylation: a chemical reaction involving the removal of a carboxyl (–COOH) group from a compound.

Dementia: significant impairment of intellectual abilities such as attention, orientation, memory, judgment, or language. By definition, dementia is not due to major depression or psychosis. Alzheimer disease is the most common cause of dementia in older adults.

Dental caries: cavities or holes in the outer two layers of a tooth—the enamel and the dentin. Dental caries are caused by bacteria that metabolize carbohydrates (sugars) to form organic acids, which dissolve tooth enamel.

Depletion–repletion study: a nutritional study designed to determine the requirement for a specific nutrient. Generally, participants are placed on a diet designed to deplete them of a specific nutrient over time. Once depletion is achieved, gradually increasing amounts of the nutrient under study are added to the diet until the individual shows evidence of sufficiency or repletion.

Dermatitis: inflammation of the skin. This term is often used to describe a skin rash.

DEXA: dual energy X-ray absorptiometry. A precise instrument that uses the energy from very small doses of X-rays to determine BMD and to diagnose and follow the treatment of osteoporosis.

Diabetes mellitus: a chronic metabolic disease, characterized by abnormally high blood glucose (sugar) levels, resulting from the inability of the body to produce or respond to insulin. Type 1 diabetes mellitus, formerly known as insulin-dependent or juvenile-onset diabetes, is usually the result of autoimmune destruction of the insulin-secreting β cells of the pancreas. The most common form of diabetes is type 2 diabetes mellitus, formerly known as noninsulin-dependent or adult-onset diabetes, which develops when the tissues of the body become less sensitive to insulin secreted by the pancreas.

Diabetic ketoacidosis: a potentially life-threatening condition characterized by ketosis (elevated levels of ketone bodies in the blood) and acidosis (increased acidity of the blood). Ketoacidosis occurs when diabetes is not adequately controlled.

Dialysis: a medical procedure to filter waste products from the blood. Dialysis is needed to perform the work of the kidneys if they can no longer function effectively. Two types of dialysis are hemodialysis and peritoneal dialysis.

Diastolic blood pressure: the lowest arterial blood pressure during the heart beat cycle, and the second number in a blood pressure reading (e.g., 120/80).

Differentiation: changes in a cell resulting in its specialization for specific functions, such as those of a nerve cell. In general, differentiation of cells leads to a decrease in proliferation.

Diffusion: a passive process, in which particles in solution move from a region of higher concentration to one of lower concentration.

Dimer: a complex of two molecules, usually proteins. Heterodimers are complexes of two different molecules, whereas homodimers are complexes of two of the same molecule.

Diuretic: an agent that increases the formation of urine by the kidneys, resulting in water loss from the individual using the diuretic.

Diverticulitis: inflammation or infection of diverticula in the colon, characterized by abdominal pain, fever, and constipation.

DNA: deoxyribonucleic acid; a double-stranded nucleic acid composed of many nucleotides. The nucleotides in DNA are each composed of a nitrogen-containing base (adenine, guanine, cytosine, or thymine), a five-carbon sugar (deoxyribose), and a phosphate group. The sequence of bases in DNA encodes the genetic information required to synthesize proteins.

Double-blind: refers to a study in which neither the investigators administering the treatment nor the participants know who is receiving the experimental treatment and who is receiving the placebo.

DRI: dietary reference intake. Refers to a set of at least four nutrient-based reference values (RDA, AI, UL, EAR), each with a specific use in defining recommended dietary intake levels for individual nutrients in the United States. The DRIs are determined by expert panels appointed by the Food and Nutrition Board of the Institute of Medicine.

DV: daily value. Refers to the dietary reference values required as the basis for declaring nutrient content on all products regulated by the US Food and Drug Administration (FDA), including nutritional supplements. The DVs for vitamins and minerals reflect the National Academy of Sciences' 1968 RDAs, and do not reflect the most up-to-date DRIs.

Dyslipidemia: a disorder of lipoprotein metabolism.

EAR: estimated average requirement. A nutrient intake value that is estimated to meet the requirement of half the healthy individuals in a particular life stage and gender group.

Echocardiography: a diagnostic test that uses ultrasound to make images of the heart. It can be used to assess the health of the valves and chambers of the heart, as well as to measure cardiac output.

Ecological study: an epidemiological study that examines the relationships between exposures and disease rates in a series of populations (e.g., different countries). Ecological studies often rely on published statistics, such as food disappearance data or disease-specific death rates.

Edema: swelling; accumulation of excessive fluid in subcutaneous tissues (beneath the skin).

Electroencephalogram (EEG): a recording of the electrical activity of the brain, used to diagnose neurological conditions such as seizure disorders (epilepsy).

Electrolytes: ionized (dissociated into positive and negative ions) salts in the body fluids. Major electrolytes in the body include sodium, potassium, magnesium, calcium, chloride, bicarbonate, and phosphate.

Electron: a stable atomic particle with a negative charge.

Electron transport chain: a group of electron carriers in mitochondria that transport electrons to and from each other in a sequence, in order to generate ATP.

Element: one of the 103 chemical substances that cannot be divided into simpler substances by chemical means, for example, hydrogen, magnesium, lead, and uranium are all chemical elements. Trace elements are chemical elements that are required in very small (trace) amounts in the diet to maintain health, for example, copper, selenium, and iodine.

Enamel: the hard, white, outermost layer of a tooth.

Endocrine system: the glands and parts of glands that secrete hormones that integrate and control the body's metabolic activity. Endocrine glands include the pituitary, thyroid, parathyroids, adrenals, pancreas, ovaries, and testes.

Endogenous: arising from within the body. Endogenous synthesis refers to the synthesis of a compound by the body.

Endotoxin: toxins released by certain bacteria.

Enzyme: a biological catalyst, that is, a substance that increases the speed of a chemical reaction without being changed in the overall process. Enzymes are vitally important to the regulation of the chemistry of cells and organisms.

Epidemiological study: a study examining disease occurrence in a human population.

Epilepsy: also known as seizure disorder. Individuals with epilepsy experience seizures, which are the result of uncontrolled electrical activity in the brain. A seizure may cause a physical convulsion, minor physical signs, thought disturbances, or a combination of symptoms.

Epithelium: layer of cells that lines a body cavity or covers an external surface of the body.

Erythropoietin: a hormone produced by specialized cells in the kidneys that stimulates the bone marrow to increase the production of red blood cells. Recombinant erythropoietin is used to treat anemia in patients with end-stage renal failure.

Esophagus: the portion of the gastrointestinal tract that connects the throat (pharynx) to the stomach.

Ester: the product of a reaction between a carboxylic acid and an alcohol involving the elimination of water. For example, a cholesterol ester is the product of a reaction between a fatty acid and cholesterol.

Estrogen: hormones that bind to estrogen receptors in the nuclei of cells and promote the transcription of estrogen-responsive genes. Endogenous estrogens are steroid hormones produced by the body. Exogenous estrogens are synthetic or natural compounds that have estrogenic activity (i.e., bind the estrogen receptor and promote estrogen-responsive gene transcription).

Etiology: the causes or origin of a disease.

Excretion: the elimination of waste from blood or tissues.

Extracellular fluid (ECF): the volume of body fluid excluding that in cells. ECF includes the fluid in blood vessels (plasma) and the fluid between cells (interstitial fluid).

Familial adenomatous polyposis: a hereditary syndrome characterized by the formation of many polyps in the colon and rectum, some of which may develop into colorectal cancer.

Fatty acid: an organic acid molecule consisting of a chain of carbon molecules and a carboxylic acid (–COOH) group. Fatty acids are found in fats, oils, and as components of a number of essential lipids, such as phospholipids and triglycerides. Fatty acids can be burned by the body for energy.

Femoral neck: a portion of the thighbone (femur). The femoral neck is found near the hip, at the base of the head of femur, which makes up the ball of the hip joint. Fractures of the femoral neck sometimes occur in individuals with osteoporosis.

Fermentation: an anaerobic process that involves the breakdown of dietary components to yield energy.

Fibrocystic breast condition (FCC): a benign (noncancerous) condition of the breasts, characterized by lumpiness and discomfort in one or both breasts.

Fortification: the addition of nutrients to foods to prevent or correct a nutritional deficiency, to balance the total nutrient profile of food, or to restore nutrients lost in processing.

Fracture: a break in a bone or cartilage, often but not always the result of trauma.

Free radical: a very reactive atom or molecule typically possessing a single unpaired electron.

Fructose: a very sweet six-carbon sugar abundant in plants. Fructose is increasingly common in sweeteners such as high-fructose corn syrup.

Gallbladder: a small sac adjacent to the liver. The gallbladder stores bile, which is secreted by the liver, and releases it into the small intestine through the common bile duct.

Gallstones: crystals formed by the precipitation of cholesterol or bilirubin in the gallbladder. Gallstones may be asymptomatic (without symptoms) or they may result in inflammation and infection of the gallbladder.

Gastroesophageal reflux disease (GERD): a condition in which stomach contents, including acid, back up (reflux) into the esophagus, causing inflammation and damage to the esophagus. GERD can lead to scarring of the esophagus, and may increase the risk of cancer of the esophagus in some patients.

Gastrointestinal: referring to or affecting the digestive tract, which includes the mouth, pharynx (throat), esophagus, stomach, and intestines.

Gene: a region of DNA that controls a specific hereditary characteristic, usually corresponding to a single protein.

Gene expression: the process by which the information coded in genes (DNA) is converted to proteins and other cellular structures. Expressed genes include those that are transcribed to messenger RNA and translated to protein, as well as those that are only transcribed to RNA (e.g., ribosomal and transfer RNAs).

Genome: all of the genetic information (encoded in DNA) possessed by an organism.

Gestation: the period of time between fertilization and birth. In humans, normal gestation is about 40 weeks.

Gluconeogenesis: the production of glucose from noncarbohydrate precursors, such as amino acids (the building blocks of proteins).

Glucose: a six-carbon sugar that plays a major role in the generation of energy for living organisms.

Glucose tolerance: the ability of the body to maintain normal glucose levels when challenged with a carbohydrate load (see Impaired glucose tolerance).

Glucoside: a glycoside that contains glucose as its carbohydrate (sugar) moiety (see Glycoside).

Glutathione: a tripeptide consisting of glutamate, cysteine, and glycine. Glutathione is an endogenous intracellular antioxidant, and is also required for some phase II biotransformation reactions.

Glycated hemoglobin: glucose-bound hemoglobin. A test for glycated hemoglobin (Hb1Ac) measures the percentage of hemoglobin that is glucose bound. As glucose remains bound to hemoglobin for the life of a red blood cell (about 120 days), Hb1Ac values reflect blood glucose control over the past 4 months.

Glycogen: a large polymer (repeating units) of glucose molecules, used to store energy in cells, especially muscle and liver cells.

Glycoside: a compound containing a sugar molecule that can be cleaved by hydrolysis to a sugar and a nonsugar component (aglycone).

Goiter: enlargement of the thyroid gland. Goiter is one of the earliest and most visible signs of iodine deficiency. The thyroid enlarges in response to persistent stimulation by thyroid-stimulating hormone (TSH). In mild iodine deficiency, this adaptive response may be enough to provide the body with sufficient thyroid hormone. However, more severe cases of iodine deficiency result in hypothyroidism. Thyroid enlargement may also be caused by factors other than iodine deficiency, especially in iodine-sufficient countries, such as the United States.

Goitrogen: a substance that induces goiter formation by interfering with thyroid hormone production or utilization.

Gout: a condition characterized by abnormally high blood levels of uric acid (urate). Urate crystals may form in joints, resulting in inflammation and pain. They may also form in the kidney and urinary tract, resulting in kidney stones. The tendency to develop elevated blood uric acid levels and gout is often inherited.

GTP: guanosine triphosphate. A high-energy molecule required for a number of biochemical reactions, including nucleic acid and protein synthesis (formation).

Hartnup disease: a genetic disorder resulting in defective absorption of the amino acid tryptophan.

HDL: high-density lipoprotein. HDLs transport cholesterol from the tissues to the liver where it can be eliminated in bile. HDL-cholesterol is considered good cholesterol, because higher blood levels of HDL-cholesterol are associated with a lower risk of heart disease.

Hematocrit: the percentage of red blood cells in whole blood.

Heme: compounds of iron complexed in a characteristic ring structure known as a porphyrin ring.

Hemodialysis: the process of removing blood from an artery, removing waste products from the blood through dialysis, and returning the blood to the body through a vein. Hemodialysis is used to treat end-stage renal failure.

Hemoglobin: the oxygen-carrying pigment in red blood cells.

Hemolysis: rupture of red blood cells.

Hemolytic anemia: anemia resulting from hemolysis (the rupture of red blood cells).

Hemorrhage: excessive or uncontrolled bleeding.

Hemorrhagic stroke: a stroke that occurs when a blood vessel ruptures and bleeds into the brain.

Hepatitis: literally, inflammation of the liver. Hepatitis caused by a virus is known as viral hepatitis. Other causes of hepatitis include toxic chemicals and alcohol abuse.

Hepatocellular carcinoma: the most common type of primary liver cancer.

Hereditary hemochromatosis: a genetic disorder that results in iron overload despite normal dietary intake of iron.

Hereditary spherocytosis: a hereditary form of anemia characterized by abnormally shaped red blood cells that are spherical and abnormally fragile. The increased fragility of these red blood cells leads to hemolytic anemia (anemia caused by the rupture of red blood cells).

Heterodimer: a dimer or complex of two different molecules, usually proteins.

Heterozygous: possessing two different forms (alleles) of a specific gene.

Histone: protein that binds to DNA and packages it into compact structures to form nucleosomes.

HIV: human immunodeficiency virus. The virus that causes AIDS.

Homocysteine: a sulfur-containing amino acid, which is an intermediate in the metabolism of another sulfur-containing amino acid, methionine. Elevated homocysteine levels in the blood have been associated with increased risk of cardiovascular disease.

Homodimer: a dimer or complex of two of the same molecules, usually a protein.

Homologous: having the same appearance, structure, or evolutionary origin.

Homozygous: possessing two identical forms (alleles) of a specific gene.

Hormone: a chemical, released by a gland or tissue, that affects or regulates the activity of specific cells or organs. Complex bodily functions, such as growth and sexual development, are regulated by hormones.

Hydrolysis: cleavage of a chemical bond by the addition of water. In hydrolysis reactions, a large compound may be broken down into smaller compounds when a molecule of water is added.

Hydroxyapatite: a calcium phosphate salt. Hydroxyapatite is the main mineral component of bone and teeth, and is what gives them their rigidity.

Hydroxylation: a chemical reaction involving the addition of a hydroxyl (–OH) group to a compound.

Hyperglycemia: an abnormally high blood glucose concentration; symptoms include increased thirst, increased urination, and general fatigue.

Hyperparathyroidism: excess secretion of parathyroid hormone by the parathyroid glands resulting in the disturbance of calcium metabolism. Symptoms may include increased blood levels of calcium (hypercalcemia), decreased blood levels of phosphorus, loss of calcium from bone, and kidney stone formation.

Hypertension: high blood pressure. Hypertension is defined by the Joint National Committee on Prevention, Detection, Evaluation and Treatment of High Blood Pressure as a systolic blood pressure of 140 mmHg or higher and/or a diastolic blood pressure of 90 mmHg or higher.

Hyperthyroidism: an excess of thyroid hormone that may result from an overactive thyroid gland or nodule, or from taking too much thyroid hormone.

Hypoglycemia: an abnormally low blood glucose concentration. Symptoms may include nausea, sweating, weakness, faintness, confusion, hallucinations, headache, loss of consciousness, convulsions, or coma.

Hypoparathyroidism: a deficiency of parathyroid hormone, which may be characterized by low blood calcium levels (hypocalcemia).

Hypothalamus: an area at the base of the brain that regulates bodily functions, such as body temperature, hunger, and thirst.

Hypothesis: an educated guess or proposition that is advanced as a basis for further investigation. A hypothesis must be subjected to an experimental test to determine its validity.

Hypothyroidism: a deficiency of thyroid hormone that is normally made by the thyroid gland, located in the front of the neck.

Idiopathic: of unknown cause.

Impaired glucose tolerance: a metabolic state between normal glucose regulation and overt diabetes. Impaired glucose tolerance is defined medically as a plasma glucose concentration between 140 and 199 mg/dL (7.8–11.0 mmol/L) 2 h after the ingestion of 75 g glucose during an oral glucose tolerance test.

Inflammation: a response to injury or infection, characterized by redness, heat, swelling, and pain. Physiologically, the inflammatory response involves a complex series of events, leading to the migration of white blood cells to the inflamed area.

Inflammatory bowel disease: a group of autoimmune diseases that affect the small and large intestines.

Insoluble: not dissolvable. With respect to bioavailability, certain substances form insoluble complexes that cannot be dissolved in digestive secretions, and therefore cannot be absorbed by the digestive tract.

Insulin: a peptide hormone secreted by the β cells of the pancreas required for normal glucose metabolism.

Insulin resistance: diminished responsiveness to insulin.

Insulin sensitive: the ability of tissues to respond to insulin.

Intervention trial: an experimental study (usually a clinical trial) used to test the effect of a treatment or intervention on a health- or disease-related outcome.

Intracellular fluid (ICF): the volume of fluid inside cells.

In vitro: literally "in glass," referring to a test or research done in the test tube, outside a living organism.

In vivo: "inside a living organism." An in vivo assay evaluates a biological process occurring inside the body.

Ion: an atom or group of atoms that carries a positive or negative electric charge as a result of having lost or gained one or more electrons.

Ion channel: a protein, embedded in a cell membrane, that serves as a crossing point for the regulated transfer of an ion or a group of ions across the membrane.

Ischemia: a state of insufficient blood flow to a tissue.

Ischemic stroke: a stroke resulting from insufficient blood flow to an area of the brain, which may occur when a blood vessel supplying the brain becomes obstructed by a clot.

Isomers: compounds that have the same numbers and kinds of atoms but that differ in the way that the atoms are arranged.

Jaundice: a yellowish staining of the skin and whites of the eyes due to increased bilirubin (a bile pigment) levels in the blood. Jaundice can be an indicator of rupture of red blood cells (hemolysis) or disease of the liver or gallbladder.

Ketone bodies: any of three acidic chemicals (acetate, acetoacetate, and β-hydroxybutyrate). Ketone bodies may accumulate in the blood (ketosis) when the body has inadequate glucose to use for energy, and must increase the use of fat for fuel. Ketone bodies are acidic, and very high levels in the blood are toxic and may result in ketoacidosis.

Kidney stones: solid masses resulting from the crystallization of minerals and other compounds found in urine. Common types of kidney stones include those composed of calcium oxalate, calcium phosphate, and urate. Kidney stones may form in the kidneys, ureters, or urinary bladder.

LDL: low-density lipoprotein. LDLs transport cholesterol from the liver to the tissues of the body. Elevated serum LDL-cholesterol is associated with increased cardiovascular disease risk.

Left ventricular hypertrophy (LVH): abnormal thickening of the wall of the left ventricle (lower chamber) of the heart muscle. The ventricles have muscular walls in order to pump blood from the heart through the arteries, but LVH occurs when the ventricle must pump against abnormally high volume or pressure loads. LVH may accompany congestive heart failure.

Lens: the transparent structure inside the eye that focuses light rays onto the retina (the nerve cells at the back of the eye).

Leukemia: an acute or chronic form of cancer that involves the blood-forming organs. Leukemia is characterized by an abnormal increase in the number of white blood cells in the tissues of the body with or without a corresponding increase of those in the circulating blood, and is classified according to the type of white blood cell most prominently involved.

Leukocytes: white blood cells. Leukocytes are part of the immune system. Monocytes, lymphocytes, neutrophils, basophils, and eosinophils are different types of leukocytes.

Lipid peroxidation: the process by which lipids are oxidatively modified; so named because lipid hydroperoxides are formed in the process.

Lipids: a chemical term for fats. Lipids found in the human body include fatty acids, phospholipids, and triglycerides.

Lipoic acid: a cofactor, essential for the oxidation of 2-oxoacids, such as pyruvate, in metabolism.

Lipoprotein(a) [Lp(a)]: a lipoprotein particle in which the protein (apolipoprotein B-100) is chemically linked to another protein apolipoprotein(a). Increased blood levels of Lp(a) are associated with an increased risk of cardiovascular diseases.

Lipoproteins: particles composed of lipids and protein that allow for the transport of lipids through the bloodstream. A lipoprotein particle is composed of an outer layer of phospholipids, which renders it soluble in water, and a hydrophobic core that contains triglycerides and cholesterol esters. Different types of lipoproteins are distinguished by their surface proteins (apoproteins), their size, and the types and amounts of lipids that they contain.

Lumbar spine: the portion of the spine between the chest (thorax) and the pelvis. It is commonly referred to as the small of the back.

Lupus: see Systemic lupus erythematosus (SLE).

Lymphocytes: leukocytes (white blood cells) that play important roles in the immune system. T lymphocytes (T cells) differentiate into cells that can kill infected cells or activate other cells in the immune system. B lymphocytes (B cells) differentiate into cells that produce antibodies.

Macrocytic anemia: low red blood cell count, characterized by the presence in the blood of larger than normal red blood cells.

Macula: a small area of the retina where vision is the sharpest. The macula is located in the center of the retina and provides central vision.

Magnetic resonance imaging (MRI): a special imaging technique that uses a powerful magnet and a computer to provide clear images of soft tissues. Tissues that are well visualized using MRI include the brain and spinal cord, abdomen, and joints.

Malabsorption syndrome: a disease or condition that results in poor absorption of nutrients from food.

Malaria: an infectious disease caused by parasitic microorganisms of *Plasmodium* species. Malaria can be spread among humans through the sting of certain types of mosquitoes (*Anopheles* sp.) or by a contaminated needle or transfusion. Malaria is a major health problem in the tropics and subtropics, affecting over 200 million people worldwide.

Malignant: cancerous.

Megaloblastic anemia: low red blood cell count, characterized by the presence in the blood of large, immature, nucleated cells (megaloblasts) that are the forerunners of red blood cells. Red blood cells, when mature, have no nucleus.

Melanin: a dark-brown pigment found in the skin.

Membrane potential: the electrical potential difference across a membrane. The membrane potential is a result of the concentration differences between potassium and sodium across cell membranes that are maintained by ion pumps. A large proportion of the body's resting energy expenditure is devoted to maintaining the membrane potential, which is critical for nerve impulse transmission, muscle contraction, heart function, and the transport of nutrients and metabolites in and out of cells.

Menstruation: the cyclic loss of blood by a woman, from her uterus (womb) when she is not pregnant. Menstruation generally occurs every 4 weeks after a woman has reached sexual maturity and before the menopause.

Meta-analysis: a statistical technique used to combine the results from different studies to obtain a quantitative estimate of the overall effect of a particular intervention or exposure on a defined outcome.

Metabolic syndrome: a combination of medical conditions that places one at risk for cardiovascular diseases and type 2 diabetes. (Metabolic syndrome is also called metabolic syndrome X, syndrome X, and insulin resistance syndrome.) Diagnostic criteria include the presence of three or more of the following conditions:

- Abdominal obesity (waist circumference: ≥ 40 inches [102 cm] for men, ≥ 35 inches [88 cm] for women)
- Elevated triglycerides (≥ 150 mg/dL)
- High blood pressure ($\geq 130/85$ mmHg)
- Glucose intolerance/insulin resistance (fasting blood glucose ≥ 110 mg/dL)
- Decreased HDL-cholesterol (< 40 mg/dL for men, < 50 mg/dL for women).

Metabolism: the sum of the processes (reactions) by which a substance is assimilated and incorporated into the body or detoxified and excreted from the body.

Metabolite: a compound derived from the metabolism of another compound is said to be a metabolite of that compound.

Metastasize: to spread from one part of the body to another. Cancer is said to metastasize when it spreads from the primary site of origin to a distant anatomical site.

Methionine: a sulfur-containing amino acid, required for protein synthesis and other vital metabolic processes. It can be obtained through the diet in protein or synthesized from homocysteine.

Methylation: a biochemical reaction resulting in the addition of a methyl group ($-CH_3$) to another molecule.

Micronutrient: a nutrient required by the body in small amounts, such as a vitamin or mineral.

Migraine headache: a type of headache thought to be related to abnormal sensitivity of blood vessels (arteries) in the brain to various triggers, resulting in rapid changes in the artery size due to spasm (constriction). Other arteries in the brain and scalp then open (dilate), and throbbing pain is perceived in the head. The tendency toward migraine appears to involve serotonin, a neurotransmitter that can trigger the release of vasoactive substances in the blood vessels.

Mineral: nutritionally significant element. Elements are composed of only one kind of atom. Minerals are inorganic, that is, they do not contain carbon as do vitamins and other organic compounds.

Mitochondria: energy-producing structures within cells. Mitochondria possess two sets of membranes, a smooth continuous outer membrane and an inner membrane arranged in folds. Among other critical functions, mitochondria convert nutrients into energy via the electron transport chain.

mmHg: millimeters of mercury. The unit of measure for blood pressure.

Moiety: a portion of something, such as a functional group of a molecule.

Mole: the fundamental unit for measuring chemical compounds (abbreviated mol). One mole equals the molecular weight of a compound in grams. The number of molecules in a mole is equal to 6.02×10^{23} (Avogadro number).

Monounsaturated fatty acid: a fatty acid with only one double bond between carbon atoms.

Multifactorial: refers to diseases or conditions that are the result of interactions between multiple genetic and environmental factors.

Multiple sclerosis (MS): an autoimmune disorder, in which the myelin sheaths of nerves in the brain and spinal cord are damaged, resulting in progressive neurological symptoms.

Mutation: a change in a gene—in other words, a change in the sequence of base-pairs in the DNA that makes up a gene. Mutations in a gene may or may not result in an altered gene product.

Myelin: the fatty substance that covers myelinated nerves. Myelin is a layered tissue surrounding the axons or nerve fibers. This sheath acts as a conduit in an electrical system, allowing rapid and efficient transmission of nerve impulses. Myelination refers to the process in which nerves acquire a myelin sheath.

Myocardial infarction (MI): death (necrosis) of heart muscle tissue due to an interruption in its blood supply. Commonly known as a heart attack, an MI usually results from the obstruction of a coronary artery by a clot in people who have coronary atherosclerosis (heart disease).

Myocarditis: an inflammation of the heart muscle.

Myoglobin: a heme-containing pigment in muscle cells that binds and stores oxygen.

Myopathy: any disease of muscle.

Natural killer (NK) cells: cytotoxic lymphocytes important for the innate immune response that kills pathogens. NK cells also have important roles in killing cancer cells.

Necrosis: unprogrammed cell death, in which cells break open and release their contents, promoting inflammation. Necrotic cell death may be the result of injury, infection, or infarction.

Neural tube defect (NTD): a birth defect caused by abnormal development of the neural tube, the structure that gives rise to the central nervous system. NTDs include anencephaly and spina bifida.

Neurodegenerative diseases: disease resulting from the degeneration or deterioration of nerve cells (neurons). Alzheimer disease and Parkinson disease are neurodegenerative diseases.

Neurological: or neurologic; involving nerves or the nervous system (brain, spinal cord, and all sensory and motor nerves).

Neuropathy: nerve damage or disease.

Neurotoxic: toxic or damaging to nervous tissue (brain and peripheral nerves).

Neurotransmitter: a chemical that is released from a nerve cell and results in the transmission of an impulse to another nerve cell or organ (e.g., a muscle). Acetylcholine, dopamine, norepinephrine, and serotonin are neurotransmitters.

Neutrophils: white blood cells that internalize and destroy pathogens, such as bacteria. Neutrophils are also called polymorphonuclear leukocytes because they are white blood cells with multilobed nuclei.

NIH: National Institutes of Health. Administered under the US Department of Health and Human Services (HHS), the NIH are more than 20 separate institutes and centers devoted to medical research.

Nitric oxide: a gaseous signaling molecule synthesized from the amino acid arginine by enzymes called nitric oxide synthases. In the vascular endothelium, nitric oxide promotes arterial vasodilation.

Nucleic acids: DNA (deoxyribonucleic acid) and RNA (ribonucleic acid); long polymers of nucleotides.

Nucleotides: subunits of nucleic acids. Nucleotides are composed of a nitrogen-containing base (adenine, guanine, cytosine, uracil, or thymine), a five-carbon sugar (ribose or deoxyribose), and one or more phosphate groups.

Nucleus: a membrane-bound cellular organelle, which contains DNA organized into chromosomes.

Obesity: a condition of increased body fat; defined as a body mass index (BMI) ≥ 30 for adults.

Observational study: a study in which no experimental intervention or treatment is applied. Participants are simply observed over time.

One-carbon unit: a biochemical term for functional groups containing only one carbon in addition to other atoms. One-carbon units transferred by folate coenzymes include methyl ($-CH_3$), methylene ($-CH_2-$), formyl ($-CH=O$), formimino ($-CH=NH$), and methenyl ($-CH=$). Many biosynthetic reactions involve the addition of a one-carbon unit to a precursor molecule.

Organelles: specialized components of cells, such as mitochondria or lysosomes, so named because they are analogous to organs.

Organic: refers to carbon-containing compounds, generally synthesized by living organisms.

Osteoarthritis: a degenerative joint condition that is characterized by the breakdown of articular cartilage (cartilage within the joint).

Osteoblasts: bone cells that are responsible for the formation of new bone mineral in the bone remodeling process.

Osteoclasts: bone cells that are responsible for the breakdown or resorption of bone in the bone remodeling process.

Osteomalacia: a disease of adults that is characterized by softening of the bones due to loss of bone mineral. Osteomalacia is characteristic of vitamin D deficiency in adults, while children with vitamin D deficiency suffer from rickets.

Osteoporosis: a condition of increased bone fragility and susceptibility to bone fracture due to a loss of bone mineral density.

Oxidant: reactive oxygen species.

Oxidation: a chemical reaction that removes electrons from an atom or molecule.

Oxidative damage: damage to cells caused by reactive oxygen species.

Oxidative stress: a condition, in which the effects of prooxidants (e.g., free radicals, and reactive oxygen and reactive nitrogen species) exceed the ability of antioxidant systems to neutralize them.

Pancreas: a small organ located behind the stomach and connected to the duodenum (small intestine). The pancreas synthesizes enzymes that help digest food in the small intestine and hormones, including insulin, that regulate blood glucose levels.

Parathyroid glands: glands located behind the thyroid gland in the neck. The parathyroid glands secrete a hormone called parathyroid hormone (PTH) that is critical to calcium and phosphorus metabolism.

Parkinson disease: a disease of the nervous system caused by degeneration of a part of the brain called the basal ganglia, as well as by low production of the neurotransmitter dopamine. Symptoms include muscle rigidity, tremors, and slow voluntary movement.

Pathogen: disease-causing agent, such as a virus or bacterium.

Peptic ulcer disease: a disease characterized by ulcers or breakdown of the inner lining of the stomach or duodenum. Common risk factors for peptic ulcer disease include the use of nonsteroidal anti-inflammatory drugs (NSAIDs) and infection with *Helicobacter pylori*.

Peptide: a chain of amino acids. A protein is made up of one or more peptides.

Peptide hormones: hormones that are proteins, as opposed to steroid hormones, which are made from cholesterol. Insulin is an example of a peptide hormone.

Peripheral neuropathy: a disease or degenerative state affecting the nerves of the extremities (arms and legs). Symptoms may include numbness, pain, and muscle weakness.

Peripheral vascular disease: atherosclerosis of the vessels of the extremities, which may result in insufficient blood flow or pain in the affected limb, particularly during exercise.

Peritoneal dialysis: a procedure, in which a special dialysis solution is introduced through a tube in the peritoneum. The dialysis solution pulls waste and extra fluid from the body, when the dialysis solution is drained through the same tube. The most common form is called continuous ambulatory peritoneal dialysis and can be performed at home without a machine.

Peritoneum: a membrane that lines the walls of the abdominal cavity.

Pernicious anemia: the end stage of an autoimmune inflammation of the stomach, resulting in destruction of stomach cells by one's own antibodies. Progressive destruction of the cells that line the stomach causes decreased secretion of acid and enzymes required to release food-bound vitamin B_{12}. Antibodies to intrinsic factor (IF) bind to IF, preventing formation of the IF–vitamin B_{12} complex, further inhibiting vitamin B_{12} absorption.

PET: positron emission tomography. A diagnostic imaging technique that uses a sophisticated camera and computer to produce images of how a person's body is functioning. A PET scan shows the difference between healthy and abnormally functioning tissues.

pH: a measure of acidity or alkalinity.

Phagocyte: a specialized cell, such as a macrophage, that engulfs and digests invading microorganisms through the process of phagocytosis.

Phagocytosis: process by which phagocytes engulf and digest invading microorganisms and foreign particles.

Pharmacokinetics: the study of the absorption, distribution, metabolism, and elimination of drugs and other compounds.

Pharmacological dose: the dose or intake level of a nutrient many times the level associated with the prevention of deficiency or the maintenance of health. A pharmacological dose is generally associated with the treatment of a disease state and considered to be a dose at least 10 times greater than that needed to prevent deficiency.

Phase I clinical trial: a clinical trial in a small group of people aimed at determining bioavailability, optimal dose, safety, and early evidence of the efficacy of a new therapy.

Phase II clinical trial: a clinical trial designed to investigate the effectiveness of a new therapy in

larger numbers of people and to further evaluate short-term side effects and safety of the new therapy.

Phenylketonuria (PKU): an inherited disorder resulting in the inability to process the amino acid, phenylalanine. If not treated, the disorder may result in learning disability. Treatment is a diet low in phenylalanine. Newborn infants are screened for PKU, in order to determine the need for treatment before brain damage occurs.

Phlebotomy: the removal of blood from a vein. Phlebotomy may be used to obtain blood for diagnostic tests or to treat certain conditions, for example, iron overload in hemochromatosis.

Phospholipids: lipids in which phosphoric acid as well as fatty acids are attached to a glycerol backbone. Phospholipids are important structural components of cell membranes.

Phosphorylation: the creation of a phosphate derivative of an organic molecule. This is usually achieved by transferring a phosphate group ($-PO_4$) from ATP to another molecule.

Physiological dose: the dose or intake level of a nutrient associated with the prevention of deficiency or the maintenance of health. A physiological dose of a nutrient is not generally greater than that which could be achieved through a conscientious diet, as opposed to the use of supplements.

Pigment: a compound that gives a plant or animal cell color by the selective absorption of different wavelengths of light.

Pituitary: a small oval gland located at the base of the brain that secretes hormones regulating growth and metabolism. The pituitary gland is divided into two separate glands, the anterior and posterior pituitary glands, which each secrete different hormones.

Placebo: an inert treatment that is given to a control group while the experimental group is given the active treatment. Placebo-controlled studies are conducted to make sure that the results are due to the experimental treatment, rather than another factor associated with participating in the study.

Placenta: the organ that connects the fetus to the pregnant woman's uterus, allowing for the exchange of oxygen, carbon dioxide, nutrients, and waste between woman and fetus.

Placental abruption: premature separation of the placenta from the wall of the uterus. Abruption is a potentially serious problem for both the woman and fetus.

Plasma: the liquid portion of blood, in which the cells are suspended. Plasma is separated from blood cells using a centrifuge. Unlike serum, plasma retains clotting factors because it is obtained from blood that is not allowed to clot.

Platelet: irregularly shaped cell fragments that assist in blood clotting.

Pneumonia: a disease of the lungs characterized by inflammation and accumulation of fluid in the lungs. Pneumonia may be caused by infectious agents (e.g., viruses or bacteria) or by inhalation of certain irritants.

Polymer: a large molecule formed by combining many similar smaller molecules (monomers) in a regular pattern.

Polymorphism: a variant form of a gene. Most polymorphisms are harmless and are part of normal human genetic variation, but some polymorphisms affect the function of the gene product (protein).

Polyp: a benign (noncancerous) mass of tissue that forms on the inside of a hollow organ, such as the colon.

Polyunsaturated fatty acid: a fatty acid with more than one double bond between carbons.

Precursor: a molecule that is an ingredient, reactant, or intermediate in a synthetic pathway for a particular product.

Pre-eclampsia: a condition characterized by a sharp rise in blood pressure during the third trimester of pregnancy. High blood pressure may be accompanied by edema (swelling) and proteinuria (protein in the urine). In some cases, untreated pre-eclampsia can progress to eclampsia, a life-threatening situation for the woman and child.

Prevalence: the proportion of a population with a specific disease or condition at a given point in time.

Prognosis: predicted outcome based on the course of a disease.

Proliferation: rapid cell division.

Prooxidant: an atom or molecule that promotes oxidation of another atom or molecule by accepting electrons. Examples of prooxidants include free radicals, reactive oxygen species, and reactive nitrogen species.

Prophylaxis: prevention; often refers to a treatment used to prevent a disease.

Prospective cohort study: an observational study in which a group of people—known as a cohort—are interviewed or tested for risk factors (e.g., nutrient intake), and then followed up at subsequent times to determine their status with respect to a disease or health outcome.

Prostaglandin: any of a class of hormone-like, regulatory molecules constructed from polyunsaturated fatty acids such as arachidonate. These molecules participate in a number of functions in the body, such as smooth muscle contraction and relaxation, vasodilation, and regulation of kidney function.

Prostate: a gland in men, located at the base of the bladder and surrounding the urethra. The prostate produces fluid that forms part of semen. If the prostate becomes enlarged it may exert pressure on the urethra and cause urinary symptoms. Prostate cancer is one of the most common types of cancer in men.

Prostate-specific antigen (PSA): a compound normally secreted by the prostate that can be measured in the blood. If prostate cancer is developing, the prostate secretes larger amounts of PSA. Blood tests for PSA are used to screen for prostate cancer and to follow up on prostate cancer treatment.

Protein: a complex organic molecule composed of amino acids in a specific order. The order is determined by the sequence of nucleic acids in a gene coding for the protein. Proteins are required for the structure, function, and regulation of the body's cells, tissues, and organs, and each protein has unique functions.

Proteoglycan: a large compound made up of protein and polysaccharide units known as glycosaminoglycans (GAGs). GAGs are polymers of sugars and amino sugars, such as glucosamine and galactosamine. Proteoglycans are integral components of structural tissues such as bone and cartilage.

Proton: an elementary particle identical to the nucleus of a hydrogen atom, which along with neutrons is a constituent of all other atomic nuclei. A proton carries a positive charge equal and opposite to that of an electron.

Psoriasis: A chronic skin condition often resulting in a red, scaly rash located over the surfaces of the elbows, knees, scalp, and around or in the ears, navel, genitals, or buttocks. Approximately 10%–15% of patients with psoriasis develop joint inflammation (psoriatic arthritis). Psoriasis is thought to be an autoimmune condition.

Pyruvate kinase deficiency: a hereditary deficiency of the enzyme pyruvate kinase. Pyruvate kinase deficiency results in hemolytic anemia.

Quartile: one-fourth of a sample or population.

Quintile: one-fifth of a sample or population.

Radiation therapy: the local use of radiation to destroy cancer cells or stop them from dividing and growing.

Randomized controlled trial (RCT): a clinical trial with at least one active treatment group and a control (placebo) group. In RCTs, participants are chosen for the experimental and control groups at random, and are not told whether they are receiving the active or the placebo treatment until the end of the study. This type of study design can provide evidence of causality.

Randomized design: an experiment in which participants are chosen for the experimental and control groups at random, in order to reduce bias caused by self-selection into experimental and control groups. This type of study design can provide evidence of causality.

RDA: recommended dietary allowance. Established by the Food and Nutrition Board of the Institute of Medicine, the RDA is the average daily dietary intake level of a nutrient sufficient to meet the requirements of nearly all healthy individuals in a specific life stage and gender group.

Reactive nitrogen species: highly reactive chemicals, containing nitrogen, that react easily with other molecules, resulting in potentially damaging modifications.

Reactive oxygen species (ROS): highly reactive chemicals, containing oxygen, that react easily with other molecules, resulting in potentially damaging modifications.

Receptor: a specialized molecule inside or on the surface of a cell that binds a specific chemical (ligand). Ligand binding usually results in a change in activity within the cell.

Recessive trait: a trait that is expressed only when two copies of the gene responsible for the trait are present.

Rectum: the last portion of the large intestine, connecting the sigmoid colon (above) to the anus (below). The rectum stores stool until it is evacuated from the body.

Redox reaction: another term for an oxidation–reduction reaction. A redox reaction is any reaction in which electrons are removed from one molecule or atom and transferred to another molecule or atom. In such a reaction one substance is oxidized (loses electrons) while the other is reduced (gains electrons).

Reduction: a chemical reaction in which a molecule or atom gains electrons.

Renal: refers to the kidneys.

Residue: a single unit within a polymer, such as an amino acid within a protein.

Resorption: the process of breaking down or assimilating something. With respect to bone, resorption refers to the breakdown of bone by osteoclasts that results in the release of calcium and phosphate (bone mineral) into the blood.

Response element: a sequence of nucleotides in a gene that can be bound by a protein. Proteins that bind to response elements in genes are sometimes called transcription factors or binding proteins. Binding of a transcription factor to a response element regulates the production of specific proteins by inhibiting or enhancing the transcription of genes that encode those proteins.

Retina: the nerve layer that lines the back of the eye. In the retina, images created by light are converted to nerve impulses, which are transmitted to the brain via the optic nerve.

Retrospective study: An epidemiological study that looks back in time. A retrospective study begins after the exposure and the disease have occurred. Most case–control studies are retrospective.

Rheumatoid arthritis: a chronic autoimmune disease, characterized by inflammation of the synovial lining of the joints. Rheumatoid arthritis may also affect other organs of the body, including the skin, eyes, lungs, and heart.

Ribonucleotide: a molecule consisting of a five-carbon sugar (ribose), a nitrogen-containing base, and one or more phosphate groups.

Rickets: often the result of vitamin D deficiency. Rickets affects children while their bones are still growing. It is characterized by soft and deformed bones, and is the result of an impaired incorporation of calcium and phosphate into the skeleton.

RNA: ribonucleic acid; a single-stranded nucleic acid composed of many nucleotides. The nucleotides in RNA are composed of a nitrogen-containing base (adenine, guanine, cytosine, or uracil), a five-carbon sugar (ribose), and a phosphate group. RNA functions in the translation of the genetic information encoded in DNA to proteins.

Ruminant: an animal that chews cud. Ruminant animals include cattle, goats, sheep, and deer.

Saturated fatty acid: a fatty acid with no double bonds between carbon atoms.

Scavenge (free radicals): to combine readily with free radicals, preventing them from reacting with other molecules.

Scurvy: a disorder caused by lack of vitamin C. Symptoms include anemia, bleeding gums, tooth loss, joint pain, and fatigue. Scurvy is treated by supplying foods high in vitamin C as well as vitamin C supplements.

Seizure: uncontrolled electrical activity in the brain, which may produce a physical convulsion, minor physical signs, thought disturbances, or a combination of symptoms.

Serotonin: 5-hydroxytryptamine. Serotonin is a neurotransmitter that may also function as a vasoconstrictor (substance that causes blood vessels to narrow).

Serum: the liquid portion of blood, in which the cells are suspended. Serum is separated from blood cells using a centrifuge. Unlike plasma, serum lacks clotting factors because it is obtained from blood that has been allowed to clot.

Short bowel syndrome: a malabsorption syndrome resulting from the surgical removal of an extensive portion of the small intestine.

Sickle cell anemia: a hereditary disease in which a mutation in the gene for one of the proteins that comprises hemoglobin results in the formation of defective hemoglobin molecules known as hemoglobin S. Individuals who are homozygous for this mutation (possess two genes for hemoglobin S) have red blood cells that change from the normal discoid shape to a sickle shape when the oxygen supply is low. These sickle-shaped cells are easily trapped in capillaries and damaged, resulting in severe anemia. Individuals who are heterozygous for the mutation (possess one gene for hemoglobin S and one normal hemoglobin gene) have increased resistance to malaria.

Sideroblastic anemia: a group of anemias that are all characterized by the accumulation of iron deposits in the mitochondria of immature red blood cells. These abnormal red blood cells do not mature normally, and many are destroyed in the bone marrow before reaching the circulation. Sideroblastic anemias can be hereditary, idiopathic (unknown cause), or caused by such diverse factors as certain drugs, alcohol, or copper deficiency.

Small intestine: the part of the digestive tract that extends from the stomach to the large intestine. The small intestine includes the duodenum (closest to the stomach), jejunum, and ileum (closest to the large intestine).

Sorbitol: the polyol (sugar alcohol) corresponding to glucose.

Spina bifida: a birth defect, also known as a neural tube defect, resulting from failure of the lower end of the neural tube to close during embryonic development. Spina bifida, the most common cause of infantile paralysis, is characterized by a lack of protection of the spinal cord by its membranes and vertebral bones.

Sprue: also known as celiac sprue and celiac disease, it is an inherited disease in which the intestinal lining is inflamed in response to the ingestion of a protein known as gluten. Treatment of celiac disease involves the avoidance of gluten, which is present in many grains, including wheat, rye, oats, and barley. Inflammation and atrophy of the lining of the small intestine lead to impaired nutrient absorption.

Status: the state of nutrition of an individual with respect to a specific nutrient. Diminished or low status indicates inadequate supply or stores of a specific nutrient for optimal physiological functioning.

Stenosis: obstruction or narrowing of a passage. Coronary stenosis refers specifically to obstruction or narrowing of a coronary artery, which supplies blood to the heart muscle (myocardium).

Steroid: a molecule related to cholesterol. Many important hormones, such as estrogen and testosterone, are steroids.

Steroid hormone receptor: a protein within a cell that binds to a specific steroid hormone. Binding of the steroid hormone changes the shape of the receptor protein and activates it, allowing it to activate gene transcription. In this way, a steroid hormone can activate the synthesis of specific proteins.

Stress fracture: a hairline or microscopic break in a bone, usually due to repetitive stress rather than trauma. Stress fractures are usually painful, and may be undetectable by X-ray. Although they may occur in almost any bone, common sites of stress fractures are the tibia (lower leg) and metatarsals (foot).

Stroke: damage that occurs to a part of the brain when its blood supply is suddenly interrupted (ischemic stroke) or when a blood vessel ruptures and bleeds into the brain (hemorrhagic stroke). A stroke is also called a cerebrovascular accident.

Subclinical: without clinical signs or symptoms; sometimes used to describe the early stage of a disease or condition, before symptoms are detectable by clinical examination or laboratory tests.

Substrate: a reactant in an enzyme-catalyzed reaction.

Supplement: a nutrient or phytochemical supplied in addition to that which is obtained in the diet.

Syndrome: a combination of symptoms that occur together and is indicative of a specific condition or disease.

Synergistic: when the effect of two treatments together is greater than the sum of the effects of the two individual treatments, it is said to be synergistic.

Synthesis: the formation of a chemical compound from its elements or precursor compounds.

Systematic review: a structured review of the literature designed to answer a clearly formulated question. Systematic reviews use systematic and explicitly predetermined methods to identify, select, and critically evaluate research relevant to the question, and to collect and analyze data from the studies that are included in the review. Statistical methods, such as meta-analysis, may be used to summarize the results of the included studies.

Systemic lupus erythematosus (SLE): a chronic autoimmune disease, characterized by inflammation of the connective tissue. SLE is more common in women than men, and the disease may result in inflammation and damage to the skin, joints, blood vessels, lungs, heart, and kidneys.

Systolic blood pressure: the highest arterial pressure measured during the heart beat cycle, and the first number in a blood pressure reading (e.g., 120 in 120/80).

Tannins: any of a large group of plant-derived compounds. Tannins tend to be bitter tasting and may function in pigment formation and plant protection.

Tetany: a condition of prolonged and painful spasms of the voluntary muscles, especially the fingers and toes (carpopedal spasm) as well as the facial musculature.

Thalassemia major: β-thalassemia is a genetic disorder that results in abnormalities of the globin (protein) portion of hemoglobin. An individual who is homozygous for the β-thalassemia gene (has two copies of the β-thalassemia gene) is said to have thalassemia major. Infants born with thalassemia major develop severe anemia a few months after birth, accompanied by pallor, fatigue, poor growth, and frequent infections. Blood transfusions are used to treat thalassemia major but cannot cure it.

Thalassemia minor: individuals who are heterozygous for the β-thalassemia gene (carry one copy of the β-thalassemia gene) are said to have thalassemia minor or thalassemia trait. These individuals are generally healthy but can pass the β-thalassemia gene to their children and are said to be carriers of the β-thalassemia gene.

Threshold: the point at which a physiological effect begins to be produced, for example, the degree of stimulation of a nerve that produces a response or the level of a chemical in the diet that results in a disease.

Thyroid: a butterfly-shaped gland in the neck that secretes thyroid hormones. Thyroid hormones regulate a number of physiological processes, including growth, development, metabolism, and reproductive function.

Thyroid follicular cancer: a cancer of the thyroid gland that constitutes about 30% of all thyroid cancers. It has a greater rate of recurrence and metastases (spreading to other organs) than thyroid papillary cancer.

Thyroid papillary cancer: the most common form of thyroid cancer, which most often affects women of childbearing age. Thyroid papillary cancer has a lower rate of recurrence and metastases (spreading to other organs) than thyroid follicular cancer.

Topical: applied to the skin or other body surface.

Total parenteral nutrition (TPN): intravenous feeding that provides patients with essential nutrients when they are too ill to eat normally.

Transcription (DNA transcription): the process by which one strand of DNA is copied into a complementary sequence of RNA.

Transcription factor: a protein that functions to initiate, enhance, or inhibit the transcription of a gene. Transcription factors can regulate the formation of a specific protein encoded by a gene.

Trans **fat:** hydrogenated or partially hydrogenated oils.

Transient ischemic attack (TIA): sometimes called a small or mini-stroke. TIAs are caused by a temporary disturbance of blood supply to an area of the brain, resulting in a sudden, brief (usually less than 1 hour) disruption in certain brain functions.

Translation (RNA translation): the process by which the sequence of nucleotides in a messenger RNA molecule directs the incorporation of amino acids into a protein.

Trauma: an injury or wound.

Tremor: trembling or shaking of all or part of the body.

Triglycerides: lipids consisting of three fatty acid molecules bound to a glycerol backbone. Triglycerides are the principal form of fat in the diet, although they are also synthesized endogenously. Triglycerides are stored in adipose tissue and represent the principal storage form of fat. Elevated serum triglycerides are a risk factor for cardiovascular disease.

Tuberculosis (TB): an infection caused by bacteria called *Mycobacterium tuberculosis*. Many people infected with TB have no symptoms because it is dormant. Once active, tuberculosis may cause damage to the lungs and other organs. Active TB is also contagious and is spread through inhalation. Treatment of TB involves taking antibiotics and vitamins for at least 6 months.

Typhoid: an infectious disease, spread by the contamination of food or water supplies with the bacterium called *Salmonella typhi*. Food and water can be contaminated directly by sewage or indirectly by flies or poor hygiene. Although rare in the United States, it is common in some parts of the world. Symptoms include fever, abdominal pain, diarrhea, and a rash. It is treated with antibiotics and intravenous fluids. Vaccination is recommended to those traveling to areas where typhoid is common.

UL: tolerable upper intake level. Established by the Food and Nutrition Board of the US Institute of Medicine, the UL is the highest level of daily intake of a specific nutrient likely to pose no risk of adverse health effects in almost all individuals of a specified age.

Ulcerative colitis: a chronic inflammatory disease of the colon and rectum. Symptoms of ulcerative colitis include abdominal pain, cramping, and bloody diarrhea.

Ultrasonography: a test in which high-frequency sound waves (ultrasound) are bounced off tissues and the echoes are converted into a picture (sonogram).

Vascular dementia: dementia resulting from cerebrovascular disease, for example, a cerebrovascular accident (stroke).

Vascular endothelium: the single cell layer that lines the inner surface of blood vessels. Healthy endothelial function promotes vasodilation and inhibits platelet aggregation (clot formation).

Vasoconstriction: narrowing of a blood vessel.

Vasodilation: relaxation or opening of a blood vessel.

Vertebral: of or pertaining to a vertebra; one of the 23 bones that make up the spine.

Vesicle: literally a small bag or pouch. Inside a cell, a vesicle is a small organelle surrounded by its own membrane.

Virulent: marked by a rapid, severe, or damaging course.

Virus: a microorganism, which cannot grow or reproduce apart from a living cell. Viruses invade living cells and use the synthetic processes of infected cells to survive and replicate.

Vitamin: an organic (carbon-containing) compound necessary for normal physiological function that cannot be synthesized in adequate amounts, and must therefore be obtained in the diet.

Xenograft: a transplant of tissue from a donor of one species to a recipient of another species.

Zollinger–Ellison syndrome: a rare disorder caused by a tumor called a gastrinoma, most often occurring in the pancreas. The tumor secretes the hormone gastrin, which causes increased production of gastric acid, leading to severe recurrent ulcers of the esophagus, stomach, and the upper portions of the small intestine.

The Linus Pauling Institute Prescription for Health

Healthy Eating

- Eat four servings (2 cups) of fruit and five servings (2½ cups) of vegetables daily, but don't include potatoes in your tally.
- To increase your intake of omega-3 fatty acids, eat fish twice weekly and consume foods rich in α-linolenic acid, such as walnuts, flaxseeds, and flaxseed or canola oil.
- Choose oils rich in unsaturated fats for cooking and salad dressings, such as soy, corn, safflower, and olive oil, and choose nuts (except Brazil nuts) for snacks.
- Reduce your intake of foods high in saturated fat, such as red meat and whole-fat dairy products (butter, whole milk, and full-fat yogurt or cheese).
- To reduce your exposure to food-borne carcinogens, avoid smoked or cured foods and charred or seared fish, meat and poultry.
- Reduce your intake of white potatoes, white flour, and white rice by substituting whole-grain products, such as whole-wheat flour and pasta, whole-grain breads and cereals, and brown rice.
- Avoid highly processed, nutrient-poor foods, such as cookies, candies, chips, crackers, soft drinks, and sugar-coated breakfast cereals, that are typically high in sugar, hydrogenated (trans) fat*, or sodium.

Healthy Lifestyle

- Aim for a healthy weight. Becoming overweight (BMI 25–29.9) or obese (BMI ≥30) increases the risk for many chronic diseases. Having too much abdominal fat (waist circumference > 40in [101.6 cm] for men and > 35in [76.2 cm] for women) also increases disease risk. If you are at risk for obesity-associated diseases, even a relatively small weight loss (10% of your current weight) can help lower your risk.

---

*The "Nutrition Facts" label of processed foods containing less than 0.5 g of *trans* fat per serving will list *trans* fat as zero (0 g), or a footnote is added stating "Not a significant source of *trans* fat." The list of ingredients of these foods will show *trans* fat as "partially hydrogenated vegetable oil" or "shortening."

- Accumulate a minimum of 30 minutes of moderate–intensity exercise most days of the week. Most people can realize additional health benefits by increasing the duration of moderate-intensity exercise to an average of 60 minutes daily or by engaging in more vigorous physical activity. To improve muscular strength and balance and minimize bone loss, include strength-building activities, such as weight lifting, at least twice a week.
- If you smoke, make every effort to quit. Even if you have smoked for many years, quitting will result in dramatically decreased risk for chronic diseases.
- Moderate alcohol consumption is associated with reduced risk for cardiovascular diseases, but increased risk for some cancers. If you drink alcohol, limit your consumption to one alcoholic drink per day for women and two for men. Avoid alcohol if you have a personal or family history of breast or colon cancer or alcoholism.

Supplements

Multivitamins/minerals. Take a multivitamin/mineral supplement with 100% of the daily value (DV) for most vitamins and essential minerals, keeping the following suggestions in mind:

- **Iron:** In general, men and postmenopausal women should take a multivitamin/mineral supplement without iron.
- **Vitamin A:** Look for a multivitamin/mineral supplement containing no more than 2500 IU (750 µg) of vitamin A or, if unavailable, a multivitamin/mineral supplement containing 5000 IU vitamin A, of which at least 50% comes from β-carotene.

Vitamin C. Aim for a daily intake of at least 400 mg. Multivitamins/minerals usually provide 60 mg of vitamin C, and five servings of fruit and vegetables provide about 200 mg. A 250-mg supplement taken twice daily will ensure near-maximal plasma concentrations in healthy people.

Vitamin D. Take 2000 IU (50 µg) of supplemental vitamin D daily. Most multivitamins/minerals 50 µg contain 400 IU vitamin D, and single-ingredient vitamin D supplements are available for additional supplementation.

Vitamin E. Take a supplement of 200 IU (133 mg) of natural source α-tocopherol (*d*-α-tocopherol) daily with a meal. If you are prone to bleeding or take anticoagulant drugs, consult your physician.

Calcium. No multivitamin/mineral supplement contains 100% of the DV for calcium. If your total calcium intake doesn't add up to 1000 mg, take an extra calcium supplement (combined with magnesium—see below) with a meal to make up the difference.

Magnesium. No multivitamin/mineral supplement contains 100% of the DV for magnesium. If you don't eat plenty of green leafy vegetables, whole grains, and nuts, you are likely not getting enough magnesium from your diet. If you add a magnesium supplement, take a combined supplement with calcium containing 133–250 mg of magnesium and 333–500 mg of calcium with a meal.

Fish oil. If you don't regularly consume fish, consider taking a 2-g fish-oil supplement several times a week. If you are prone to bleeding or take anticoagulant drugs, consult your physician.

Lipoic acid and L-carnitine. Healthy adults over the age of 50 may consider a daily supplement of 200–400 mg of α-lipoic acid and 500–1000 mg of acetyl-L-carnitine.

Index

Page numbers in *italics* refer to illustrations or tables